FAQs in Pediatric Infectious Diseases

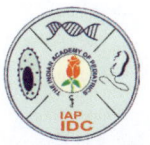

FAQs in Pediatric Infectious Diseases

Chief Editors

Ritabrata Kundu
Professor of Pediatrics
Institute of Child Health
Kolkata, West Bengal, India
E-mail: rkundu22@gmail.com

Digant D Shastri
Chief Consultant Pediatrician and CEO
Killol Children Hospital
NICU and Vaccination Center
Surat, Gujarat, India
E-mail: drdigant@hotmail.com

Editor

Jaydeep Choudhury
Associate Professor
Institute of Child Health
Kolkata, West Bengal, India
E-mail: drjaydeep_choudhury@yahoo.co.in

Academic Editors

Vijay N Yewale
Consultant Pediatrician
Dr Yewale Multispecialty Hospital
for Children
Navi Mumbai, Maharashtra, India
E-mail: vnyewale@gmail.com

Abhay K Shah
Senior Consultant Pediatrician
Ahmedabad, Gujarat, India
E-mail: drabhaykshah@yahoo.com

AJ Chitkara
Head
Department of Pediatrics
Max Superspeciality Hospital
Shalimar Bagh, New Delhi, India
E-mail: drajchitkara@gmail.com

Publication Editor

Kheya Ghosh Uttam
Assistant Professor
Institute of Child Health
Kolkata, West Bengal, India
E-mail: kheyauttam@yahoo.co.in

IAP National Publication House, Gwalior

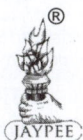

JAYPEE BROTHERS MEDICAL PUBLISHERS (P) LTD
New Delhi • London • Philadelphia • Panama

Jaypee Brothers Medical Publishers (P) Ltd

Headquarters
Jaypee Brothers Medical Publishers (P) Ltd
4838/24, Ansari Road, Daryaganj
New Delhi 110 002, India
Phone: +91-11-43574357
Fax: +91-11-43574314
Email: jaypee@jaypeebrothers.com

Overseas Offices

J.P. Medical Ltd
83, Victoria Street, London
SW1H 0HW (UK)
Phone: +44-2031708910
Fax: +02-03-0086180
Email: info@jpmedpub.com

Jaypee-Highlights Medical Publishers Inc.
City of Knowledge, Bld. 237, Clayton
Panama City, Panama
Phone: +1 507-301-0496
Fax: +1 507-301-0499
Email: cservice@jphmedical.com

Jaypee Medical Inc
The Bourse
111 South Independence Mall East
Suite 835, Philadelphia, PA 19106, USA
Phone: +1 267-519-9789
Email: jpmed.us@gmail.com

Jaypee Brothers Medical Publishers (P) Ltd
17/1-B Babar Road, Block-B, Shaymali
Mohammadpur, Dhaka-1207
Bangladesh
Mobile: +08801912003485
Email: jaypeedhaka@gmail.com

Jaypee Brothers Medical Publishers (P) Ltd
Bhotahity, Kathmandu, Nepal
Phone: +977-9741283608
Email: kathmandu@jaypeebrothers.com

Website: www.jaypeebrothers.com
Website: www.jaypeedigital.com

© 2014, Jaypee Brothers Medical Publishers

The views and opinions expressed in this book are solely those of the original contributor(s)/author(s) and do not necessarily represent those of editor(s) of the book.

All rights reserved. No part of this publication may be reproduced, stored or transmitted in any form or by any means, electronic, mechanical, photocopying, recording or otherwise, without the prior permission in writing of the publishers and the author.

All brand names and product names used in this book are trade names, service marks, trademarks or registered trademarks of their respective owners. The publisher and author are not associated with any product or vendor mentioned in this book.

Medical knowledge and practice change constantly. This book is designed to provide accurate, authoritative information about the subject matter in question. However, readers are advised to check the most current information available on procedures included and check information from the manufacturer of each product to be administered, to verify the recommended dose, formula, method and duration of administration, adverse effects and contraindications. It is the responsibility of the practitioner to take all appropriate safety precautions. Neither the publisher nor the author(s)/editor(s) assume any liability for any injury and/or damage to persons or property arising from or related to use of material in this book.

This book is sold on the understanding that the publisher is not engaged in providing professional medical services. If such advice or services are required, the services of a competent medical professional should be sought.

Every effort has been made where necessary to contact holders of copyright to obtain permission to reproduce copyright material. If any have been inadvertently overlooked, the publisher will be pleased to make the necessary arrangements at the first opportunity.

Inquiries for bulk sales may be solicited at: jaypee@jaypeebrothers.com

FAQs in Pediatric Infectious Diseases
First Edition: **2014**
ISBN 978-93-5152-159-4
Printed at Rajkamal Electric Press, Kundli, Haryana.

Dedicated to

*All our readers
who have constantly encouraged us
to bring out books
on pediatric infectious diseases*

Contributors

Abhay K Shah
Senior Consultant Pediatrician
Ahmedabad, Gujarat, India

Ajay Kalra
Erstwhile Professor
Department of Pediatrics
SN Medical College
Ex-Head of Department
Institute of Medical Sciences
Agra, Uttar Pradesh, India

AK Prasad
Former University Professor and Head
Respiratory Virology
V Patel Chest Institute
Delhi, India
Medical Microbiology
Delhi University, Delhi, India
Chairman, Influenza Foundation of India
Member
Asia Pacific Alliance for the Control of Influenza (APACI) Ltd

Alok Kumar Deb
Scientist—'D', Epidemiology Division
National Institute of Cholera and Enteric Diseases
Kolkata, West Bengal, India

Anand Shandilya
Director, Dr Anand's Hospital for Children
Mumbai, Maharashtra, India

Anju Aggarwal
Associate Professor of Pediatrics
University College of Medical Sciences
and Guru Tegh Bahadur Hospital
New Delhi, India

Ashok Rai
Director
Surya Superspeciality Hospital and
Associated Max Heart Center
Director, Indian Institute of Cerebral
Palsy and Handicapped Children
Varanasi, Uttar Pradesh, India

Atul A Kulkarni
Consultant Pediatrician
Department of Pediatrics
Ashwini Sahakari Rugnalaya and
Research Center
Solapur, Maharashtra, India

Baldev S Prajapati
Professor
GCS Medical College,
Hospital and Research Center
Ahmedabad, Gujarat, India

Devdeep Mukherjee
Senior Resident
Institute of Child Health
Kolkata, West Bengal, India

Dhanya Dharmapalan
Consultant Pediatrician
Dr Yewale's Multispeciality Hospital
for Children
Vashi, Navi Mumbai, Maharashtra, India

Dhritobrata Das
Consultant Pediatric Cardiologist
Apollo Gleneagles Hospital
Kolkata, West Bengal, India

Digant D Shastri
Chief Consultant Pediatrician and CEO
Killol Children Hospital
NICU and Vaccination Center
Surat, Gujarat, India

Ira Shah
Consultant
Pediatric Infectious Diseases and
Hepatology
Nanavati Hospital
Mumbai, Maharashtra, India
Associate Professor and In-Charge
Pediatric HIV Clinic
TB Clinic and Pediatric Liver Clinic
BJ Wadia Hospital for Children
Mumbai, Maharashtra, India

Janani Sankar
Senior Consultant
Kanchi Kamakoti CHILDS Trust Hospital
Chennai, Tamil Nadu, India

Jayati Sengupta
Consultant Pediatric Nephrologist
Institute of Child Health
Kolkata, West Bengal, India

Jaydeep Choudhury
Associate Professor
Institute of Child Health
Kolkata, West Bengal, India

K Dhanalakshmi
Senior Registrar
Kanchi Kamakoti CHILDS Trust Hospital and The Child Trust Medical Research Foundation
Chennai, Tamil Nadu, India

Ketan Shah
Consultant Pediatrician
Ketan Children Hospital
Shankheswar Complex
Surat, Gujarat, India

Kheya Ghosh Uttam
Assistant Professor
Institute of Child Health
Kolkata, West Bengal, India

M Govindraj
Professor and Medical Superintendent
Indira Gandhi Institute of Child Health
Bengaluru, Karnataka, India

Malathi Sathiyasekaran
Consultant Pediatric Gastroenterologist
KKCTH, SMF and Apollo Hospital
Chennai, Tamil Nadu, India

Monjori Mitra
Associate Professor
Institute of Child Health
Kolkata, West Bengal, India

Narendra Rathi
Consultant Pediatrician
Rathi Children Hospital
Akola, Maharashtra, India

Nigam Prakash Narain
Professor of Pediatrics
Patna Medical College
Patna, Bihar, India

Niranjan Mohanty
Professor and Head
Department of Pediatrics
Shri Ramachandra Bhanj Medical College
Cuttack, Odisha, India

Nupur Ganguly
Associate Professor
Department of Pediatric Medicine
Institute of Child Health
Kolkata, West Bengal, India

P Ramachandran
Professor of Pediatrics
Sri Ramachandra University
Chennai, Tamil Nadu, India

Parang Mehta
Consultant Pediatrician
Surat, Gujarat, India

Patima R Shah
Professor
Adani Medical College
Bhuj, Gujarat, India

Rajal B Prajapati
Professor
Smt NHL Municipal Medical College
Sheth VS General Hospital
Ahmedabad, Gujarat, India

Rajniti Prasad
Associate Professor
Department of Pediatrics
Institute of Medical Sciences
Banaras Hindu University
Varanasi, Uttar Pradesh, India

Raju C Shah
Professor and Head
GCS Medical College
Ahmedabad, Gujarat, India

Ritabrata Kundu
Professor of Pediatrics
Institute of Child Health
Kolkata, West Bengal, India

Contributors

Rohit Agrawal
Director and Consultant Pediatrician
Chandrajyoti Children Hospital
Visiting Consultant
Kohinoor Hospital
Mumbai, Maharashtra, India

S Balasubramanian
Senior Consultant Pediatrician
Kanchi Kamakoti CHILDS Trust
Hospital and The Child Trust Medical
Research Foundation
Chennai, Tamil Nadu, India

Sandipan Dhar
Associate Professor
Department of Pediatric Dermatology
Institute of Child Health
Kolkata, West Bengal, India

Sangeeta Sharma
Head of Pediatrics
LRS Institute Tuberculosis and
Respiratory Diseases
New Delhi, India

Sanjay K Ghorpade
Director and Professor of Pediatrics
Postgraduate Institute of Pediatrics and
Niramay Hospital and Research Center
Sadar Bazar, Maharashtra, India

Santanu Bhakta
Assistant Professor
Institute of Child Health
Fellow in Pediatric Pulmonology
Kolkata, West Bengal, India

Subhasish Bhattacharya
Professor of Pediatrics
Calcutta Medical College
Kolkata, West Bengal, India

Suhas V Prabhu
Visiting Pediatric Consultant
PD Hinduja National Hospital and
Medical Research Center
Mumbai, Maharashtra, India

Sumanth Amperayani
Senior Registrar
Kanchi Kamakoti CHILDS Trust
Hospital and The Child Trust Medical
Research Foundation
Chennai, Tamil Nadu, India

Tanu Singhal
Consultant
Pediatrics and Infectious Diseases
Kokilaben Dhirubhai Ambani Hospital
and Medical Research Institute
Mumbai, Maharashtra, India

Upendra Kinjawadekar
Consultant Pediatrician and
Neonatologist
Kamalesh Mother and Child Hospital
Navi Mumbai, Maharashtra, India

Vijay N Yewale
Consultant Pediatrician
Dr Yewale Multispecialty Hospital for
Children
Navi Mumbai, Maharashtra, India

Foreword

It give me immense pleasure to present this book *FAQs in Pediatric Infectious Diseases* published under the banner of Indian Academy of Pediatrics, Infectious Diseases Chapter. There are many standard textbooks on various aspects of infection in children. At time, it gets very difficult for a busy practicing doctor to find the right information from the textbooks. This book provides only the salient points that will help in day-to-day management in children. I congratulate the editorial board and the present chairperson and secretary of the chapter to take up this effort. It is also laudable that this chapter has kept its continuity in publishing every year. My special thank goes to Dr Ritabrata Kundu, Dr Digant D Shastri, Dr Abhay K Shah, Dr Jaydeep Choudhury and Dr Kheya Ghosh Uttam, for their tireless efforts to bring out this book. My thank also goes to the authors who have taken their valuable time to contribute in this book. I hope the book will be useful to the practitioners for whom it is published and become their desk companion.

Vijay N Yewale
President, IAP 2014

Foreword

It is a proud privilege for me to write Foreword for this book *FAQs in Pediatric Infectious Diseases* in the capacity of Chairperson of IAP Infectious Diseases Chapter. Publishing academic books has been legacy of IAP Infectious Diseases Chapter and as a continuation of the tradition after successful publication of First Edition of *Textbook of Pediatric Infectious Diseases* in 2012 publishing a book which is quite handy and helps our members to find out their query on the spot while being busy in the OPD without referring to a bulky textbook was thought of. Seeing the popularity received to earlier publications from ID Chapter motivated us to envisage a project of publishing a book which can address common queries which arise while dealing with patients with infectious diseases in "Frequently Asked Questions (FAQs)" format under ID Chapter Chairperson's Action Plan 2013.

The literal meaning of FAQ is "listed questions and answers, all supposed to be commonly asked in some context, and pertaining to a particular topic" and here in this book all important issues pertaining to infectious diseases have been illustrated through 45 well-written chapters in the form of frequently asked questions. Besides being evidence based, the book is thoroughly written keeping up time with the advancements in the pediatric subspecialty. More than 50 faculty from different parts of country have contributed. It is a great venture where experts have tried their best to answer commonly asked questions. I am sure that the hard work of the editorial board and also of experts will be most useful to readers.

Friends, the job that looks doable was not at all that simple task. Firstly, to enlist important clinical conditions, to draft FAQ related to these conditions and then to get precise evidence-based answers from various contributors. All in all, it requires consistent communication, periodic reminders and editing of the received manuscripts. Executing all these issues with our busy professional schedule is definitely a difficult task. But our sincere, dedicated editorial team members have been successful to implement this very swiftly and efficiently within short time period of 10 months. Without untiring effort of the team, this dream of mine would have remained unfulfilled. My heartfelt compliments, congratulations and thanks to the entire team.

It gives me immense pleasure to present this novel book for the academic need of pediatrician colleagues and I am sure that it will serve as desk top ready reckoner for its readers. I wish all of you very happy reading.

Digant D Shastri
Chairperson, 2013
IAP Infectious Diseases Chapter

Prologue

Greetings from IAP Infectious Diseases Chapter.

It is a matter of great honor and pleasure for me to write a prologue for *FAQs in Pediatrics Infectious Diseases*, a publication of IAP Infectious Diseases Chapter.

Infectious diseases contribute a major chunk of cases in our day-to-day practice. In spite of availability of morden therapeutic and preventive modalities, thousands of children die in our resource poor country because of various infections.

Infectious Disease Chapter of Indian Academy of Pediatrics is one of the most active chapters known for its various scientific publications. Such type of publications has definitely made a positive impact as far as the rational management and prevention of the infectious diseases are concerned. In continuation of our established legacy and tradition, we have decided to come out with *FAQs in Pediatric Infectious Diseases* which can serve the purpose of desk top ready reckoner during busy hours of routine practice. Experts and stalwarts with national and international reputation have contributed to this project initiated by ID Chapter as per Action Plan, 2013. We are sure, this book will have a phenomenal impact in our understanding of various aspects of childhood infections. We express our gratitude to all the contributors, editors, Chairman (ID Chapter 2013) and office bearers of Indian Academy of Pediatrics, for their cooperation and contribution for the proposed project.

We are sure, this book will be very useful, handy tool in our day-to-day practice.

We wish all of you happy reading and happy learning.

Abhay K Shah
Honorary Secretary
IAP ID Chapter, 2012–13

Preface

IAP Infectious Diseases Chapter has added another feather in its cap *FAQs in Pediatric Infectious Diseases*. These frequently asked questions have been collected from discussions in various forums. Busy pediatric practitioners often find it difficult to get the answer to the questions in the midst of bulky texts. This time we have taken up the common diseases, which we encounter in our daily life. The questions have been selected in the manner, which covers basic knowledge about the disease, its diagnosis and management. The book intends to give an outline of the way one should encounter the disease. Infections in this book have been broadly classified into various systems and also according to the causative organisms. Care has been taken to include infections, that are common in our country and also emerging and re-emerging infections such as pertussis, rickettsia, brucella and leptospira.

IAP Infectious Diseases Chapter has been striving to uplift the knowledge and academics amongst the pediatrician of this country. This time, our effort has been directed not only to the pediatricians but also to the general physicians who are still the first line caregiver of the ailing children of our country. The busy general practitioners will find it very handy for their day-to-day work. The students may utilize this book for ready reference.

Editorial Board

Acknowledgments

We are grateful to the chairperson and members of Executive Board of Indian Academy of Pediatrics Infectious Diseases Chapter, for giving us the humble task of bringing out the *FAQs in Pediatric Infectious Diseases*.

Our sincere thanks to the various contributors, for their tireless efforts to submit the articles.

We are also thankful to Dr Vijay N Yewale (President, IAP 2014), for his cooperation and active help.

Like every year, we are indebted to Dr Prabal Chandra Neogi and Mr Somnath Mukherjee, for the secretarial assistance.

Thanks also go to M/s Jaypee Brothers Medical Publishers (P) Ltd, New Delhi, India, especially to Shri Jitendar P Vij (Group Chairman), Mr Ankit Vij (Managing Director), Mr Tarun Duneja (Director-Publishing), Ms Samina Khan and the whole team in Delhi. We also appreciate the help extended by Mr Sandeep Gupta, Mr Sabyasachi Hazra and others of Kolkata Branch of M/s Jaypee Brothers Medical Publishers (P) Ltd.

All attempts have been made to acknowledge the sources of information. Inadvertent omission, if any, is regretted.

Contents

SECTION 1: SPECIFIC INFECTIONS

PART A: BACTERIAL INFECTIONS

1. ***Staphylococcus aureus*** — 3
   Vijay N Yewale, Dhanya Dharmapalan

2. **Group A Streptococcus** — 12
   Santanu Bhakta

3. **Diphtheria** — 23
   Anju Aggarwal

4. **Pertussis** — 28
   Rohit Agrawal

5. **Meningococcus** — 33
   Raju C Shah, Pratima R Shah

6. **Cholera** — 43
   Alok Kumar Deb

7. **Brucella** — 51
   Sanjay Krishna Ghorpade

8. ***Mycoplasma pneumoniae*** **and** ***Chlamydia*** — 60
   Baldev S Prajapati, Rajal B Prajapati

9. **Rickettsia** — 66
   Atul Kulkarni

10. **Leptospira** — 72
    Janani Sankar

PART B: VIRAL INFECTIONS

11. **Measles** — 77
    Ketan H Shah

12. **Mumps** — 85
    Ashok Rai

13. **Rubella** — 89
    P Ramachandran

14. **Non-polio Enteroviruses** — 94
    Dhanya Dharmapalan

15. **Herpes Simplex** — 98
    Niranjan Mohanty

16. **Varicella** — 102
    Parang Mehta

17.	**Epstein-Barr Virus** *S Balasubramanian, Sumanth Amperayani, K Dhanalakshmi*	107
18.	**Influenza and Parainfluenza** *AK Prasad*	111
19.	**Respiratory Syncytial Virus** *M Govindraj*	118
20.	**Dengue** *Jaydeep Choudhury*	121
21.	**Rabies** *Jaydeep Choudhury*	134
22.	**Viral Hepatitis** *Malathi Sathiyasekaran*	143
23.	**Chikungunya** *Rajniti Prasad*	154

PART C: FUNGAL AND PROTOZOAL INFECTIONS

24.	**Common Fungi** *Kheya Ghosh Uttam*	157
25.	**Kala-azar** *Nigam P Narain*	165
26.	**Malaria** *Jaydeep Choudhury*	171
27.	**Amebiasis and Giardiasis** *Ajay Kalra*	178

SECTION 2: SYSTEMIC INFECTIONS

28.	**Bacterial Meningitis** *Digant D Shastri*	185
29.	**Encephalitis** *Abhay K Shah*	190
30.	**Upper Respiratory Infections** *Nupur Ganguly*	199
31.	**Community Acquired Pneumonia** *Upendra Kinjawadekar, Jaydeep Choudhury*	206
32.	**Infective Endocarditis** *Dhritobrata Das*	212
33.	**Acute Gastroenteritis** *Devdeep Mukherjee*	218
34.	**Urinary Tract Infection** *Jayati Sengupta, Kheya Ghosh Uttam*	227

35. **Enteric Fever** 233
   Monjori Mitra

36. **Intra-abdominal Infections** 242
   Suhas V Prabhu

37. **Bone and Joint Infections** 245
   Narendra Rathi

38. **Skin and Soft Tissue Infections** 249
   Sandipan Dhar

39. **Tuberculosis** 256
   Sangeeta Sharma

40. **Congenital Infections** 267
   Anand K Shandilya

41. **Primary Immunodeficiency** 285
   Subhasish Bhattacharyya

42. **Sepsis Syndrome** 290
   Tanu Singhal

43. **Febrile Neutropenia** 297
   Kheya Ghosh Uttam

44. **Lymphadenitis** 301
   Ritabrata Kundu

45. **HIV Infection** 305
   Ira Shah

Index *319*

SECTION 1:
SPECIFIC INFECTIONS

Part A: Bacterial Infections
1. *Staphylococcus aureus*
2. Group A *Streptococcus*
3. Diphtheria
4. Pertussis
5. *Meningococcus*
6. Cholera
7. *Brucella*
8. *Mycoplasma pneumoniae* and *Chlamydia*
9. Rickettsia
10. *Leptospira*

Part B: Viral Infections
11. Measles
12. Mumps
13. Rubella
14. Non-polio Enteroviruses
15. Herpes simplex
16. Varicella
17. Epstein-Barr Virus
18. Influenza and Parainfluenza
19. Respiratory Syncytial Virus
20. Dengue
21. Rabies
22. Hepatitis Viruses
23. Chikungunya

Part C: Fungal and Protozoal Infections
24. Common Fungi
25. Leishmaniasis
26. Malaria
27. Amebiasis and Giardiasis

PART A: BACTERIAL INFECTIONS

1

Staphylococcus aureus

Vijay Yewale, Dhanya Dharmapalan

1. How is *Staphylococcus aureus* transmitted in community and hospital environment?

Staphylococcus aureus is transmitted by various routes.

Contact with infected persons

Open draining lesions are abundant in staphylococci and direct contact helps transmit these bacteria to other personnel or vehicles of infection.

Contact with asymptomatic carriers

Staphylococcus is ubiquitous in nature and 30% of the population carries it without any symptoms. Colonization increases the risk of infection. Nose, skin, hair, nail, axillae and perineum are the usual sites where *Staphylococcus* colonize, the anterior nasal vestibule being the most prominent site.

Vertical transmission to infant can occur due to colonization of groins or vaginal sites. Horizontal transmission by direct contact by asymptomatic carriers is extremely significant in neonates and young infants who are handled frequently.

Airborne spread

Airborne spread may contribute to nasal colonization and respiratory infections. Desquamated skin scales dispersed into air by movements like bed-making can contribute to airborne transmission.

Contact with contaminated objects

Fomites play an important role in transmission. Objects which are repeatedly handled like toys, remote control, taps, doorknobs, telephone handles, hand towels, etc. are important vehicles for transmission among household contacts. Overcrowding and sports personnel where there is sharing of same towel, also play a role in transmission.

Some nonporous fomites have shown more pronounced and greater period of transmissibility (even for more than 8 weeks after contamination) than porous fomites and metal fomites.

Contact with pets

Infection of pets or transient carriage by pets can transmit infections in households to children by direct contact, licking or indirectly by the shared home environment.

Transmission in healthcare settings

The transmission in healthcare setting occurs from an exogenous source via the hands of the health workers, medical devices and equipments and the hospital environment. It has been widely accepted that improving hand hygiene can cause significant reduction in the transmission. Airborne transmission during procedures like bed-making may contribute to nasal colonization. Methicillin resistant *Staphylococcus aureus* (MRSA) is known to be an endemic in healthcare settings, which employ poor infection control measures mostly predisposed by understaffing.

2. What are the various localized and invasive infections caused by *Staphylococcus aureus*?

Localized infections

Localized infections by staphylococci result by breaching the host defense barriers. Skin is the most common portal of entry. Direct invasion of skin and adjacent tissues leads to a spectrum of localized infections like:
- Folliculitis (infection of hair follicle)
- Furuncle(boil), carbuncle (infection of epidermis)
- Acute paronychia (infection of lateral nail folds)
- Abscess (suppuration within dermis and deeper skin tissues)
- Bullous impetigo (infection of epidermis)
- Cellulitis (extension of infection into the subcutaneous tissue)
- Secondary infections of surgical and traumatic wounds are most likely due to *Staphylococcus*
- Omphalitis (infection of umbilical stump in neonates). The initial local cellulitis around umbilicus seen in babies with risk factors like chorioamnionitis, preterm, low weight babies, if untreated, can easily disseminate and cause severe septicemia.

The skin lesions caused by community acquired MRSA have been described as spontaneous tender red lesions which progress to develop a necrotic center. However, it is clinically very difficult to differentiate between methicillin-susceptible *Staphylococcus aureus* (MSSA) and MRSA.

Invasive infections

The invasive infections are caused by colonization, invasion across epithelial barriers, and evasion of host defenses and destruction of the host tissues.

Respiratory System

Primary staphylococcal pneumonia can occur in young infants. There is usually intense neutrophilic infiltration, necrosis, leading to pneumatocele (thin-walled air-filled cysts) and abscess formation. Rupture of subpleural abscess may result in pyopneumothorax while rupture of abscess into large bronchus can cause bronchopleural fistula.

Other rare respiratory infections caused by staphylococci are exudative pharyngitis, otitis media and chronic sinusitis.

Central nervous system

It is an important etiological agent for brain abscess. The common predisposing factors are cyanotic congenital heart diseases and chronic ear infection. Purulent meningitis may accompany staphylococcal brain abscess. Staphylococcal meningitis may occur following neurological interventions like shunts, craniotomy, etc. or trauma.

Cardiovascular system

Staphylococcus aureus is a predominant cause of acute bacterial endocarditis of both native and prosthetic valves and device. It has been postulated that the increasing incidence of staphylococcal endocarditis could be secondary to more invasive surgical procedures being performed for correction of congenital heart disease.

Musculoskeletal infection

Staphylococcus is the most important etiological agents in muskuloskeletal infections like septic arthritis, osteomyelitis and pyomyositis.

Sequelae like avascular necrosis of epiphysis, limb length discrepancy, and pathologic fracture can occur, especially in longer duration of presenting symptoms, neonates, hip joint involvement, MRSA infection and delayed administration of appropriate antibiotics.

3. What are the toxin-mediated syndromes of *Staphylococcus*?

The toxin-mediated staphylococcal infections occur solely due to toxins produced either in vivo as in toxic shock syndrome and staphylococcal scalded skin syndrome or via the vector that delivers it to host as in food poisoning.

Toxic shock syndrome (TSS)

It is a life, threatening severe illness manifested by fever, rash, diarrhea, hypotension, desquamation and multisystem failure. The manifestation is related to an infection or colonization with a toxin (TSST-1) producing strain of *Staphylococcus aureus*. Any foreign material like nasal packing, tampon used during menstruation, etc. should be removed immediately. Management includes vasopressors, supportive therapy and antitoxin antimicrobials like clindamycin and linezolid. Since TSS is thought to be a superantigen-mediated disease, intravenous immunoglobin can be an adjuvant therapy.

Staphylococcal scalded skin syndrome

staphylococcal exfoliative or epidermolytic toxin produced by the organism can cause an extensive blistering exfoliative dermatitis called staphylococcal scalded skin syndrome (SSSS) or Ritter's disease. It generally affects the infants and young children and may begin with fever and poor feeding. There is intense erythema with formation of large fragile blisters and peeling of the epithelial layer of the skin. There is absence of mucosal involvement. The complications caused include hypothermia, dehydration, and secondary infections.

Food poisoning

Though *Staphylococcus* can be destroyed by pasteurization, its heat resistance depends on the type of food it contaminates. It is highly salt tolerant and can easily thrive in products like cheese. Since skin is the biggest reservoir of staphylococci, contamination often occurs from direct contact or through respiratory droplets of the food handlers. Improper cooking or consumption of improperly stored or refrigerated food are other causes of food poisoning. Within 1–6 hours of ingestion of contaminated food, the child presents with sudden onset of nausea, vomiting, abdominal pain and diarrhea.

4. What are the features of coagulase-negative staphylococcal infection?

Coagulase-negative staphylococci (CONS) except the *S. saprophyticus* cause primarily nosocomial infections. Infections caused by CONS are indolent with a subacute and sometimes even a chronic course. The capability of producing biofilm appears to play a central role in their virulence.

Since majority of the coagulase-negative staphylococci are part of the normal flora of human skin, the dilemma arises in the differentiation of the true pathogen from the contaminant.

CONS cause the following infections:

Neonatal septicemia

CONS are leading cause of late onset septicemia, particularly in the preterm and low birthweight babies. This is due to the innate immunodeficient state, prolonged neonatal intensive case unit (NICU) stay and the need for invasive procedures in these babies. Transmission mostly occurs horizontally and endemic strains may be circulated for a long time in NICU via the hands of health workers. The clinical features are subtle due to the low virulence though more virulent strains are associated with severe thrombocytopenia.

Pediatric oncology patients and bone marrow recipients

- CONS is the most commonly isolated pathogen (30–40%) in blood stream infections in pediatric cancer patients. It is related to more intense chemotherapy regimens, increased use of indwelling catheters and alterations in cellular and humoral immunity. Most of the serious infections occur in the induction period.
- Post bone marrow transplant, many early infections are associated with the indwelling central venous catheter. Graft versus host disease is an additional risk factor for bacteremic infections.

Indwelling medical devices

Children with indwelling medical devices such as central venous catheters, cerebrospinal fluid shunts, peritoneal dialysis catheter, prosthetic valves or joints, vascular grafts and prostheses, hemodialysis shunt, pacemaker, etc. are prone for colonization with CONS.

5. What is meant by MSSA, MRSA and VRSA? What are the management guidelines?

MSSA and MRSA

Based on the susceptibility to antimicrobials, *Staphylococcus aureus* are grouped as MSSA—Methicillin-susceptible *Staphylococcus aureus* and MRSA—Methicillin-resistant *Staphylococcus aureus*.

MRSA is further classified based on the epidemiology, antimicrobial susceptibility and molecular characteristics into:
- Healthcare-associated MRSA (HA-MRSA)
- Community-acquired MRSA (CA-MRSA).

Molecular typing shows that different staphylococcal chromosome cassette (SCC) mec types are associated with HA-MRSA (SCC mecA I-III) and CA-MRSA (SCC mecA IV–V).

HA-MRSA are resistant to all beta-lactamase resistant beta-lactam and cephalosporins while CA-MRSA although resistant to all beta-lactam antimicrobials are susceptible to drugs like trimethoprim-sulfamethoxazole, fluoroquinolones, gentamycin and doxycycline.

HA-MRSA are predisposed by hospitalization within the previous year, antimicrobial use in recent three months, prolonged hospital stay, presence of intravascular or peritoneal catheters and tracheal tubes, increased number of surgical procedures or frequent contact with person with one or more preceding risk factors. CA-MRSA is labeled in those MRSA infections which are devoid of the above risk factors.

VRSA

There are reports of Vancomycin-resistant *Staphylococcus aureus* (VRSA) or vancomycin-resistant strains. The definition used by CDC for classification of staphylococci isolates are vancomycin-susceptible: MIC or minimum inhibitory concentration less than or equal to 2 µg/mL; Vancomycin-intermediate *S. aureus* (VISA) vancomycin MIC = 4-8 µg/mL and Vancomycin-resistant *S. aureus* (VRSA): vancomycin MIC >16 µg/mL. Fortunately, all VRSA and VISA are susceptible to one or more of the available antimicrobials like linezolid, daptomycin, tigecycline. The other agents which can be used are teicoplanin, trimethoprim-sulfamethoxazole, tetracycline, rifampin (usually in combination therapy), and chloramphenicol.

Management

Staphylococcal infections should be treated with the most specific antistaphylococcal antimicrobial agents. In general, community-acquired staphylococcal infections in an immunocompetent child are caused by MSSA and should be treated with cloxacillin. Other agents used to treat MSSA infections include clindamycin, cephalexin, cefadroxil, cefuroxime, co-amoxyclav.

The treatment of choice for invasive MRSA is vancomycin. In children who are allergic or unable to tolerate vancomycin, the drugs used are, clindamycin, linezolid, teicoplanin, daptomycin and trimethoprim-sulfamethaxazole. Linezolid, a bacteriostatic drug achieves better concentration in lung tissue but should be avoided when a bacteremic illness is being treated.

6. How do we manage skin and soft tissue infection caused by community-acquired *Staphylococcus*?

An important step in the management of the skin and soft tissue infections like furunculitis, abscesses, etc. whether caused by MSSA or MRSA is adequate drainage and, if necessary, debridement.

Topical antibiotics like mupirocin may be applied for cutaneous infections like boils, impetigo. Most community-acquired infections respond to cloxacillin or first generation cephalosporins like cefadroxil or cephalexin.

Treatment with oral clindamycin or trimethoprim-sulfamethaxazole and rifampin may be considered in areas with high prevalence of CA-MRSA.

In infections which require hospitalization, clindamycin or vancomycin is indicated. Clindamycin may be rendered ineffective in presence of macrolide–lincosomide recognized by D-test. In this test, the clindamycin and erythromycin discs are placed together on a culture plate. The zone of inhibition around clindamycin resembles a letter 'D' instead of 'O' due to flattening on the side towards erythromycin due to inducible lincosomide resistance.

Linezolid, is useful for severe refractory MRSA infections but should be reserved for serious infections because of emerging resistance to linezolid. Similarly, the newer parenteral antibiotics like daptomycin and tigecycline should be used extremely judiciously for serious infections.

In case of recurrent episodes of skin or soft tissue infections, the patient and close contacts should be treated with 2% mupirocin local application in the anterior nares for seven days.

7. How to manage Staphylococcal pneumonia and its complications?

Attempts should be made to isolate the pathogen for drug susceptibility from either pleural fluid or blood. Staphylococci isolated from community acquired pneumonia are fortunately to a large scale methicillin sensitive.

Therefore, cloxacillin is the first choice of therapy. Alternatives may be first generation cephalosporins like cefazolin and cefuroxime. Cloxacillin is found to be superior to vancomycin in MSSA infections and hence, the later should be avoided to prevent drug resistance. In suspected staphylococcal pneumonia, where microbiological diagnosis is not established and other etiology is not ruled out, amoxyclav or cefuroxime may be used.

Vancomycin/linezolid can be used to treat MRSA pneumonia. However, linezolid appears to have a better concentration in the respiratory epithelial cells and may be superior to vancomycin. Linezolid also has antitoxin effect.

Complications in children include pleural effusion, empyema, lung abscess, pneumatocele and cavitary/necrotising pneumonia.

Parapneumonic effusion may resolve with antibiotics alone. Systemic antibiotics with cloxacillin and physiotherapy with postural drainage is the initial treatment of choice for lung abscess. Empyema in young children should be drained to prevent dissemination of infection and long-term sequelae such as pleural fibrosis. Closed tube thoracostomy drainage is the treatment of choice. In event of failure, thoracoscopy and formal thoracotomy with either decortication or open drainage may be employed. Some retrospective studies suggest that an early VATS (video-assisted thoracoscopic surgery) or thoracotomy leads to shorter hospitalization. Incomplete drainage may result into partial response and should not be misinterpreted as drug resistance.

8. What are the various control measures of staphylococcal infection?

Hand hygiene

Hand hygiene plays one of the most important roles in the control of staphylococcal infections as the principal mode of transmission appears to be contaminated hands of personnel. Hands should be washed thoroughly with soap and water or with the use of alcohol hand antiseptics which contain either isopropanol, ethanol, n-propanol, or a combination of two of these products.

Personal protection

Apart from hand hygiene by covering wounds with draining pus with clean and dry bandages, sharing of contaminated towels, clothing, razors etc. should be avoided.

Screening for MRSA in healthy carriers in a community is extremely challenging and may be undertaken in case of an outbreak from a crowded place like schools, hostels, etc.

In healthcare settings:
- Hand cleansing either with proper wash or alcohol in between touching of patients, medical devices and also after removal of gloves
- Screening and isolation of patients suspected with MRSA and treatment on confirmation
- Identification of carriage in health settings and among close contacts of CA-MRSA and decolonization with mupirocin application in the anterior nares for five days. They should, in addition, use hand hygiene measures to eliminate transmission by contact
- Judicious management of staphylococcal infections by incision and drainage of pus and prevention of delayed resolution of infection, thereby reducing the selecting out antibiotic-resistant staphylococci. Also, rational use of antimicrobials will overall reduce the selection pressure of antibiotics
- Implementation of infection control policy in the healthcare setting for surveillance, detection, control and prevention of nosocomial infections
- Education for increased awareness about staphylococcal infection among the healthcare workers.

Antistaphylococcal vaccine

Currently, there is no vaccine available against *Staphylococcus* strains. However, there are at least seven vaccine and immunotherapy candidates against *S. aureus* in the developmental phase targeting both active and passive immunization.

Further Reading

1. Albrich WC, Harbarth S. Health-care workers: source, vector, or victim of MRSA? Lancet Infect Dis. 2008;8·289-30.
2. Alshammary A, Hervas-Malo M, Robinson JL. Pediatric infective endocarditis: Has *Staphylococcus aureus* overtaken viridans group streptococci as the predominant etiological agent? Can J Infect Dis Med Microbiol. 2008;19(1):63-8.
3. Centers for Disease Control and Prevention " VRSA/VISA" Web site http://www.cdc.gov/HAI/organisms/visa_vrsa/visa_vrsa.html (Accessed November, 24, 2010).
4. Chuang YY, Huang YC, Lin TY. Toxic shock syndrome in children: epidemiology, pathogenesis, and management. Paediatr Drugs. 2005;7(1):11-25.
5. Davis MF, Iverson SA, Baron P, et al. Household transmission of meticillin-resistant *Staphylococcus aureus* and other staphylococci. Lancet Infect Dis 2012;12(9):703-16.
6. Desai R, Pannaraj PS, Agopian J, Sugar CA, Liu GY, Miller LG. Survival and transmission of community-associated methicillin-resistant *Staphylococcus aureus* from fomites. Am J of Infect Control. 2011;39 (3):219-25.
7. Elston DM. Methicillin-Sensitive and Methicillin-Resistant *Staphylococcus aureus*: Management Principles and Selection of Antibiotic Therapy. Dermatol Clin 2007;25:157-64.
8. Gates RL, Caniano DA, Hayes JR, Arca MJ. Does VATS provide optimal treatment of empyema in children? A systematic review. J Pediatr Surg. 2004;39(3):381-6.

9. Gold HS, Pillai SK. Antistaphylococcal agents. Infect Dis Clin North Am. 2009; 23(1):99-131. doi: 10.1016/j.idc.2008.10.008.
10. Huda T, Nair H, Theodoratou E, et al. An evaluation of the emerging vaccines and immunotherapy against staphylococcal pneumonia in children. BMC Public Health. 2011;11(Suppl 3):S27.
11. Karambelkar GR, Agarkhedkar SR, Karwa DS, Singhania SS, Mane SV. Disease pattern and bacteriology of childhood pneumonia in WesternIndia. Int J Pharm Biomed Sci. 2012;3(4): 177-80.
12. Katsibardi K, Papadakis V, Harisiadi A, Haidas S, Polychronopoulou S. Infections in pediatric patients with acute lymphoblastic leukemia during the entire course of treatment. Arch Hellen Med. 2009;26(3):366-73.
13. Landgraf M, Destro MT. Staphylococcal Food Poisoning. Foodborne Infections and Intoxications, 4th edition 2013.p.389-400.
14. Marchant EA, Boyce GK, Sadarangani M, Lavoie PM. Neonatal Sepsis due to Coagulase-Negative Staphylococci. Clin Dev Immunol. 2013;586076.
15. Moran GJ, Amii RN, Abrahamian FM, Talan DA. Emerg Infect Dis. 2005; 11(6):928-30.
16. Skova R, Christiansenb K, Dancerc SJ, et al. Update on the prevention and control of community-acquired meticillin-resistant *Staphylococcus aureus* (CA-MRSA). Int J Antimicrob Agents, 2012;39(3):193-200.
17. Sukswai P, Kovitvanitcha D, Thumkunanon V, Chotpitayasunondh T, Sangtawesin V, Jeerathanyasakun Y. Acute hematogenous osteomyelitis and septic arthritis in children: clinical characteristics and outcomes study. J Med Assoc Thai. 2011;94(Suppl 3):S209-16.
18. Tekkök IH, Erbengi A. Management of brain abscess in children: review of 130 cases over a period of 21 years. Child's Nervous System. 1992;8(7):411-6.

2
Group A Streptococcus

Santanu Bhakta

1. What is the epidemiology of Group A Streptococcus (GAS) infection?

Overall, the epidemiology of GAS infection is complex. Group A streptococci are gram-positive coccoid-shaped bacteria that tend to grow in chains. Humans are the natural reservoir of GAS. It is highly communicable and can produce disease in normal individual of all ages. While disease in neonates is uncommon, probably due to transmitted maternal antibody, this organism commonly produces two main types of diseases.

Pharyngeal infection

Pharyngeal infection is very common in children between 5 to 15 years of age. They can spread via salivary droplets and nasal discharge and close proximity helps in transmission. Incubation period for pharyngitis is 2–5 days. If untreated, GAS has the potential to be an important upper respiratory tract pathogen causing outbreaks, especially in day care settings like schools, military barracks, crèche, etc. Chronic pharyngeal carriers of GAS rarely transmit to others.

Skin infection

Streptococcal skin infection (impetigo, pyoderma) occurs throughout the year in warmer climates. GAS cannot penetrate intact skin and thus, colonization of healthy skin by GAS precedes development of impetigo. Then it invades the breached skin like traumatic wounds, insect bites, burns, etc. to produce impetigo. Although, impetigo-serotypes may colonize throat, spread via skin to skin is usual and not via respiratory tract. Fingernails and perianal regions harbor GAS and important in spreading impetigo as we see multiple cases in same family. Both pharyngitis and impetigo occur in crowded homes and poor hygienic conditions.

Invasive GAS infections

The incidence of severe invasive GAS infections including bacterimia, streptococcal toxic shock syndrome, necrotizing fasciitis has increased in recent years and attacks very young and older persons. Risk factors include varicella, HIV infection, intravenous drug use, chronic pulmonary and cardiac disease. Severe invasive disease rarely follows GAS pharyngitis and is believed to be mostly through skin and mucous membrane though the portal of entry is unknown in 50% cases. Two types commonly associated with pharyngitis, rarely cause skin infections and those commonly associated with skin infections, rarely cause pharyngitis. A few of the pharyngeal strains (M type 12) have been associated with glomerulonephritis, but more of the skin strains (M types 49, 55, 57 and 60) have been considered nephritogenic. A few of the pharyngeal serotypes, but none of the skin strains, have been associated with acute rheumatic fever. M types 1, 3, 12, and 28 have been the most common isolates from patients with shock and multiorgan failure.

2. **What are the common manifestations of Group A Streptococcus infection?**

The most common infections caused by GAS, involves the respiratory tract and skin and soft tissues. In upper respiratory tract infection (URTI), it is an important cause for acute pharyngitis and pneumonia is rare. In skin and soft tissue infection, it is responsible for impetigo. Other manifestations are as follows:

Scarlet fever

Scarlet fever, caused by erythrogenic toxin-producing GAS, manifested by fever with characteristic rash appearing 24–48 hours after fever along with pharyngitis. Age distribution, mode of transmission and other epidemiological features are same as GAS pharyngitis.

Impetigo

Impetigo (or pyoderma) is of two clinical types; bullous, and more common, nonbullous. It is a superficial infection of skin occurring mostly in face and extremities and regional lymphadenitis is common. Bullous impetigo is less common and occurs mostly in neonates and young infants. Face, buttocks, trunk and perineum are mostly affected.

Erysipelas

Erysipelas is a relatively rare acute GAS infection of the deeper layer of skin and underlying connective tissue. Onset is abrupt and affected skin is swollen, red and very tender with systemic manifestation of fever.

Perianal dermatitis

Perianal dermatitis is a distinct clinical entity with well-demarcated perianal erythema, anal pruritus, painful defecation and blood-streaked stools. They are very tender but systemic manifestations are unusual.

Vaginitis

Vaginitis is a common in prepubertal girls manifested as serous discharge, marked erythema and irritation of vulvar area with dysuria.

Severe invasive GAS infection

Severe invasive GAS infection is defined by isolation of GAS from a normally sterile body site. It includes three overlapping clinical syndromes. The first is streptococcal toxic shock syndrome. The second is GAS necrotizing fasciitis characterized by extensive local necrosis of skin and soft tissues. The third is the group of focal and systemic infections that do not meet the criteria for toxic shock syndrome or necrotizing fasciitis and includes bacteremia with no identified focus. It may be in the form of meningitis, pneumonia, peritonitis, puerperal sepsis, osteomyelitis, suppurative arthritis, myositis, and surgical wound infections.

3. What is streptococcal toxic shock syndrome?

It is a type of severe invasive disease produced by GAS and differentiated from other types of invasive GAS infections by the presence of shock and multiorgan system failure early in the course of the infection. Following are the criteria:

Case definition of streptococcal toxic shock syndrome (streptococcal TSS)

I. Isolation of group A Streptococcus

- A. From a sterile site (blood, CSF, Peritoneal fluid, tissue biopsy specimen)
- B. From a nonsterile body site (throat, sputum, vagina, open surgical wound, superficial skin lesion)

II. Clinical signs of severity

- A. Hypotension
- B. Clinical and laboratory abnormalities (requires two or more of the following) signs:
    - i. Renal impairment
    - ii. Coagulopathy
    - iii. Liver abnormalities
    - iv. Acute respiratory distress syndrome
    - v. Extensive tissue necrosis, i.e., necrotizing fasciitis
    - vi. Erythematous rash

Definite Case = An illness fulfilling criteria IA and IIA and IIB
Probable Case = An illness fulfilling criteria IB and IIA and IIB

> Pain is the most common initial symptom of streptococcal TSS, abrupt in onset and severe.
> Fever is the most common early sign, although hypothermia may be present in patients with shock. Eighty percent of patients have clinical signs of soft tissue infection, such as localized swelling and erythema. Blood cultures are positive in 60% of cases. Renal impairment is very common and important component of streptococcal TSS. Persons of all ages are affected; most do not have predisposing underlying diseases. This is in sharp contrast to previous reports of GAS bacteremia, in which patients were either under 10 or over 60 years of age, and most had underlying conditions such as cancer, renal failure, leukemia, or severe burns, etc. The pathogenic mechanisms responsible for severe, invasive GAS infections, like streptococcal toxic shock syndrome is yet to be defined completely, but an association with streptococcal pyrogenic exotoxins A, B, and C has been suggested, which act as superantigens, and stimulate an intense activation and proliferation of T lymphocytes and macrophages resulting in the production of large quantities of cytokines. These cytokines are capable of producing shock and tissue injury, and are believed to be responsible for many of the clinical manifestations of severe, invasive GAS infections.

4. What are the suppurative and nonsuppurative complications of Streptococcal infection? Give a brief description of each.

Suppurative complication from GAS infection may occur due to spread of the infection to the adjacent structures because of inadequate treatment and can give rise to cervical lymphadenitis, peritonsilar abcess, retrophryngeal abscess, mastoiditis, sinusitis and otitis media.

The non-suppurative complications are acute rheumatic fever, acute poststreptococcal glomerulonephritis, poststreptococcal reactive arthritis and pediatric autoimmune neuropsychiatric disorders associated with *Streptococcus pyogenes* (PANDAS).

Acute rheumatic fever

Acute rheumatic fever is a nonsuppurative complication of group A beta hemolytic streptococcal (GABHS) sore throat. It usually occurs 2-4 weeks after streptococcal pharyngitis. It affects joints, skin, subcutaneous tissue, brain and heart. Except heart, all other effects are reversible, needing only symptomatic relief during the episodes. Cardiac complications are significant in absence of secondary prophylaxis and culminate into chronic and life-threatening valvular heart disease. Prevalence of acute rheumatic fever and rheumatic heart disease (RHD) in Indian population varies from 0.5/1000 to 11/1000 in various studies. Not all of the serotypes of GAS can cause rheumatic fever. Acute rheumatic fever can occur only after an infection of the upper respiratory tract. Patients with acute rheumatic fever almost always have serologic evidence of a recent GAS infection. Antimicrobial therapy that eliminates GAS from the pharynx also prevents initial episodes of acute rheumatic fever, and long-term, continuous prophylaxis that prevents GAS pharyngitis also prevents recurrences of acute rheumatic fever. Carditis and resultant chronic rheumatic heart disease are the most serious manifestations of acute rheumatic fever and account for essentially all of the associated morbidity and mortality.

Acute poststreptococcal glomerulonephritis (APSGN)

Acute glomerulonephritis can occur after a GAS infection of either the upper respiratory tract or the skin. This is a classic example of the acute nephritic syndrome characterized by the sudden onset of gross hematuria, edema, hypertension, and renal insufficiency. Acute poststreptococcal glomerulonephritis is one of the most common glomerular causes of gross hematuria in children and is a major cause of morbidity in GAS infection. Although epidemics of nephritis have been described in association with both throat (serotype 12) and skin (serotype 49) infections, this disease is most commonly sporadic. Early systemic antibiotic therapy for streptococcal throat and skin infections does not eliminate the risk of acute poststreptococcal glomerulonephritis. APSGN is most common in children aged 5–12 years and uncommon before the age of 3 years. The typical patient develops symptoms 1–2 week after an antecedent streptococcal pharyngitis or 3–6 weeks after a streptococcal pyoderma. Complete recovery occurs in more than >95% of children with APSGN. Recurrences are extremely rare.

Poststreptococcal reactive arthritis

It is a syndrome characterized by the onset of acute arthritis following an episode of GAS pharyngitis in a patient whose illness does not otherwise fulfill the Jones criteria for the diagnosis of acute rheumatic fever. Though it usually involves the large joints, in contrast to the arthritis of acute rheumatic fever, it may involve small peripheral joints as well as the axial skeleton and is typically non-migratory. In contrast to the arthritis of acute rheumatic fever, poststreptococcal reactive arthritis does not respond dramatically to therapy with aspirin or other nonsteroidal anti-inflammatory agents. A small proportion of patients with poststreptococcal reactive arthritis may go on to develop valvular heart disease. Therefore, these patients should be carefully observed for several months for the subsequent development of carditis.

Pediatric autoimmune neuropsychiatric disorders associated with streptococcus pyogenes (PANDAS)

PANDAS have been used to describe a group of neuropsychiatric disorders (particularly obsessive-compulsive disorders, tic disorders, and Tourette syndrome) for which a possible relationship with GAS infections has been suggested.

5. What is the diagnostic test for Group A streptococcal pharyngitis?

Diagnostic studies for GAS pharyngitis are not indicated for children less than 3 years old because acute rheumatic fever is rare and the classic presentation of streptococcal pharyngitis are uncommon in this age group. Selected children less than 3 years old who have other risk factors, such as an older sibling with GAS infection, may be considered for testing.

Swabbing the throat and testing for GAS pharyngitis by rapid antigen detection test (RADT) and/or culture should be performed because the clinical features alone do not reliably discriminate between GAS and viral pharyngitis except when overt viral features like rhinorrhea, cough, oral ulcers, and/or hoarseness are present. In children and adolescents, negative RADT tests should be backed up by a throat culture. Positive RADTs do not necessitate a back-up culture because they are highly specific (>95%).

Anti-streptococcal antibody titers are not recommended in the routine diagnosis of acute pharyngitis as they reflect past but not current events.

Diagnostic testing or empiric treatment of asymptomatic household contacts of patients with acute streptococcal pharyngitis is not routinely recommended.

6. What is the treatment of streptococcal pharyngitis?

GAS is the most common bacterial cause of acute pharyngitis, responsible for 20–30% in children. Accurate diagnosis of streptococcal pharyngitis followed by appropriate antimicrobial therapy is important for the prevention of acute rheumatic fever; for the prevention of suppurative complications (e.g. peritonsillar abscess, cervical lymphadenitis, mastoiditis, and possibly, other invasive infections); to improve clinical symptoms and signs; for the rapid decrease in contagiousness; for reduction in transmission of GAS to family members, classmates, and other close contacts of the patient; to allow for the rapid resumption of usual activities.

Patients with acute GAS pharyngitis should be treated with an appropriate antibiotic at an appropriate dose for duration likely to eradicate the organism from the pharynx (usually 10 days). Based on their narrow spectrum of activity, infrequency of adverse reactions, and modest cost, penicillin or amoxycillin is the recommended drug of choice for those non-allergic to these agents.

Treatment of GAS pharyngitis in penicillin-allergic individuals should include a first generation cephalosporin (for those not anaphylactically sensitive) for 10 days, clindamycin or clarithromycin for 10 days, or azithromycin for 5 days (Table 1).

Clinicians caring for patients with recurrent episodes of pharyngitis associated with laboratory evidence of GAS pharyngitis consider that they may be experiencing more than one episode of bona fide streptococcal pharyngitis at close intervals, but they should also be alert to the possibility

Table 1: Antibiotic regimens recommended for group A streptococcal pharyngitis

Drug, route	Dose or Dosage	Duration or Quantity
For individuals without penicillin allergy		
Penicillin V, oral	Children: 250 mg twice daily or 3 times daily; adolescents and adults: 250 mg 4 times daily or 500 mg twice daily	10 d
Amoxycillin, oral	50 mg/kg once daily (max = 1000 mg); alternate: 25 mg/kg (max = 500 mg) twice daily	10 d
Benzathine penicillin G, intramuscular	< 27 kg: 600,000 U; $\geq$ kg: 1,200,000 U	1 dose
For individuals with penicillin allergy		
Cephalexin, oral	20 mg/kg/dose twice daily (max = 500 mg/dose)	10 d
Cefadroxil, oral	30 mg/kg once daily (max = 1 g)	10 d
Clindamycin, oral	7 mg/kg/dose 3 times daily (max = 300 mg/dose)	10 d
Azithromycin, oral	12 mg/kg once daily (max = 500 mg)	5 d
Clarithromycin, oral	7.5 mg/kg/dose twice daily (max = 250 mg/dose)	10 d

Source: Shulman T, et al. Clinical Practice Guideline for the Diagnosis and Management of Group A Streptococcal Pharyngitis: 2012 Update by the Infectious Diseases Society of America by Stanford

that the patient may actually be a chronic pharyngeal GAS carrier who is experiencing repeated viral infections. If a physician suspects that "ping-pong" spread of infections is the explanation for multiple recurrent episodes of infections within a family, it may be helpful to obtain throat swabs from all family contacts simultaneously, and to treat those for whom culture or RADT results are positive. There is no credible evidence that family pets are reservoirs for GAS pharyngitis or that they contribute to familial spread.

7. How to manage acute rheumatic fever?

Management of acute rheumatic fever consists of diagnosis and treatment.

Diagnosis

Because no clinical or laboratory finding is pathognomonic for acute rheumatic fever, Jones criteria (Table 2) is used to aid in diagnosis and to limit over-diagnosis. The criteria, revised in 1992 by the American Heart Association (AHA) are intended only for the diagnosis of the initial attack of acute rheumatic fever and not for recurrences. Diagnosis is based on recognition of major and minor criteria supported by evidence of preceding streptococcal infection.

Table 2: Diagnosis of rheumatic fever

Clinical and laboratory criteria	Supportive evidence of preceding streptococcal infection (essential except for diagnosis of Chorea)
Major criteria (more specific) • Carditis • Polyarthritis • Chorea • Subcutaneous nodule • Erythema marginatum	Antistreptolysin O ASO titer: >333 unit for children and 250 for adults. Anti-deoxyribonuclease B (normal values AntiDNase B titer 1:60 unit in preschool, 1:480 units in school children and 1:340 in adults)
Minor criteria (less specific) • Fever • Polyarthralgia • ESR. CRR polymorphouuclear leukocytosis (follow standard laboratory values) • * ECG prolonged PR interval	**History of (within previous 45 days)** • streptococcal sore throat • scarlet fever • positive throat culture • positive rapid streptococcal antigen detection test

* Normal upper range—PR Interval: 3–12 years: 0.16 sec; 12–14 year: 0.18 sec; >17y:0.20 sec

Source: Consensus Guidelines on Pediatric Acute Rheumatic Fever and Rheumatic Heart Disease; Working group on Pediatric acute Rheumatic fever and Cardiology chapter of IAP These Guidelines were formulated at National Consultative Meeting on 20th May, 2007, IMA Hall, New Delhi, under IAP Vision 2007.

First episode: Two major or one major and two minor criteria plus supportive evidence of previous Streptococcal throat infection.

Recurrence in a patient without established heart disease: Two major or one major and two minor criteria plus supportive evidence of previous streptococcal throat infection.

Recurrence in a patient with established heart disease: Two minor criteria and supportive evidence of previous streptococcal throat infection.

Rheumatic chorea and insidious onset rheumatic carditis: No requirement of other major manifestations or supportive evidence of streptococcal sore throat infection.

Treatment

According to clinical status, treatment for pain relief should be given (codeine or paracetamol till diagnosis is confirmed and aspirin after the diagnosis is confirmed). Hospitalization is needed for moderate to severe carditis, severe arthritis or chorea. Rest is individualized according to symptoms. For arthritis, rest for two weeks is adequate. Carditis without congestive heart failure (CHF) needs 4–6 weeks of rest. In cases of CHF, rest must be continued till the CHF is controlled. Appropriate diet is a must for a growing child with cardiac involvement. Total duration of anti-inflammatory therapy after the diagnosis of acute rheumatic fever is established, must be 12 weeks. Aspirin and steroids are primarily used to control inflammation. Naproxen and methylprednisolone can be used alternatively. Mild chorea is treated with quite environment, and sedatives like oral phenobarbitone or diazepam. If there is no response, then one may use haloperidol (0.25–0.5 mg/kg/d), sodium valproate (15 mg/kg/day), or carbamazepine (7–20 mg/kg/d) may be used.

Management of cardiac complication should be done according to the case (CHF, atrial fibrillation, valvular heart disease, etc.).

8. What are the guidelines for prophylaxis of acute rheumatic fever?

Secondary prevention of rheumatic fever is defined as the continuous administration of specific antibiotics to patients with a previous attack of rheumatic fever, or documented rheumatic heart disease (RHD). The purpose is to prevent colonization or infection of the upper respiratory tract with group A beta-hemolytic streptococci and the development of recurrent attacks of rheumatic fever. Secondary prophylaxis should be started only after establishing the diagnosis of acute rheumatic fever. Isolated ASO titer is not a criteria to start secondary prophylaxis. After surgery or intervention, secondary prophylaxis should be continued (Table 3).

Table 3: Drugs recommended for secondary prophylaxis

Drugs	Dose	Sore-throat treatment (duration)	Secondary prophylaxis (interval)*
Benzathine Penicillin G (deep 1M inj)	1.2 million unit (>27 kg) after sensitivity test (AST) 0.6 million unit (<27 kg) (after sensitivity test) Contraindication: Penicillin allergy	single dose** single dose**	21 d 15 d
Penicillin V (oral)	Children: 250 mg qid Adult: 500 mg qid Contraindication: Penicillin allergy	10 d 10 d	twice a day twice a day
Azithromycin (oral)	12.5 mg/kg/day once daily	5 d	not recommended
Cephalexin (oral)	15–20 mg/kg dose bid	10 d	not recommended
Erythromycin (oral)	20 mg/kg/dose max 500 mg Contraindication: Liver disorder	not recommended	twice a day

* see text for duration of secondary prophylaxis and references
** only one dose is sufficient for GABHS pharyngitis

Source: Consensus Guidelines on Pediatric Acute Rheumatic Fever and Rheumatic Heart Disease; Working group on Pediatric acute Rheumatic fever and Cardiology chapter of IAP These Guidelines were formulated at National Consultative Meeting on 20th May, 2007, IMA Hall, New Delhi, under IAP Vision 2007

Duration of secondary prophylaxis
  i. No carditis: 5 years/18 years of age, whichever is longer.
  ii. Mild to moderate carditis and healed carditis: 10 years/25 years of age, whichever is longer.
  iii. Severe disease or post intervention patients: Lifelong. One may opt for secondary prophylaxis up to the age of 40 years.

Further Reading

1. Barnham M. Invasive streptococcal infections in the era before the acquired immune deficiency syndrome: a 10 years' compilation of patients with streptococcal bacteraemia in North Yorkshire. J Infect Dis. 1989;18:231-48.
2. Braunstein H. Characteristics of group A streptococcal bacteremia in patients at the San Bernardino County Medical Center. Rev Infect Dis. 1991;13:8-11.
3. Carapetis JR, Brown A, Wilson NJ, Edwards KN. On behalf of the Rheumatic Fever Guidelines Writing Group. An Australian guideline for rheumatic fever and rheumatic heart disease: an abridged outline eMJA. 2007;186:581-6.
4. Dillon HC. Impetigo contagiosa: suppurative and nonsuppurative complication. Clinical, bacteriologic and epidemiologic characteristics of impetigo. Am J Dis Child. 1968;115:530-41.
5. Francis J, Warren RE. Streptococcus pyogenes bacteraemia in Cambridge: a review of 67 episodes. Q J Med. 1988; 256:603-13.
6. Gemmell CG, Peterson PK, Schmeling D, Kim Y, Mathews J, Wannamaker L, et al. Potentiation of opsonization and phagocytosis of *Streptococcus pyogenes* following growth in the presence of clindamycin. J Clin Invest. 1981;67:1249-56.
7. Holm S. Fatal group A streptococcal infections. Presented at the 89th Conference of the American Society for Microbiology; New Orleans, LA;1989.
8. Johnson DR, Stevens DL, Kaplan EL. Epidemiologic analysis of group A streptococcal serotypes associated with severe systemic infections, rheumatic fever, or uncomplicated pharyngitis. J Infect Dis. 1992;166:374-82.
9. Kohler W, Gerlach D, Knoll H. Streptococcal outbreaks and erythrogenic toxin type A. Zbl Bakt Hyg. 1987;266:104-15.
10. Kumar R, Raizada A, Aggarwal AK, Ganguly NK. A community based rheumatic fever/rheumatic heart disease cohort: twelve year experience. Indian Heart J 2002:54:54-8.
11. Kumar R, Thakur JS, Aggarwal A, Ganguly NK. Compliance of secondary prophylaxis for controlling rheumatic fever and rheumatic heart disease in a rural area of Northern India. Indian Heart J 1997;49: 283-88.
12. Nair PM, Philip E, Bahuleyan CG, Thomas M, Shanmugham JS, Saguna Bai NS. The first attack of acute rheumatic fever in childhood: clinical and laboratory profile. Indian Pediatr. 1990;27:241-6.
13. Report of expert consultation on rheumatic fever and rheumatic heart disease 29 October-1November 2001. World Health Organization. Available from: URL: http://www.who.int/cardio vascular diseases/resources/en/cvd_trs 923.pdf. Accessed February, 2008
14. Sanyal SK, Berry AM, Duggal S, Hooja V, Ghosh S. Sequelae of the initial attack of acute rheumatic fever in children from north India. A prospective 5-year follow-up study. Circulation. 1982;65:375-79.

15. Shulmam T, et al. Clinical Practice Guideline for the Diagnosis and Management of Group A Streptococcal Pharyngitis: Update by the Infectious Diseases Society of America; Stanford; 2012.
16. Stevens DL, Bryant AE, Hackett SP. Antibiotic effects on bacterial viability, toxin production and host response. Clin Infect Dis 1995;20(Suppl 2):S154-7.
17. Stevens DL. Invasive group A *Streptococcus* infections. Clin Infect Dis. 1992; 14:2-13.
18. Stevens DL, Maier KA, Mitten JE. Effect of antibiotics on toxin production and viability of *Clostridium perfringens*. Antimicrob Agents Chemother. 1987; 31:213-8.
19. Stevens DL, Yan S, Bryant AE. Penicillin-binding protein expression at different growth stages determines penicillin efficacy in vitro and in vivo: an explanation for the inoculum effect. J Infect Dis. 1993;167:1401-5.
20. Streptococcus. Nelson Textbook of Pediatrics, 18th edition; WB Saunders, Philadelphia; 2008.
21. Yan S, Bohach GA, Stevens DL. Persistent acylation of high-molecular weight Penicillin-binding proteins by penicillin induces the post-antibiotic effect in *Streptococcus pyogenes*. J Infect Dis. 1994;170:609-14.
22. Yan S, Mendelman PM, Stevens DL. The in vitro antibacterial activity of ceftriaxone against *Streptococcus pyogenes* is unrelated to penicillin-binding protein. FEMS Microbiol Lett 1993;110:313-18.

3

Diphtheria

Anju Aggarwal

1. What is the epidemiology of diphtheria?

The usual causative organism for diphtheria is *Corynebacterium diphtheriae*. It is a gram positive bacterium. There are 4 biotypes of this bacteria, i.e, *mitis, intermedius, belfanti* and *gravis*. These strains become toxigenic by acquiring a bacteriophage. It inhabits the human mucous membranes and skin. It is carried in the respiratory tract and spreads by respiratory droplets or from skin secretions. It may be a commensal in respiratory tract in endemic areas. The disease is seen in children less than 5 years or up to 15 years. Now it is occurring in elderly people due to falling immunity. For last 10 years, spurt of cases have been reported from Ahmedabad, Dibrugarh and most parts of northern India. These have occurred in elder children and adults. According to WHO, India accounts for 19-84% of global burden from 1998 to 2008.

C. diphtheriae spread is primarily by airborne respiratory droplets, direct contact with respiratory secretions of symptomatic individuals, or exudate from infected skin lesions. Asymptomatic respiratory tract carriage is important in transmission. It can remain viable in dust or on fomites for up to 6 months. Mortality remains 10-20%, due to respiratory collapse or cardiac problems. There is no race or sex predilection.

Virulence of the organism lies in its ability to produce the potent 62 kD polypeptide exotoxin, which inhibits protein synthesis and causes local tissue necrosis. Within the first few days of respiratory tract infection (usually in the pharynx), a dense necrotic coagulum of organisms, epithelial cells, fibrin, leukocytes and erythrocytes forms, advances, and becomes a gray-brown, leather-like adherent pseudomembrane (*Diphthera is a Greek term for leather*). Removal is difficult and reveals a bleeding edematous submucosa. Paralysis of the palate and hypopharynx is an early local effect of diphtheritic toxin. Toxin absorption can lead to systemic manifestations: kidney tubule necrosis, thrombocytopenia, cardiomyopathy, and/or demyelination of nerves. Because the latter two complications can occur 2-10 weeks after mucocutaneous infection, the pathophysiology in some cases is suspected to be immunologically mediated.

2. How to recognize it and what are the differential diagnoses?

Most common presentation is focus of infection on tonsils or pharynx in about 90% of the patients; next comes nasal and laryngeal diphtheria. After an average incubation period of 2-4 days, local signs and symptoms of inflammation develop. Child is febrile.

Tonsils and pharynx

Tonsillar and pharyngeal diphtheria are the most common; symptoms begin with a sore throat, usually in the absence of systemic complaints. Fever malaise, dysphagia and headache are not prominent features.

In nonimmune individuals, membrane formation can be seen after the 2-days to 5-days incubation period and grows to involve the pharyngeal walls, tonsils, uvula and soft palate. The membrane may extend to the larynx and trachea, causing airway obstruction and eventual suffocation. Leather-like adherent membrane, extension beyond the faucial area, relative lack of fever, and dysphagia help differentiate diphtheria from exudative pharyngitis due to *Streptococcus pyogenes* and Epstein-Barr virus. Edema and lymphadenopathy develops. Marked edema of the neck may lead to a bull-neck appearance with a distinct collar of swelling; the patient throws the head back to relieve pressure on the throat and larynx. Swallowing may be made difficult by unilateral or bilateral paralysis of the muscles of the palate. If toxin production is unopposed by antitoxin and severe disease occurs, early localized signs and symptoms give way to circulatory collapse, respiratory failure, stupor, coma, and death.

Larynx

Initially present as laryngotracheobronchitis. There is hoarseness of voice and severe respiratory tract obstruction.

Nasal diphtheria

It may present as a common viral upper respiratory tract infection. A foul odor may develop. This form of diphtheria is most common in infants.

Cutaneous diphtheria

It is usually localized to areas of previous mild trauma or bruising. There is pain, tenderness, and erythema at the site of infection progresses to ulceration with sharply defined borders and formation of a brownish-gray membrane. Local disease may persist for weeks to months. Extremities are affected more often than the trunk or head. Pain, tenderness, erythema, and exudate are typical. Local hyperesthesia or hypoesthesia is unusual.

Additional sites

Additional sites of infection have included the external ear, the eye (usually the palpebral conjunctivae), and the genital mucosa. Rare sporadic cases of endocarditis have been reported, usually due to nontoxigenic strains. Septicemia caused by *C. diphtheriae* is rare but universally fatal. Differential diagnosis includes epiglottis, herpes simplex virus infection and impetigo.

3. What are the various modalities for diagnosis of diphtheria?

Diagnosis is mainly clinical. Culture of bacteria remains the gold standard for diagnosis. Specimens for culture should be obtained from the throat and nose and any other mucocutaneous lesion. A portion of membrane with exudates should be cultured. Laboratory should know about suspicion of diphtheria because isolation of *C. diphtheriae* requires special culture media containing tellurite agar or specially enriched Loeffler, Hoyle, Mueller, or Tinsdale medium.

Evaluation of a direct smear using gram stain or Albert stain or specific fluorescent antibody is unreliable. Diagnostic tests used to confirm diphtheria infection combine isolation of *C. diphtheriae* on cultures with toxigenicity testing (which can be performed using the Elek test). Toxigenicity tests are not readily available in many clinical microbiology laboratories. PCR test may be available in few reference laboratories.

4. How to treat a case of diphtheria?

Supportive care

Mechanical ventilation is required if there is airway obstruction by the diphtheritic membrane and parapharyngeal edema. Critical care is required for complications as myocarditis or palatal palsy or neuropathy. Droplet precautions are required till cessation of therapy or culture negativity. Bed rest is essential during the acute phase of disease, usually for ≥2 weeks until the risk for symptomatic cardiac damage has passed, with a return to physical activity guided by the degree of toxicity and cardiac involvement. Cutaneous wounds are cleaned thoroughly with soap and water.

Specific antitoxin

It is the mainstay of therapy and should be administered on the basis of clinical diagnosis. Because it neutralizes only free toxin, antitoxin efficacy diminishes with elapsed time after the onset of mucocutaneous symptoms. Antitoxin is administered as a single empirical dose of 20,000–120,000 U based on the degree of toxicity, site and size of the membrane, and duration of illness. Antitoxin is probably of no value for local manifestations of cutaneous diphtheria, but its use is prudent because toxic sequelae can occur. Commercially available intravenous immunoglobulin preparations contain low titers of antibodies to diphtheria toxin; their use for therapy of diphtheria is not proven or approved. Antitoxin is not recommended for asymptomatic carriers.

Antimicrobial therapy

It includes penicillins or erythromycin. Antibiotics decrease or stop toxin production, treat localized infection, and prevent transmission of the organism to contacts. Only erythromycin or penicillin is recommended; erythromycin is marginally superior to penicillin for eradication of nasopharyngeal carriage. Appropriate therapy is erythromycin (40–50 mg/kg/day divided every 6 hour by mouth [PO] or intravenously [IV]; maximum 2 g/day), aqueous crystalline penicillin G (100,000–150,000 U/kg/day divided every 6 hour IV or intramuscularly [IM]), or procaine penicillin (25,000–50,000 U/kg/day divided every 12 hour IM) for 14 days. Treatment with erythromycin is repeated if either culture yields *C. diphtheria* after completion of therapy.

Household contacts

Household contacts and people who have had intimate respiratory or habitual physical contact with a patient are closely monitored for illness through the 7-day incubation period. Cultures of the nose, throat, and any cutaneous lesions are performed. Antimicrobial prophylaxis is presumed effective and is administered regardless of immunization status, using erythromycin (40–50 mg/kg/day divided qid PO for 10 days; maximum 2 g/day) or a single injection of benzathine penicillin G (600,000U IM for patients <30 kg, 1,200,000 U IM for patients ≥30 kg). Diphtheria toxoid vaccine, in age-appropriate form, is given to immunized individuals who have not received a booster dose within 5 years. Children who have not received their 4th dose should be vaccinated. Those who have received fewer than 3 doses of diphtheria toxoid or who have uncertain immunization status are immunized with an age-appropriate preparation on a primary schedule.

5. **How to follow up a child after treatment? How a carrier state is managed?**

Repeat cultures are performed at a minimum of 2 weeks after completion of therapy in patients and carriers; if results are positive, an additional 10-day course of oral erythromycin should be administered and follow-up cultures performed. When an asymptomatic carrier is identified, the following steps are taken, antimicrobial prophylaxis is administered for 7–10 days. An age-appropriate preparation of diphtheria toxoid is immediately administered if the patient has not received a booster injection within 1 year. Individuals are placed in strict isolation (respiratory tract colonization) or contact isolation (cutaneous colonization only) until at least 2 subsequent cultures, taken 24 hours apart after cessation of therapy, demonstrate negative results.

6. **What could be the complications of diphtheria?**

   i. Respiratory tract obstruction by pseudomembranes may require bronchoscopy or intubation and mechanical ventilation.

ii. Toxic cardiomyopathy occurs in 10–25% of patients. It usually occurs in 2nd and 3rd weeks but can be seen in 1st week of illness. There is tachycardia out of proportion to fever. A prolonged PR interval and changes in the ST-T wave on an electrocardiographic tracing are relatively frequent findings; dilated and hypertrophic cardiomyopathy detected by echocardiogram has been described. Single or progressive cardiac dysrhythmias can occur, including 1st, 2nd, and 3rd degree heart block. Temporary transvenous pacing may improve outcomes. Recovery from toxic myocardiopathy is usually complete, although survivors of more severe dysrhythmias can have permanent conduction defects.
iii. Toxic neuropathy parallels the severity of primary infection and are multiphasic in onset. Acutely or 2–3 weeks after onset of oropharyngeal inflammation, it is common for hypesthesia and local paralysis of the soft palate to occur. Weakness of the posterior pharyngeal, laryngeal, and facial nerves may follow, causing a nasal quality in the voice, difficulty in swallowing, and risk for aspiration. Cranial neuropathies characteristically occur in the 5th week, leading to oculomotor and ciliary paralysis, which can cause strabismus, blurred vision, or difficulty with accommodation. Symmetric polyneuropathy has its onset 10 days to 3 months after oropharyngeal infection and causes principally motor deficits with diminished deep tendon reflexes. Complete neurologic recovery occurs by 2–3 weeks after onset of illness, rarely after that.

7. What should be the policy of vaccination in a patient suffering from diphtheria?

Diphtheria disease might not confer immunity. Persons recovering from diphtheria should begin or complete active immunization with diphtheria toxoid during convalescence. Child should receive active immunization as per schedule 6 weeks after the acute illness.

Further Reading
1. John TJ. Resurgence of diphtheria in India in the 21st century. Indian J Med Res. 2008;128:669-70.
2. Nath B, Mahanta TG. Investigation of an outbreak in Borborooah block of Dirbrugarh district, Assam. Indian J Community Med. 2010;35:436-8.
3. Sharma NC, Banavaliker JN, Ranjan R, Kumar R. Bacteriological and epidemiological characteristics of diphtheria cases in and around Delhi – A retrospective study. Indian J Med Res. 2007;126:545-52.
4. World Health Organization. Immunization, surveillance, assessment and monitoring. Available from: http://www.who.int/entity/immunization_monitoring/data/incidence_series.xls (Accessed October, 2010)

4

Pertussis

Rohit Agrawal

1. What is the epidemiology of pertussis in children and adolescents?

Pertussis is caused by the bacterium *Bordetella pertussis* which is transmitted from infected person to susceptible individuals through droplets. Before vaccines became widely available, pertussis was one of the commonest childhood diseases worldwide.

Worldwide, it is estimated that there are 30–50 million pertussis cases and about 300,000 deaths per year. According to WHO 2008 estimates, around 16 million (95% in developing countries) cases of disease occurred worldwide and around 195,000 had died due to this disease. Pertussis is increasingly reported from older children, adolescents and adults. According to one serological study from US, 21% (95% confidence interval [CI]: 13–32%) of adults with prolonged cough had pertussis. The pertussis burden is believed to be substantially more than the number of reported cases; approximately 600,000 cases are estimated to occur annually just among adults.

In India, the incidence of pertussis declined sharply after launch of Universal Program of Immunization (UIP). Prior to UIP, India reported 200,932 cases and 106 deaths in the year 1970 with a mortality rate of <0.001%. During the year 1987, the reported incidence was about 163,000 cases which came down to 40, 508 in 2010 and 39, 091 in 2011 reflecting a decline of about 75% . Amongst different states, AP, MP, Jharkhand, WB and Bihar reported the maximum cases in 2010. In 2010, only 6 and in 2011, a total of 11 deaths were reported.

On the other hand, according to infectious disease data available at WHO, India reported a total of 35, 217 cases of pertussis in 2011, whereas from 2000 to 2010, the total number of reported cases ranged from 30,088 in 2006 to 60,385 in 2009.

A substantial portion of pertussis disease seen in the last decade is attributable to the increased reports of pertussis infection in adolescents and adults. Adolescents and adults are the significant sources of transmission of *B. pertussis* to unvaccinated young infants. Newborn babies are more susceptible, vulnerable and at risk for infection while adolescents and adults act as reservoir. There is no data on the incidence of adolescent and adult pertussis in India but is perceived to be significant, especially in those states where childhood immunization coverage is good and reduced natural circulation of pertussis leads to infrequent adolescent boosting.

Also, the routine immunization coverage in India is poor (60%), further increasing the prevalence of the disease. Lack of adequate reporting of cases with poor disease surveillance system reflects in above figures, which represents only the tip of iceberg.

2. How to recognize it?

Recognition of pertussis is essentially clinical. Clinically, the course is divided in three distinct stages:

Stage 1—**Catarrhal Stage** (1-2 weeks): Characterized by insidious onset of coryza, sneezing, low grade fever, occasional cough.

Stage 2—**Paroxysmal Stage** (1-6 weeks): At this stage, pertussis is suspected. Cough occurs in bouts or paroxysms of numerous rapid cough episodes apparently due to difficulty in expelling the thick mucus from the tracheobronchial tree. At the end of the paroxysm long inspiratory effort is followed by a whoop. In between episodes, child looks apparently well. During the episodes of cough, the child may become cyanosed, followed by vomiting, exhaustion and seizures. Apneic episodes may be life threatening following cough. Apnea is more common in neonates and in infant less than six months of age. Cough increases for 1-2 weeks, remains static for next 2-3 weeks and decreases over next 10 weeks. Absence of whoop or post-tussive vomiting does not rule out clinical diagnosis of pertussis.

Stage 3—**Convalescence Stage**: It is a period of gradual recovery. Children may continue to whoop even up to 6 months.

WHO definition of pertussis consists of—

Cough lasting ≥ 2 weeks with at least one of following symptoms:
- Paroxysms of cough
- Inspiratory whoop
- Post-tussive vomiting without other apparent cause.

Disease can occur in partially immunized children with modified course and altered features.

3. How pertussis is diagnosed?

Diagnosis of pertussis is essentially clinical which can be suspected on the basis of history and clinical examination and is confirmed by culture, genomics and serology.
- Elevated white blood cells count with lymphocytosis is commonly encountered. The absolute lymphocyte counts of 10,000 or higher may be seen with 70% sensitivity. It is one of the commonest causes of lymphocytic leukemoid reaction. Neonates and young infants have greater elevation of WBC counts (30,000-60,000 per microliter). Normal WBC count does not rule out pertussis.
- Culture is gold standard for the diagnosis. *B. pertussis* isolated in the catarrhal stage is diagnostic. A saline nasal swab or swab from the

posterior pharynx is to be preferred. The swab should be taken using Dacron or calcium alginate and not cotton and has to be plated on the selective (Bordet-Gangou) medium. A cough plate can be used sometimes. Results may take as long as two weeks. Culture positivity depends on the stage of the disease and the yield is highest during the first 3–4 weeks of illness. Cultures are difficult to perform and are not recommended in the clinical practice as the yield is poor because of previous vaccination, antibiotic use, diluted specimen and faulty collection and transportation of specimen.

- Polymerase chain reaction (PCR): It is rapid and most sensitive in early disease stages, but sensitivity decreases with illness duration. They are expensive and not easily available. Usually not recommended in routine practice.
- Serological tests to detect antibodies (IgG and IgA) against pertussis toxin or filamentous hemagglutinin can be used for diagnosis. Serum antibodies generally increase during first few weeks after onset of cough and then decline during the convalescent phase, also recent immunization may alter serological assessment. A single result of a high titer of IgG against pertussis toxin (>100–125 U/mL on ELISA) is highly sensitive and specific for diagnosis.
- Chest X-ray is little help and abnormal in only 20–25%. (poor sensitivity). Abnormalities if present are in the form collapse/consolidation usually more on right middle and lower lobes.
- Direct fluorescent antigen testing: Not easily available, poor sensitivity and specificity, routinely not recommended.

4. What could be the complication of pertussis?

Young infants are at highest risk of complications. Common complication and cause of mortality in pertussis are due to secondary pneumonia and apneic spells. Neurological complications include seizures (1 in 100) and encephalopathy (1 in 300) due to hypoxia or due to toxin itself or cerebral hemorrhage. Other complications include otitis media, anorexia and dehydration. Pneumothorax, rib fractures, epistaxis, subdural hematoma, hernia and rectal prolapse are the other complications that develop as a result of pressure effects of severe paroxysms. Complications are less in adults. They may present with loss of bladder control (28%).

5. How to treat a case of pertussis?

Being a bacterial disease, antibiotics have a role to play, but are effective if started early in the course of illness. Unfortunately, most patients are diagnosed late and the antibiotics are not very helpful to relieve the symptoms, but therapy can help to reduce the patient's ability to spread the disease to others.

Macrolides are drug of choice. Erythromycin 40–50 mg/kg/day in 6 hourly divided doses for 2 weeks is the drug of choice. Alternatively, azithromycin in dose of 10 mg/kg for 5 days in children less than 6 months and for children older than 6 months 10 mg/kg on day 1 followed by 5 mg/kg from day 2–5 is recommended and tolerated better than erythromycin. Clarithromycin in the dose of 15 mg/kg in two divided doses for 7 days can also be used. Co-trimoxazole is another choice to be given for 14 days in 8 mg/kg/day of trimethoprim in two divided doses.

Steroids play no role in management of pertussis.

Cough sedatives may be used in older children to relieve the symptoms, whereas bronchodilators have a questionable role.

Other supportive management includes maintenance of hydration and nutrition, avoidance of trigger factors such as passive smoking; humidified oxygen and assisted ventilation as and if required.

6. How to manage the contacts?

Pertussis is highly transmissible illness with secondary attack rates up to 80% in susceptible household contacts who are exposed to index case during the period of infectiousness (first four weeks of illness). Post exposure prophylaxis of contacts has, however, not shown to reduce the incidence of culture confirmed cases. In most clinical instances, the diagnosis is mainly presumptive. Hence, routine post-exposure prophylaxis should be restricted to high-risk groups such as neonates, unimmunized/partially immunized young infants and children with other comorbidities. All other contacts should be placed on surveillance and antibiotics may be started at the appearance of first respiratory symptom in the same therapeutic regime.

7. What should be the policy of vaccination in a patient suffering from pertussis?

It is essential to immunize even those recovering from pertussis, as natural disease does not offer complete protection. Two types of pertussis vaccines are available: whole-cell (wP) vaccines based on killed *B. pertussis* organisms, and acellular (aP) vaccines based on highly purified, selected components of this agent.

The standard dose of pertussis vaccine is 0.5 mL; this is administered intramuscularly in the anterolateral thigh of children aged <12 months and in the deltoid muscle in older age groups. The standard primary vaccination schedule is three primary doses at 6, 10 and 14 weeks and two boosters at 15–18 months and 4–6 years. Early completion of primary immunization is desirable as there is no maternal antibody for protection against pertussis. The booster should be given ≥6 months after the last primary dose. The last dose of the recommended primary series should be completed by the age of 6 months. All infants, including those who are HIV positive, should be immunized against pertussis.

Schedule for catch up vaccination: Three doses at 0, 1 and 6 months interval should be offered. The 2nd childhood booster is not required if the last dose has been given beyond the age of 4 years.

Recommendations for adolescents and adults: Immunity against pertussis following primary/booster wP/aP vaccination wanes over the next 4–12 years. Hence, offering *Tdap* vaccine instead of Td/TT vaccine to all children/adolescents/adults who can afford to use the vaccine in the schedule discussed below.

In those children who have received all three primary and the two booster doses of *DTwP/DTaP*, *Tdap* should be administered as a single dose at the age of 10–12 years. Catch up vaccination is recommended till the age of 18 years.

A single dose of *Tdap* may also be used as replacement for Td/TT booster in adults of any age if they have not received *Tdap* in the past. *Tdap* can now be given regardless of time elapsed since the last vaccine containing tetanus toxoid or diphtheria toxoid.

Only aP-containing vaccines should be used for vaccination in those aged >7 years. Admittedly, there is no data on the incidence of pertussis disease and *B. pertussis* infection among adolescents and adults in India, but is perceived to be significant, especially in those states where childhood immunization coverage is good and reduced natural circulation of pertussis leads to infrequent adolescent boosting just like in developed countries.

Though there is no conclusive evidence in favor of cocooning strategy, the available data indicate that a decreased risk of infection in newborns can be achieved with the immunization of all family members who could have a strict contact with a newborn (cocoon strategy). Maternal immunization, particularly of pregnant women may be an effective approach to protect very young infants and neonates. Hence, immunization of pregnant women with a single dose of *Tdap* during the second trimester of pregnancy may be beneficial.

Further Reading

1. Centers for Disease Control and Prevention. Epidemiology and Prevention of Vaccine-Preventable Diseases. In: Atkinson W, Wolfe S, Hamborsky J (Eds). 12th edition, second printing. Washington DC: Public Health Foundation, 2012.
2. Cortese MM, Bisgard KM. Pertussis. In: Wallace RB, Kohatsu N, Kast JM (eds). Maxcy-Rosenau-Last Public Health and Preventive Medicine, 5th Edition. The McGraw-Hill Companies, Inc; 2008:111-4.
3. Marconi GP, Ross LA, Nager AL. An upsurge in pertussis: epidemiology and trends. Pediatr Emerg Care. 2012;28(3):215-9.
4. Updated Recommendations for the Use of Tetanus Toxoid, Reduced Diphtheria Toxoid and Acellular Pertussis (Tdap) Vaccine from the Advisory Committee on Immunization Practices. 2010. MMWR. 2011;60(01):13-5.
5. Walsh PF, Kimmel L, Feola M, Tran T, Lim C, De Salvia L, et al. Prevalence of *Bordetella pertussis* and *Bordetella parapertussis* in infants presenting to the emergency department with bronchiolitis. J Emerg Med. 2011;40(3):256-61.
6. Wendelboe AM, Njamkepo E, Bourillon A, et al. Transmission of *Bordetella pertussis* to young infants. Pediatr Infect Dis J. 2007;26:293-9.

5
Meningococcus

Raju C Shah, Pratima R Shah

1. What is the epidemiology of meningococcal disease in our country?

As far back as 1805, there was outbreak of meningitis in Geneva. Scientist could identify organisms for that outbreak in 1887 as Meningococci. In 1996, world's biggest outbreak of meningococcal disease was reported from Africa leading to more than 20,000 deaths. In India, first outbreak of meningococcal disease was reported from Rajasthan in 1983, but could not be conformed due to paucity of lab facilities. India has documented three main outbreak of this disease since 1930 at an interval of approximately 20 years and small isolated outbreak in-between. Cases in all these outbreaks were first reported from New Delhi. Out of all these the largest epidemic began in winter of 1984, which peaked in 1985 with 6,133 cases and 799 deaths was due to meningococcal A. All these reported cases were from seven major hospitals only, so the total number could not be assessed. Even the conservative estimates suggest it to be almost double in number. In the same year, there are published reports of smaller outbreak from Chandigarh, Agra and Mumbai also. During 1985 to 87 outbreak of meningococcal meningitis was reported from south Gujarat (Surat) also with 197 cases and 34 deaths. National Institute of Communicable Diseases (NICD) in those years received reports of cases from all over country.

In 1989, outbreak of disease reported from three districts of Andhra Pradesh namely Vishakhapattanam, Vijayanagar and Srikakulam. Total of 475 cases were reported with 108 deaths. In the same year Odisha reported total of 2,957 cases with 344 deaths from three districts Kalahandi, Kendujhar and Phulbani. State of Madhya Pradesh reported 250 cases with 75 deaths. Etiological agent in all these three states was meningococcal type A.

Again in the winter of 2004 onwards cases of meningococcal infection reported from New Delhi. There were reports of 444 cases and 62 deaths in 2005 and peak in 2006 with case reports of 867. In year 2008, Meghalaya reported outbreak of meningococcal disease with 2,000 cases and 260 deaths and in 2009 Tripura 277 cases and 60 deaths.

In 2010–2011 again, there was small outbreak of meningococcal A in New Delhi with 603 cases and 16 deaths, and 137 cases and 4 deaths in 2010 and

2011 respectively. Total number of cases reported by National Center for Disease Control (NCDC) from India in outbreak years is as follows in Table 1.

Table 1: Cases reported by National Center for Disease Control

Year	Total No. of cases	Total No. of deaths
2005	8,367	485
2006	3,438	312
2010	6,547	341
2011	3,224	245

As per National Health Profile 2011 report, number of cases reported in year 2010 were 6,855 with 367 deaths and in year 2011 were 6,629 with 464 deaths.

All these outbreaks reported in last century and in this century, were meningococcal A epidemics. Serogroups B and C play its role in sporadic disease cases only. During 2004 to 2006 epidemics of New Delhi, majority of cases (44%) and deaths (62%) were in adolescent and young adult aged between 15 to 29 years. During 2005 peak attack rate of outbreak was 13.23/100,000.

NCDC, New Delhi carried out surveillance study from samples received from various hospitals of New Delhi from 2005 to 2011, numbers of positive cases were as follows in Table 2.

Table 2: Number of positive cases as per National Center for Disease Control

Year	Sample tested	Positive
2005	625	85
2006	10,500	194
2007	273	43
2008	289	34
2009	183	8
2010	121	2
2011	65	1

The epidemic cycles in India especially in New Delhi occur every 15–20 year as against 5–10 years cycles seen in meningococcal belt of Africa. It is similar to the other African countries surrounding the meningococcal belt. Almost all the epidemics peaked in the dry winter months in the north of country. Epidemiological burden of meningococcal disease outside the outbreaks is not possible to quantify in India as very little or no data is available. Studies since 1990 in non-outbreak setting have detected little meningococcal disease.

2. **How do you recognize meningococcal infection?**

Invasive meningococcal disease has wide spectrum of presentation from asymptomatic to fatal infection.

It can present as:
- Acute mild meningococcemia presented as bacteremia without shock
- Fulminant meningococcemia bacteremia with shock, without meningitis
- Meningitis and shock
- Meningitis alone
- Chronic benign meningococcemia (adults).

3. How to recognize and confirm meningococcal disease?

Symptoms and signs of meningitis
- Sudden onset of intense headache
- High fever
- Stiff neck
- Nausea and vomiting
- Photophobia
- Neurological signs like confusion, lethargy, delirium, coma, and/or convulsions
- Infants may have illness without any stiff neck and onset could be slow.

Meningococcemia
- Abrupt onset
- Fever
- Shock
- Petechial rash or purpura may not be obvious initially and meningeal symptoms are usually absent
- Rapid circulatory collapse.

Physical examination should include an examination for
- Meningeal rigidity, stiff neck, Kernig's or Brudzinski's signs
- Neurological signs, such as decreased awareness; localized neurological symptoms are unusual
- Purpura, sometimes extensive and necrotic, usually localized to the extremities, or generalized, cutaneous or mucosal (conjunctival) are often associated with meningococcal disease; purpura is a basic symptom of meningococcemia
- Lowered blood pressure and symptoms of shock
- Shock associated with purpura indicates fulminating meningococcemia, the most severe form of meningococcal disease
- Focal infection, such as arthritis, pleuritis or pneumonia, pericarditis, episcleritis.

In infants (under one year of age), the clinical features of meningitis are often atypical and may be difficult to recognize. The onset is not always rapid. In addition to fever, inconsolable irritability and screaming, failure to feed, vomiting, lethargy, convulsions or hypotonia may be presenting features. Stiff neck may be absent, bulging fontanelle may be observed.

The bacterial meningitis may result in brain damage, hearing loss or learning disability in 10–20% of survivors.

Standard case definition of meningococcal meningitis (WHO Guidelines)

Suspected case of acute meningitis

- Sudden onset of fever (>38.5°C rectal or 38.0°C axillary), with stiff neck
- In patients under one year of age, a suspected case of meningitis occurs when fever is accompanied by a bulging fontanelle.

Probable case of bacterial meningitis

- Suspected case of acute meningitis as defined above, with
- Turbid CSF.

Probable case of meningococcal meningitis

- Suspected case of either acute or bacterial meningitis as defined above, with
- Gram stain showing gram-negative diplococcus, or
- Ongoing epidemic, or
- Petechial or purpural rash.

Confirmed case of meningococcal meningitis

Suspected or probable case as defined above, with either
- Positive CSF antigen detection for *N. meningitidis*, or
- Positive culture of CSF or blood with identification of *N. meningitides*.

4. What are the sequelae and common complications of meningococcal infection?

Compartmentalized metastatic infections, such as arthritis or pericarditis, can develop; the latter is caused mainly by serogroup C. The pericarditis that occurs in the first few days of meningococcal disease may demonstrate the organism. Late onset pericarditis, one to two weeks after infection, may contain no organisms. Arthritis occurs commonly during active meningococcal infection. There may be late onset arthritis, after resolution of meningococcal infection. Less commonly, septic purulent arthritis may occur spontaneously in the absence of meningococcal disease elsewhere. Cellulitis and endophthalmitis have been found occasionally. Additionally, primary meningococcal conjunctivitis, pneumonia, sialadenitis, adnexitis, or pelvic inflammatory disease have been reported. Meningococcal infections in the upper or lower airways, genitals and anus differ from invasive disease as they develop without preceding bacteremia. Meningococcal pneumonia is uncommon and generally occurs in immunocompromised or elderly patients.

Most untreated cases of meningococcal meningitis and/or septicemia are fatal. Even with appropriate care, up to 10% of patients die, typically within 24–48 hours of the onset of symptoms. In the meningitis belt of Africa, fatality from Meningococcal A disease has been estimated at 10–15%, although higher rates have been seen in some settings. Approximately, 10% to 20% of survivors of meningococcal meningitis are left with permanent sequelae, such as mental retardation, deafness, epilepsy, or other neurological disorders.

5. How to manage meningococcal disease?

Meningococcal disease (either meningitis or septicemia) is potentially fatal and should always be viewed as a medical emergency:
- Admission to a hospital or health center is necessary for diagnosis (lumbar puncture and CSF examination) and for treatment.
- Antimicrobial therapy is essential and should be combined with supportive treatment.
- As contagiousness of patients is moderate and disappears quickly following antimicrobial treatment, isolation of the patient is not necessary except probably during the first 24 hours of illness.

Antimicrobial therapy

Antimicrobial treatment must be instituted as soon as possible after the lumbar puncture has been carried out. Many antimicrobials are active against meningococci in vitro, but only those that sufficiently penetrate the cerebrospinal space and are affordable should be used. The range of antibiotics used for treatment includes penicillin, ampicillin, chloramphenicol and ceftriaxone. Chloramphenicol is a good and inexpensive choice. The third generation cephalosporins—ceftriaxone and cefotaxime are preferred and still very effective.

Supportive therapy

Fluid and electrolyte balance should be monitored and fluid replaced accordingly. When required, anticonvulsants or antiemetics may be administered. Severe forms of the disease including coma, shock and purpura should be treated in an intensive care unit by well-trained physicians.

6. How to prevent meningococcal infection?

Meningoccal disease is potentially preventable through avoiding close contact with cases or carriers of the disease, vaccination and/or chemoprophylaxis.

Prevention of transmission

Transmission of *N. meningitidis* occurs from person to person, usually from a nasopharyngeal carrier rather than from a patient, through contact with respiratory droplets or oral secretions. Contagiousness rapidly disappears in patients after starting antibiotic therapy.

Meningococcal vaccines

Currently available meningococcal vaccines include polysaccharide vaccines and polysaccharide-protein conjugate vaccines against meningococci of serogroups A, C, W135 and Y. Conjugate vaccines are more immunogenic and also induce immunological memory. Serogroup B vaccines are based on protein (outer membrane vesicles) extracted from selected outbreak strains, but they are not widely available. A multicomponent Meningococcal B (MenB) vaccine (recombinant, adsorbed) was licensed in January 2013 by Europian regulatory authorities and in august 2013 by Australian authorities.

Polysaccharide vaccines

Meningococcal polysaccharide vaccines consist of purified, heat-stable, lyophilized capsular polysaccharides from meningococci of the respective serogroup. They are available in bivalent (A, C), trivalent (A, C, W135), and quadrivalent (A, C, W135,Y) formulations.

Meningococcal polysaccharide vaccines are administered as a single dose to persons >2 year old, in a dose of 0.5 mL given subcutaneously preferably in the deltoid region. Adverse reactions are mild like 1–2 days of pain and redness at the site of injection, (occurring in 4–56% of vaccine recipients) and transient fever (in < 5%). Systemic allergic reactions (e.g. urticaria, wheezing, rash) occur in < 0.1/100,000 vaccine doses and anaphylaxis has been documented in < 0.1/100,000 vaccine recipients. Neurological reactions (e.g., seizures, anesthesias, and paresthesias) have also been observed infrequently. The only contraindication for use of this vaccine is previous severe allergic reaction. It can be administered to pregnant women and immunodeficient individuals.

Efficacy of the polysaccharide vaccine

Polysaccharide vaccines are regarded as T-cell independent antigens and elicit serum bactericidal antibodies (SBA) responses in the absence of T cell involvement. Hence, these vaccines tend to be immunogenic in older children and adults, but fail to be as immunogenic in young children. This age-related response is likely to reflect intrinsic B-cell maturation. Plain polysaccharide vaccines are not licensed for use in children under the age 2 years.

When different serogroups of meningococcal polysaccharide are administered together as bivalent, trivalent or quadrivalent vaccines, independent group-specific immune responses are obtained. Such vaccines are also used successfully in outbreak control, but they do not seem to have any significant impact on meningococcal carriage in the nasopharynx.

After 3–5 years, one booster dose may be given to persons considered to be at continued risk of exposure including health workers. However, on repeated use of polysaccharide vaccine hyporesponsiveness to vaccine antigen develops and therefore efficacy declines. This is one of the greatest disadvantage of polysaccharide vaccine.

Conjugate vaccines

The meningococcal conjugate vaccines licensed for use are currently monovalent (A or C) or quadrivalent (A, C, W135, Y) and also include a combination vaccine based on *Haemophilus influenzae* type b and *Neisseria meningitides* serogroup C vaccines (Hib Men C). All meningococcal conjugate vaccines have been found to be safe with only mild adverse effects like redness, swelling and pain at the site of injection or fever and irritability usually lasting 1 to 3 days.

Monovalent serogroup C conjugate vaccines (MenC conj vaccines)

These vaccines contain 10 g of group C oligosaccharide conjugated to 12.5-25.0 g of the carrier (diphtheria toxoid, CRM-197, or tetanus toxoid); MenC conjugate vaccines are licensed for children aged >2 months, adolescents and adults. Infants aged 2-11 months are given 2 doses (0.5 mL per dose) with at least 2 months between the doses, followed by a booster dose about one year later. The possible need for boosters is not yet established for individuals >1 year of age.

Efficacy of MenC conj vaccine
Though, Men C vaccination provides robust short-term protection, antibody titers wane over time with only 8-25% of the children who received 3 dose primary scedule showing protective titers (rSBA titers >1:8 at 4 year of age). However, ten years of adequate surveillance in some countries like England, Wales, has shown large reductions in meningococcal serogroup C disease as a result of MenC conjugate vaccine introduction in England and Wales, Australia, Canada and Netherlands, inspite of gradual decline in antibody titers. This has been attributed to the development of herd immunity as a result of reduced nasopharyngeal carriage.

Monovalent serogroup a conjugate vaccine (MenA conj vaccine)

MenA conjugate vaccine, licensed in 2010, is a lyophilized vaccine containing 10 gram of group A polysaccharide conjugated to 10-33 gram tetanus toxoid, with alum as adjuvant and thiomersal as preservative. It is recommended for use in children and adults from 1-29 years of age, as a single intramuscular dose. Need for booster is not established as yet. It has been used in various areas of the African meningitic belt.

Quadrivalent meningococcal conjugate vaccines

In 2005, a quadrivalent (A, C, W135, Y-D) meningococcal conjugate vaccine was introduced, containing 4 gram of each of the serogroup polysaccharides, which are individually conjugated to diphtheria toxin as carrier protein. A single dose (0.5 mL intramuscular) is recommended from 2-55 years of age and 2 doses between 9 months and 23 months. A second quadrivalent vaccine, conjugated to CRM-197 (A, C, W135, Y-CRM) became available in 2010 containing 10 gram of polysaccharide A and 5 gram of each of the polysaccharides C, W135 and Y. No adjuvants or preservatives are added (single dose formulations). In Canada and the United States, both these vaccines are recommended for routine administration to adolescents aged 11-18 years and those with high risk in the age group from 2-55 years. In immunodeficient individuals, repeat doses of the quadruvalent vaccine have been proposed, though consensus is not yet established. The conjugate vaccine A,C,W135,Y-D had comparable immunogenicity to the quadrivalent polysaccharide vaccine.

Most side effects are mild, though a risk of Guillain-Barre syndrome (GBS) is expected in 1 in 1 million vaccine recipients. Hence, it is recommended that people who have previously been diagnosed with GBS should not receive this vaccine unless they are at increased risk of Meningococcal disease.

Efficacy of quadrivalent conjugate vaccine
A large study involving 2,907 children from 2-10 years, concluded that both the quadrivalent conjugate vaccines were immunogenic and well tolerated. The response to A, C, W135, Y-CRM was statistically non-inferior to A, C, W135, Y-D for all groups, but statistically superior for groups C, W135, and Y. Overall, the effectiveness of the vaccines has been estimated to range from 80 to 85% after 3-4 years of vaccination.

Conjugate vaccine is superior to plain polysaccharide vaccine as there is no hyporesponsiveness in repeated doses, lowers carriage rate, has booster effect and provides hard immunity.

Serogroup B vaccines (MenB vaccines)

Progress in the development of vaccines against serogroup B has been slow, owing to several reasons : 1) native B polysaccharide contains epitopes that potentially cross-react with human antigens; 2) it is poorly immunogenic; 3) other potential antigen targets of group B meningococci are highly diverse. Some vaccines based on the outer membrane vesicles (OMV) of specific outbreak strains were developed and have been used to control serogroup B disease in Cuba, New Zealand, Norway, Latin American countries and France. The OMV vaccines are immunogenic, but have certain drawbacks like need for multiple doses with short lasting protection. Several sub-capsular proteins, including factor H binding protein, Neisserial adhesin A, and Neisseria-heparin binding antigen have been identified as antigens and vaccines targeting these antigens are being currently undergoing clinical trials.

Recently in January 2013 conjugated Men B vaccine has been licensed by Europian licensing agency and in August 2013 Australian licensure agency for use which contains recombinant *Neisseria meningitidis* group B NHBA fusion protein, Recombinant *Neisseria meningitidis* group B NadA protein, Recombinant *Neisseria meningitidis* group B fHbp fusion protein and outer membrane vesicles (OMV) from *Neisseria meningitidis* group B strain NZ98/254 produced in *E. coli* cells by recombinant DNA technology, adsorbed on aluminum hydroxide (0.5 mg Al^{3+}), NHBA (Neisseria Heparin Binding Antigen), NadA (Neisserial adhesin A), fHbp (factor H binding protein).

WHO recommendation for meningococcal vaccination

WHO classifies countries into three groups based on the incidence of invasive meningococcal disease. Countries with incidence of >10 cases/100,000 population/year are labeled as high endemic and those with rates 2–10 cases/100,000 population/year are labeled as intermediate endemic. In both these group of countries, WHO recommends introduction of large scale vaccination programs in the form of routine immunization and supplementary immunization programs.

On the contrary, those countries with low incidences (< 2 cases/1000,000/year), meningococcal vaccines are recommended for only high-risk individuals, such as children and young adults residing in closed communities, (e.g. boarding schools or military camps), laboratory workers at risk of exposure to meningococci, travelers to high-endemic areas, individuals suffering from immunodeficiency, including asplenia, terminal complement deficiencies, or advanced HIV infection.

Conjugate vaccines are preferred over polysaccharide vaccines due to their potential for herd protection and their increased immunogenicity, especially in children < 2 year of age. Polysaccharide vaccines can be used to control outbreaks in resource poor countries.

Vaccination policy in the country

Meningococcal vaccine is only recommended to be given to:
- Haj pilgrims and other travelers visiting the countries where meningococcal disease is a major problem or where outbreaks are occurring.
- High risk groups, e.g. children living in orphanages, jail inmates, soldiers in barracks, etc.
- Routine vaccination of the population at large is not recommended except during epidemic situations.

Chemoprophylaxis

The aim of chemoprophylaxis is to prevent secondary cases by eliminating nasopharyngeal carriage. Chemoprophylaxis has been considered for control of meningococcal disease but it has several limitations, and its use should be limited to special circumstances. To be effective in preventing secondary cases, chemoprophylaxis must be initiated as soon as possible (i.e. not later than 48 hours after diagnosis of the case).

Special circumstances for which chemoprophylaxis are appropriate

In non-epidemic settings, chemoprophylaxis should be restricted to close contacts of a case, which are defined as:
- Household members (i.e. persons sleeping in the same dwelling as the case); institutional contacts who shared sleeping quarters (i.e. for boarding school pupils, room-mates; for military camps, persons sharing

a barrack); nursery school or childcare center contacts (i.e. children and teachers who share a classroom with the case).
- Others who have had contact with the patient's oral secretions through kissing or sharing of food and beverages.

In addition, in areas where household contacts routinely receive prophylaxis, chemoprophylaxis should also be given to the patient with meningococcal disease upon discharge from the hospital provided the patient's illness was treated with antibiotics (e.g. penicillin), which do not eliminate the organism from the nasopharynx. Table 3 shows the recommended drugs for chemoprophylaxis.

Table 3: Recommended drugs for chemoprophylaxis

Generic name	Dose (adults)	Dose (children)	Route	Duration
Rifampicin	600 mg/12h	10 mg/kg/12h	Oral	2 days
Ciprofloxacin	500 mg	Not given	Oral	Single dose
Ofloxacin	400 mg	Not given	Oral	Single dose
Ceftriaxone	250 mg	<15 year – 125 mg	IM	Single dose
Azithromycin	500 mg	10 mg/kg	Oral	Single dose

Further Reading

1. Al-Tawfiq JA, Clarke TA, Memish ZA, et al. Meningococcal disease: the organism, clinical presentation, and worldwide epidemiology. J Travel Med. 2010;17:3-8.
2. Choudhry A, et al. Meningococcal disease in India, 2005-2011: A Surveillance Study. Int J Med Public health. 2012:2:28-36.
3. EMA. Authorization details for bexsero. Available at: http://www.ema.europa.eu/ema/index.jsp?curl=pages/medicines/human/medicines/002333/human_med_001614.jspandmid=WC0b01ac058001d124. Accessed August 7, 2013.
4. EMA. EU Member States. Available at: http://www.ema.europa.eu/ema/index.jsp?curl=pages/partners_and_networks/general/general_content_000219.jspandmid=WC0b01ac058003174e. Accessed August 7, 2013.
5. Manchanda V, Gupta S, Bhalla P. Meningococcal disease: history, epidemiology, pathogenesis, clinical manifestations, diagnosis, antimicrobial susceptibility and prevention. Ind J of Med Microbiol 2006;24 (1):7-19.
6. Sinclair D, Preziosi MP, John TJ, Greenwood B. The epidemiology of meningococcal disease in India. Trop Med Int Health. 2010;15:1421-35.
7. Sunil Gupta, Arti Bahl. Meningococcal Disease : Need to remain alert. CD Alert. 2009:13-3:1-8.
8. Vaccines WHO assessed on 20.08.13. Available at: http://www.who.int/ith/vaccines/meningococcal/en/index.html.
9. Yewale V, Choudhary P, Thacker N. Meningococcal vaccines, IAP Guide Book on Immunization. 2009-11:135-41.

6. Cholera

Alok Kumar Deb

1. What is the epidemiology of cholera?

Historically, cholera has been endemic in the Ganges and Brahmaputra delta regions. The state of West Bengal in India, together with neighboring Bangladesh, is often called the "homeland of cholera". Since 1817, six out of seven cholera pandemics emerged from the Indian subcontinent; only the ongoing seventh pandemic originated in Indonesia in 1961.

Cholera is a grossly under-reported disease. The estimated global burden is around 3–5 million cases and 1,00,000–1,30,000 deaths per year, most of which occurs in the developing world due to lack of access to clean water and proper sanitation systems. Increasing urbanization, cross-border travels, social and political unrest and natural disasters also result in its spread and persistence. For example, devastating natural disasters perhaps caused a 30% increase in reported cholera cases in 2005 compared with 2004, while the 2010 outbreak of cholera in Haiti after a gap of 100 years illustrated the introduction of cholera through human activities from a distant geographic source. Contrary to popular belief, cholera has been found to be a significant contributor to morbidity in the pediatric population in India and other developing countries where cholera is endemic.

2. What is the pathogenesis of cholera?

Cholera is caused by *Vibrio cholerae*, a gram-negative, facultatively anaerobic rod in the family Vibrionaceae. Among >200 serogroups of *Vibrio cholerae* based upon their somatic (O) surface antigens, only O1 and O139 serogroups produce a potent enterotoxin, called "cholera toxin" that causes cholera. The O1 serogroup has three serotypes (Ogawa, Inaba and Hikojima) and two biotypes (classical and El Tor). Currently, most cases are caused by the El Tor biotype that usually results in milder infections. Recently, some new variant strains of El Tor have been associated with more severe disease.

The cholera toxin has two subunits—the B subunit binds onto the intestinal epithelial cells while the A subunit enters into the epithelial cells and increases intracellular cAMP. This blocks absorption of sodium and chloride by microvilli and promotes secretion of water into intestinal lumen, causing watery diarrhea. The fluid loss mainly occurs in the duodenum and upper jejunum. The colon is less sensitive to the toxin and still can absorb some fluid; however, the large volume of secreted water overwhelms its absorptive capacity.

Cholera is usually transmitted through fecal-contaminated drinking water, food, fruits and vegetables and utensils washed with contaminated water. Due to a short incubation period (2 hours to 5 days), the number of cases can rise extremely quickly. A relatively high infectious dose (10^3 to 10^6 organisms in water or 10^2 to 10^4 organisms in food) is required to produce clinical disease as the organism is very susceptible to the acidity of the stomach. Thus, drugs or conditions that decrease gastric acidity increase the risk of infection, as also occurs with blood group O.

Most people excrete *V. cholerae* in the feces and vomitus during diarrhea and for a few days after recovery. A few individuals carry the organism in the gall bladder for several months. Rare long-term carriers have also been reported. Organisms survive in feces for up to 50 days, in soil for up to 16 days and on fingertips for 1 to 2 hours. *V. cholerae* is susceptible to many common disinfectants such as 0.05% sodium hypochlorite, 70% ethanol, 2% glutaraldehyde, 8% formaldehyde, 10% hydrogen peroxide and iodine-based disinfectants.

3. What are the clinical features?

About 75% of infected people remain asymptomatic. However, the pathogens stay in their feces for 7 to 14 days and their shedding may infect other individuals. Less than 20% of symptomatic cases develop typical cholera with signs of moderate or severe dehydration; others are of mild or moderate severity, indistinguishable clinically from other types of acute diarrhea. The symptoms mostly include a sudden onset of effortless high volume watery diarrhea, often followed by vomiting. Abdominal cramps and fever may also accompany in some children. The characteristic "rice water" stool may not be found in milder cases. The clinical signs correspond to the patient's degree of dehydration on presentation (Table 1).

Other signs may also help in assessing the dehydration status, e.g. dryness of tongue, decreased urine output, sunken anterior fontanelle in infants, weak or absent pulse, cold and moist extremities and fast breathing (in absence of cough or chest indrawing) due to acidosis. The assessment of dehydration is often difficult in children with severe undernutrition, which may alter many of the signs described in Table 1 (e.g. general conditions, sunken eyes and diminished skin turgor).

4. How is cholera diagnosed?

Cholera can be diagnosed clinically (as suspected cases) or by laboratory methods (as confirmed cases). During outbreaks, a clinical diagnosis using WHO standard case definition is usually sufficient, along with sporadic testing. In endemic areas, although signs and symptoms of severe cholera may be unmistakable, the diagnosis is only confirmed by identifying the bacteria in stool sample. According to WHO, a case of cholera should be

Table 1: Assessment of dehydration status in children with acute diarrheal diseases

Dehydration status	Estimated fluid deficit	Clinical assessment criteria	Treatment plan
Severe	More than 10% of body weight	At least two of the following signs: • Lethargic/unconscious • Sunken eyes • Skin pinch goes back very slowly • Unable to drink/drinks poorly	WHO treatment plan C: • IV fluid • ORS • Antibiotics
Some	5–10% of body weight	At least two of the following signs: • Restless/irritable • Sunken eyes • Skin pinch goes back slowly • Drinks eagerly, thirsty	WHO treatment plan B: • ORS/HAF • Antibiotics (selective cases)
No	Less than 5% of body weight	Not enough sign to classify as "some" or "severe" dehydration	WHO treatment plan A: • ORS/HAF

suspected in an area where (a) the disease is not known to be present and a patient aged 5 years or more develops severe dehydration or dies from acute watery diarrhea, or (b) there is a cholera epidemic and a patient aged 5 years or more develops acute watery diarrhea, with or without vomiting. However, infants and young children bear the greatest burden of cholera in endemic areas.

Confirmation of cholera requires demonstration of presence of *V. cholerae* in stools/rectal swabs (a transport media such as Cary-Blair media may be used, if required) through various laboratory procedures, such as (a) observing the organism's characteristic motility during direct, bright-field or dark-field microscopic examination of the feces; the addition of specific antibodies stops this motility, (b) isolation of the organism from distinctive yellow colonies grown on selective thiosulfate-citrate-bile salts-sucrose (TCBS) agar and serotyping using specific antisera, (c) identification through immunofluorescence, polymerase chain reaction (PCR) assay and other intensive methods. Whenever possible, microbiological confirmation of cholera should also accompany testing for antimicrobial sensitivity patterns.

A new rapid diagnostic test (dipstick), claimed to have sensitivity and specificity of more than 90%, may allow quick bedside testing even in remote areas. Such rapid identification may also decrease death rates during cholera outbreaks. Till this test is fully validated, WHO suggests that all samples tested positive with this rapid test be re-tested using classic laboratory procedures for confirmation.

5. What is the fluid management of a child suffering from cholera?

The mainstay of cholera treatment is replacement and maintenance of fluid and electrolyte losses through timely, adequate and appropriate rehydration, using oral rehydration salts solution (ORS), various home available fluids (HAF) and intravenous (IV) fluid replacement therapy according to the stage of dehydration (Table 1). Antibiotics in severe cases and zinc supplements are also recommended.

Oral rehydration salts solution (ORS)

Based on the glucose-facilitated sodium, and hence, water absorption mechanism in the small intestine, which remains intact in secretory diarrhea such as cholera, ORS can adequately treat about 80% of cholera patients. Even when IV therapy is indicated, ORS should be used together whenever possible. The amount of ORS to be administered depends on the dehydration status. In "some" dehydration, the deficit of water is 50-100 mL/kg of body weight. If the child's weight is known, approximately 75 mL of ORS per kg should be given in the first four hours. If the weight is unknown, the amount can be determined using the child's age (Table 2), although this approach is less precise.

These estimates only provide a rough guide; the actual amount depends on the extent of thirst, stool losses and dehydration. In general, children should receive as much ORS as they want, with one teaspoonful every 1-2 minutes for children below 2 years of age, and frequent sips from a cup for older children. If the child vomits, stop ORS for 10 minutes and then resume more slowly. For breastfed children, continue breastfeeding along with ORS. For non-breastfed infants below 6 months of age, also give 100-200 mL of clean water during the first 4 hours.

Home available fluids (HAF)

In absence of ORS and when there is no dehydration, HAFs can also be used, although they are less efficient than ORS for treating dehydration. These may include soups, cereal gruels, cereal-salt solutions, or home-made sugar-and-salt solutions. However, commercial soups and sweetened commercial fruit drinks or soft drinks as well as plain glucose solution should be avoided as their high concentrations of salt, sucrose or glucose may lead to hypernatremia, osmotic diarrhea or both. On the other hand, giving only plain water is less effective and may lead to hyponatremia.

Table 2: Oral fluid requirements during first four hours of rehydration

Age	< 4 months	4–11 months	1–2 years	> 2–4 years	5–14 years	≥ 15 years
Weight (kg)	< 5	5–7.9	8–10.9	11–15.9	16–29.9	≥30
ORS (mL)	200–400	400–600	600–800	800–1200	1200–2200	2200–4000

Cholera

Intravenous (IV) therapy

Intravenous administration of fluids is indicated for children with severe dehydration and in situations when oral rehydration cannot be done, e.g. very rapid stool loss, severe repeated vomiting, paralytic ileus, glucose malabsorption, and the child is unable to drink. Ringer's lactate is the preferred IV fluid; normal (0.9%) saline or half-normal saline with 5% glucose can be used in its absence. Oral potassium supplements may be required (e.g. in case of paralytic ileus), as these fluids have inadequate or no potassium. Early institution of ORS and feeding will also provide sufficient potassium and glucose.

Infants are given IV fluid as 30 mL/kg in the first hour, followed by 70 mL/kg in the next 5 hours (i.e. 100 mL/kg in 6 hours). The rate for older children and adults is 30 mL/kg within 30 minutes, followed by 70 mL/kg in the next 2.5 hours (i.e. 100 mL/kg in 3 hours). After administering the first 30 mL/kg, if the radial pulse is still very weak and rapid, a second infusion of 30 mL/kg should be given at the same rate. Small amounts of ORS solution should also be given by mouth (about 5 mL/kg/hour) as soon as the patient is able to drink.

When IV rehydration is not possible and the patient cannot drink, ORS can be given by nasogastric tube (size 6-8 French for a child, 12-18 French for an adult). However, this is contraindicated in unconscious patients. The child's head should be kept slightly raised to prevent regurgitated fluid from entering the lungs. If severely dehydrated, administer about 120 mL of ORS per kg of body weight over 6 hours (i.e. 20 mL/kg/hour). This rate should be reduced if there is repeated vomiting or increasing abdominal distension.

The child needs careful monitoring during rehydration process. Increasing stool losses or repeated vomiting will require more fluid. If the child develops puffy eyelids, a sign of "overhydration", fluid should be stopped, although, breastfeeding and provision of plain water should continue. The dehydration status should be reassessed at least every 4 hours of oral therapy or hourly for IV therapy. Treatment plans should change (or continue) accordingly.

6. What antibiotics are used for treatment?

Antibiotics are indicated in severe cases of cholera and should be started even without bacteriologic confirmation. They reduce the stool volume, decrease shedding of organism and shorten the duration of diarrhea, but it cannot obviate the need for fluid replacement. Since, antimicrobial resistance of *V. cholerae* is of great concern, especially in cholera-endemic areas, the choice of antibiotic should follow local susceptibility pattern. In Indian subcontinent, where 60-90% of clinical isolates show resistance to furazolidone, TMP-SMX and erythromycin, preferred antibiotics for childhood cholera may include single oral dose of Doxycycline (2-4 mg/kg), azithromycin (20 mg/kg) or ciprofloxacin (20 mg/kg).

Role of other drugs

Oral zinc supplementation as 20 mg of elemental zinc per day (10 mg/day if below 6 months of age) for 14 days reduces the severity and duration of diarrhea and prevents further occurrences in the next few months. Antidiarrheals including anti-motility drugs (e.g. loperamide, diphenoxylate, codeine), adsorbents (e.g. kaolin), live bacterial cultures (e.g. *Lactobacillus*, *Streptococcus faecium*) and charcoal do not offer any benefits, and may have dangerous side-effects. Thus, no drug besides antibiotics and zinc for treatment of diarrhea or vomiting should be given.

7. What should be the policy for prevention of cholera?

Equally important to the treatment of cholera is the prevention of future infections. Since cholera spreads via the fecal-oral route, preventive measures mostly consist of providing clean water and proper sanitation. Boiling and chlorination of water can help kill the bacteria. It is important to educate people about maintaining hygiene including hand washing with soap at appropriate times and food hygiene, and proper disposal and/or sterilization of infectious waste. Patient's bedding and clothing can be disinfected by stirring them for 5 minutes in boiling water. Bedding including mattresses can also be disinfected by thorough drying in the sun. Chemoprophylaxis using appropriate antibiotics can be offered selectively for close contacts of the patient, especially for those at higher risk. Mass chemoprophylaxis for a community, however, is not recommended since it has no effect on spread of cholera and may contribute to antimicrobial resistance.

There is a long history of development of vaccines against cholera, with varied success. Currently, an oral cholera vaccine (against both O1 and O139 cholera) of demonstrated safety and effectiveness is available for those aged one year and above. Two doses of 1.5 mL are given 14 days apart. However, use of this vaccine in both endemic and epidemic situations requires further assessment. For international travelers, vaccination is no longer required since the risk of contracting cholera is very small.

Further Reading

1. Ali M, Lopez AL, You YA, et al. The global burden of cholera. Bull WHO. 2012;90:209-218A.
2. Azman AS, Rudolph KE, Cummings DA, Lessler J. The incubation period of cholera: a systematic review. J Infect. 2013;66:432-8.
3. Azurin JC, Kobari K, Barua D, et al. A long-term carrier of cholera: Cholera Dolores. Bull WHO. 1967;37:745-9.
4. Barua D. History of cholera. In: Barua D, Greenough WB III, (eds). Cholera. New York: Plenum Medical Book Co; 1992. 1-36.
5. Bharati K, Ganguly NK. Cholera toxin: A paradigm of a multifunctional protein. Indian J Med Res. 2011;133:179-87.
6. Centers for Disease Control and Prevention. Laboratory methods for the diagnosis of epidemic dysentery and cholera [WHO/CDS/CSR/EDC/99/8/EN]. CDC, Atlanta: USA;1999.

7. Cholera. The Center for Food Security and Public Health, Iowa State University. January 2004. http://www.cfsph.iastate.edu/Factsheets/pdfs/cholera.pdf. Accessed June 17, 2013.
8. Cholera vaccines: WHO Position Paper. Weekly Epidemiol Rec. 2010;85:117-128.
9. Deen JL, von Seidlein L, Sur D, et al. The high burden of cholera in children: comparison of incidence from endemic areas in Asia and Africa. PLoS Negl Trop Dis. 2008;2 (e)173.
10. Faruque SM, Sack DA, Sack RB, Colwell RR, Takeda Y, Nair GB. Emergence and evolution of Vibrio cholerae O139. PNAS. 2003; 100:1304-9.
11. Ganguly NK, Kaur T. Mechanism of action of cholera toxin and other toxins. Indian J Med Res. 1996;104:28-37.
12. Ghosh-Banerjee J, Senoh M, Takahashi T, et al. Cholera toxin production by the El Tor variant of Vibrio cholerae O1 compared to prototype El Tor and classical biotypes. J Clin Microbiol. 2010;48(11):4283-6.
13. Graves PM, Deeks JJ, Demicheli V, Jefferson T. Vaccines for preventing cholera: killed whole cell or other subunit vaccines (injected). Cochrane Database of Systematic Reviews. 2010; Issue 8. Art. No.: CD000974. DOI: 10.1002/14651858. CD000974.pub2.
14. Harris JB, Khan AI, LaRocque RC, et al. Blood group, immunity, and risk of infection with *Vibrio cholerae* in an area of endemicity. Infect Immun. 2005;73:7422-7.
15. Hoshino K, Yamasaki S, Mukhopadhyay AK, et al. Development and evaluation of a multiplex PCR assay for rapid detection of toxigenic *Vibrio cholerae* O1 and O139.FEMS. Immunol Med Microbiol. 1998;20:201-7.
16. Kaper JB, Morris JG Jr., Levine MM. Cholera. Clin Microbiol Rev. 1995;8:48-86.
17. Kaper JB. *Vibrio cholerae* vaccines. International Symposium on Vaccine Development and Utilization. Rev Infec Dis.1989;11:S568-3.
18. Longini IM Jr., Nizam A, Ali M, et al. Controlling endemic cholera with oral vaccines. PLoS Med. 2007;4:e336.
19. Nato F, Boutonnier A, Rajerison M, et al. One-Step Immunochromatographic Dipstick Tests for Rapid Detection of *Vibrio cholerae* O1 and O139 in Stool Samples. Clin Vaccine Immunol. 2003;10:476-8.
20. Pierce NF, Banwell JG, Gorbach SL, Mitra RC, Mondal A. Convalescent carriers of *Vibrio cholerae*: Detection and detailed investigation. Ann Intern Med. 1970;72(3):357-64.
21. Ramamurthy T, Bhattacharya SK (eds). Epidemiological and molecular aspects on cholera, 1st ed. New York: Humana Press, Springer Science+Business Media; 2010.
22. Reveiz L, Chapman E, Ramon-Pardo P, et al. Chemoprophylaxis in contacts of patients with cholera: systematic review and meta-analysis. PLoS One. 2011;6:e27060.
23. Sack D, Sack RB, Nair GB, Siddique AK. Cholera. Lancet.2004;363:223-33.
24. Sur D, Deen JL, Manna B, et al. The burden of cholera in the slums of Kolkata, India: data from a prospective, community based study. Arch Dis Child. 2005;90:1175-81.
25. Sur D, Lopez AL, Kanungo S, et al. Efficacy and safety of a modified killed-whole-cell oral cholera vaccine in India: an interim analysis of a cluster-randomised, double-blind, placebo-controlled trial. Lancet. 2009;374:1694-702.
26. Tuite AR, Tien J, Eisenberg M, Earn DJ, Ma J, Fisman DN. Cholera epidemic in Haiti, 2010: using a transmission model to explain spatial spread of disease and identify optimal control interventions. Ann Intern Med. 2011;154:593-601.

27. WHO/UNICEF Joint Statement. Clinical management of acute diarrhea. The United Nations Children's Fund/World Health Organization; 2004. WHO/FCH/CAH/04.7.
28. World Health Organization. Cholera, 2005. Wkly Epidemiol Rec. 2006;81:297-307.
29. World Health Organization. Cholera Fact sheet No.107, July 2012. Available from: http://www.who.int/mediacentre/factsheets/fs107/en/. Accessed June 12, 2013.
30. World Health Organization. Cholera surveillance and number of cases. Geneva: WHO; 2007. Available from: http://www.who.int/topics/cholera/surveillance/en/index.html. Accessed June 12, 2013.
31. World Health Organization. Prevention and control of cholera outbreaks: WHO policy and recommendations. Global Task Force on Cholera Control. Available from:http://www.who.int/cholera/technical/prevention/control/en/index2.html. Accessed June 20, 2013.
32. World Health Organization. The treatment of diarrhea: A manual for physicians and other senior health workers. WHO/FCH/CAH/05.1. Geneva: WHO; 2005.
33. World Health Organization. Zinc supplementation in the management of diarrhea. e-Library of Evidence for Nutrition Actions (eLENA). Available from: http://www.who.int/elena/titles/bbc/zinc_diarrhoea/en/. Accessed June 20, 2013.
34. Yamazaki W, Seto K, Taguchi M, Ishibashi M, Inoue K. Sensitive and rapid detection of cholera toxin-producing *Vibrio cholerae* using a loop-mediated isothermal amplification. BMC Microbiology. 2008;8:94.
35. Zuckerman JN, Rombo L, Fisch A. The true burden and risk of cholera: implications for prevention and control. Lancet Infect Dis. 2007;7:521-30.

7
Brucella

Sanjay Krishna Ghorpade

1. How *Brucella* is transmitted?

Transmission is usually from infected animals to human. There are some evidences of human to human transmission also.

The routes of spread are:
  i. *Food-borne infections:* Infection takes place indirectly by the ingestion of raw milk or dairy products (cheese) from infected animals. Fresh raw vegetables grown on soil and water contaminated with the excreta of infected animals may also serve as a source of infection.
  ii. *Contact infection:* Most commonly, infection occurs by direct contact with infected tissues, abraded skin, mucosa, conjunctiva (mucocutaneous route), blood, urine, vaginal discharge, aborted fetuses, etc.
  iii. *Air-borne infections:* The environment of a cowshed may be heavily infected. Few people living in such an environment can expose to inhalation of infected dust or aerosols. *Brucella* may be inhaled in aerosol form in slaughter houses and laboratories, so these infections are notified as occupational.
  iv. *Transplacental infections:* Neonatal and congenital infections with these organisms have also been described. These have been transmitted transplacentally from breast milk, and through blood transfusions.
  v. *Person-to-person infection:* This is extremely rare. Occasional cases have been reported in which circumstantial evidence suggests close personal or sexual contact as the route of transmission. Of more potential significance is transmission through blood donation or tissue transplantation. Bone marrow transfer in particular carries a significant risk. It is advisable that blood and tissue donors be screened for evidence of brucellosis and positive reactors with a history of recent infection be excluded. Transmission to attendants of brucellosis patients is most unlikely but basic precautions should be taken.

2. When do you suspect Brucellosis?

Brucellosis is a systemic illness that can be very difficult to diagnose in children without a history of animal or food exposure. Human brucellosis usually manifests as an acute or subacute febrile illness, which may persist, and progress to a chronically incapacitating disease with severe complications.

Complaints may persist for weeks or months in absence of specific treatment. Symptoms can be acute or insidious in nature and are usually nonspecific, beginning 2–4 weeks after inoculation. The clinical features of brucellosis depend on the stage of the disease, and the organs and systems involved. Although the clinical manifestations do vary, the classic triad of fever, arthralgia/arthritis, and hepatosplenomegaly can be demonstrated in most patients. Some patients present as a fever of unknown origin.

Brucella has been reported to compromise the central and peripheral nervous system, gastrointestinal, hepatobiliary, genitourinary, musculoskeletal, cardiovascular, and integumentary systems. Despite major ongoing controversies in the taxonomy of *Brucella* species, the bulk of human disease is caused by two species: *B. melitensis* and *B. abortus*. On physical examination, the most common findings are hepatomegaly and splenomegaly, which occur in about one-third of patients. Lymphadenopathy is seen in about 10% of patients.

i. *Gastrointestinal and hepatobiliary manifestations:* Liver is the most commonly involved organ. Abdominal pain, constipation, hepatomegaly, jaundice and splenomegaly are also seen.

ii. *Osteoarticular manifestations:* Sacroiliitis, spondylitis, peripheral arthritis, and osteomyelitis account for over half of the focal complications. The most common osteoarticular finding in children is monoarticular arthritis (usually of the knees and hips).

iii. *Cardiovascular manifestations*: Endocarditis with the aortic valve being the most commonly affected structure and multiple valve involvement being common within this subset of patients. It is the most serious complication, accounting for 5% total mortality rate of human *Brucella* infections. Cardiac murmur is rare.

iv. *Genitourinary manifestations:* Glomerulonephritis, orchiepididymitis and renal abscesses can be found in 10% of cases.

v. *Neurological manifestations*: This includes peripheral neuropathies, chorea, meningoencephalitis, transient ischemic attacks, psychiatric manifestations, and cranial nerve compromise.

vi. *Skin manifestations*: Erythematous papular lesions, purpura, dermal cysts and Stevens-Johnson syndrome.

vii. *Pulmonary manifestations*: These include pleural effusion and pneumonias, can be found in up to 16% of complicated cases of brucellosis.

viii. *Congenital and neonatal manifestations*: Neonatal and congenital infections with these organisms have also been described. The signs and symptoms associated with brucellosis are vague and not pathognomonic.

3. What is the long-term sequel if not properly managed?

Osteoarticular complications (sacroiliitis, spondylitis, peripheral arthritis and osteomyelitis) account for over half of the focal complications. Endocarditis with the aortic valve being the most commonly affected structure. Multiple valve involvement being common within this subset of patients is the most serious complication, accounting for most of the 5% total mortality rate in human brucellosis.

Genitourinary complications (orchiepididymitis, glomerulonephritis, and renal abscesses) can be found in around 10% of patients. Neurological complications include peripheral neuropathies, chorea, meningoencephalitis, transient ischemic attacks, psychiatric manifestations and cranial nerve compromise. Mucocutaneous complications include erythematous papular lesions, purpura, dermal cysts, and Stevens-Johnson syndrome. Pulmonary complications including pleural effusions and pneumonias can be found in up to 16% of complicated cases of brucellosis.

Before the use of antimicrobial agents, the course of brucellosis was often prolonged and may have led to death. Since the institution of specific therapy, most deaths are due to specific organ system involvement (e.g. endocarditis) in complicated cases. The prognosis after specific therapy is excellent if patients are compliant with the prolonged therapy.

4. What is the common differential diagnosis?

Brucellosis may be confused with other infections such as tularemia, cat scratch disease, typhoid fever and fungal infections due to histoplasmosis, blastomycosis, or coccidioidomycosis. Infections caused by *Mycobacterium tuberculosis*, atypical mycobacteria, *Rickettssia*, and *Yersinia* can present in a similar fashion to brucellosis.

5. How to diagnose brucellosis?

A history of exposure to animals or ingestion of unpasteurized dairy products is very helpful. A definitive diagnosis is made by recovering the organism from blood culture, bone marrow aspiration, or other tissues. Routine laboratory examinations of the blood are not helpful; thrombocytopenia, neutropenia, anemia, or pancytopenia may occur. Leukocytosis is observed in about 9% of patients and if found, focal complications should be excluded. Leukopenia (11% of patients) and thrombocytopenia (10% of patients) are seen in similar frequencies. Anemia is seen more frequently, affecting 26% of patients.

Culture

Blood culture is the gold standard in the diagnosis of bacterial infections, including brucellosis. Although the biphasic Ruiz-Castañeda system is the traditional method for the isolation of *Brucella* spp. from clinical samples, it has now largely been replaced by automated culture systems, such as the lysis centrifugation method with increased sensitivity and reduced culture times. The sensitivity of blood culture depends on several factors, particularly the phase of the disease and previous use of antibiotics. For instance, in acute cases, the sensitivities of the Ruiz-Castañeda method and lysis-centrifugation have been reported as high as 80% and 90%, respectively, but as low as 30% and 70%, respectively, in chronic cases.

Although automated culture systems and the use of the lysis-centrifugation method have shortened the isolation time from weeks to days, it is prudent to alert the clinical microbiology laboratory that brucellosis is suspected. Isolation of the organism still may require as long as 4 weeks from a blood culture sample. Caution is also advised when using automated bacterial identification systems, because isolates have been misidentified as other gram-negative organisms (*Haemophilus influenzae* type b).

Bone marrow cultures may provide a higher sensitivity, yield faster culture times, and may be superior to blood cultures when evaluating patients with previous antibiotic use. *Brucella* can also be cultured from pus, tissue samples, and cerebrospinal, pleural, joint, or ascitic fluid. Since brucellosis constitutes one of the most common laboratory-acquired infections, special care should be taken when using the lysis-centrifugation method to avoid infection from contaminated aerosols.

Serodiagnosis

Agglutination tests

The serum agglutination test (SAT) detects antibodies against *B. melitensis, B. abortus* and *B. suis*. This method does not detect antibodies against *B. canis* because this organism lacks the smooth lipopolysaccharide. In the absence of culture facilities, the diagnosis of brucellosis traditionally relies on serological testing with a variety of agglutination tests such as the Rose Bengal test, the serum agglutination test, and the antiglobulin or Coombs' test.

In general, the Rose Bengal test is used as a screening test, and positive results are confirmed by the serum agglutination test. These agglutination tests are based on the reactivity of antibodies against smooth lipopolysaccharide. These antibodies tend to persist in patients long after recovery; therefore, in endemic areas, high background values could occur that may affect the diagnostic value of the test (Prozone effect). In addition, the prozone effect can give false negative result in the presence of high titers of antibodies, to avoid this serum that is being tested should be diluted to ≥ 1:320. Furthermore, the *Brucella* smooth lipopolysaccharide antigen tends to show cross reactivity with other gram-negative bacteria such as *Yersinia enterocolitica* 0:9, *Vibrio cholerae, Escherichia coli* 0:157, and *Francisella tularensis*, increasing the possibility of false-positive results.

No single titer is ever diagnostic, but most patients with acute infections have titers of ≥1:160. Low titers may be found early in the course of the illness, requiring the use of acute and convalescent sera testing to confirm the diagnosis. Because patient with active infection have both an immunoglobulin M (IgM) and an IgG response and the SAT measures the total quantity of agglutinating antibodies, the total quantity of IgG is measured by treatment of the serum with 2-mercaptoethanol. It is important to remember that all titers must be interpreted in light of a patient's history and physical examinations. Coombs' test may be more suitable for confirmation of brucellosis in relapsing patients or patients with persisting disease.

Enzyme-linked Immunosorbent Assay (ELISA)
ELISA has become increasingly popular as a well-standardized assay for brucellosis. The sensitivity of ELISAs prepared in the laboratory may be high, especially when the detection of specific IgM antibodies is complemented with the detection of specific IgG antibodies. The specificity of ELISA, however, seems to be less than that of the agglutination tests. Since ELISA for *Brucella* is based on the detection of antibodies against smooth lipopolysaccharide, the cut-off value may need adjustment to optimize specificity when used in endemic areas, and this may influence sensitivity.

Rapid point-of-care assays
Rapid tests such as the fluorescent polarization immunoassay (FPA) for brucellosis and the immunochromatographic *Brucella* IgM/IgG lateral flow assay (LFA) a simplified version of ELISA, have great potential as point-of-care tests. The FPA test is done by incubation of a serum sample with *Brucella* O-polysaccharide antigen linked to a fluorescent probe. The sensitivity of this test at the selected cut-off value is 96% for culture-confirmed brucellosis, and the specificity was determined to be 98% for samples from healthy blood donors.

The LFA uses a drop of blood obtained by fingerpick, does not require specific training. It is easy to interpret, and can be used at the bedside. The components are stabilized and do not require refrigeration for transportation or storage. The sensitivity and specificity of LFA are high (more than 95%), and the test can be used at all stages of disease. Another useful application for these tests is to screen the contacts of brucellosis patients.

Molecular detection
Polymerase chain reaction (PCR) is a convenient tool for the diagnosis of human brucellosis that may improve sensitivity compared with culture. As per various studies, PCR is found to be 100% sensitive and 98.3% specific to *Brucella* species, compared with 70% sensitivity for blood culture. PCR could be particularly useful in patients with specific complications such as neurobrucellosis, or other localized infections, since serological testing often fails in such patients. Relapsing brucellosis is another diagnostic challenge in which PCR could prove to be useful.

Other applications of PCR
PCR also appears to be useful in species differentiation and biotyping of isolates. PCR amplification of these variable repeats is more robust than classic typing methods for species and biovar identification. PCR was recently used to assess treatment efficacy.

Sonography abdomen
Microabscesses are seen in spleen and liver *Brucella* infection.

6. What is the treatment?

Prolonged antimicrobial therapy is imperative for achieving a cure. Relapses generally are not associated with development of *Brucella* resistance but rather with premature discontinuation of therapy. Monotherapy is associated with a high rate of relapse; combination therapy is recommended. Many antimicrobial agents are active in vitro against the *Brucella* species, but the clinical effectiveness does not always correlate with these results. Doxycycline is the most useful antimicrobial agent and when combined with an aminoglycoside, is associated with the fewest relapses (Table 1).

Table 1: Recommended therapy for the treatment of brucellosis

Age and Condition	Antimicrobial agent	Dose	Route	Duration
≥ 8 year	Doxycycline +	2–4 mg/kg/day; maximum 200 mg/day	PO	6 weeks
	Rifampin	15–20 mg/kg/day; maximum 600–900 mg/day	PO	6 weeks
	Doxycycline +	2–4 mg/kg/day; maximum 200 mg/day	PO	6 weeks
	Streptomycin or	15–30 mg/kg/day; maximum 1g/day	IM	2 weeks
	Gentamicin	3–5 mg/kg/day	IM/IV	2 weeks
<8 year	Alternative: Trimethoprim-sulfamethoxazole (TMP-SMZ)	TMP (10 mg/kg/day; Maximum 480 mg/day) and SMZ (50 mg/kg/day; maximum 2.4 g/day)	PO	4–8 weeks
	+ Rifampin	15–20 mg/kg/day	PO	6 weeks
Meningitis, Osteomyelitis, Endocarditis	Doxycycline +	2–4 mg/kg/day; Maximum 200 mg/day	PO	4–6 months
	Gentamicin +	3–5 mg/kg/day	IV	2 weeks
	Rifampin	15–20 mg/kg/day; Maximum 600–900 mg/day	PO	4–6 months

Treatment failures with beta-lactam antimicrobial agents, including the 3rd generation cephalosporins, may be due to the intracellular nature of the organism. Agents that provide intracellular killing are required for eradication of this infection. Similarly, it is apparent that prolonged treatment is the key to prevent disease relapse. Relapse is confirmed by isolation of *Brucella* within weeks to months after therapy has ended and is usually not associated with antimicrobial resistance.

The onset of initial antimicrobial therapy may precipitate a Jarisch-Herxheimer-like reaction, presumably due to a large antigen load, It is rarely severe enough to require corticosteroid therapy.

Evaluation of immunomodulation with levamisole plus conventional therapy in the management of chronic brucellosis has shown mixed results. Although initial reports of the addition of interferon alfa 2a to standard therapy in allergic patients seemed somewhat promising, this has not led to any practical application. Currently, extended treatment with standard drug combinations should be given to those patients with persisting signs and symptoms of recurrent disease.

Additionally, when treating focal infections, careful attention must be given to the penetration and activity of the drug in the particular tissue involved, and the choice and duration of therapy must be individualized, with prolonged treatment in cases with specific complications such as endocarditis or central nervous system involvement. The more effective doxycycline-streptomycin combination is preferred in patients with more severe disease, such as spinal involvement, and the duration of therapy may be prolonged. Abscesses and specific focalized forms of brucellosis including endocarditis, cerebral, epidural, or splenic abscess might require surgical interventions since these forms are resistant to antibiotics.

Further Reading

1. Abdoel TH, Smits HL. Rapid latex agglutination test for the serodiagnosis of human brucellosis. Diagn Microbiol Infect. Dis. 2007;57:123–8.
2. Agasthya AS, Isloor S, Prabhudas K. Brucellosis in high risk group individuals. [Journal Article]. Indian J Med Microbiol. 2007;25(1):28-31.
3. Almuneef M, Memish ZA. Persistence of *Brucella* antibodies after successful treatment of acute brucellosis in an area of endemicity. J Clin Microbiol. 40:2313.
4. Almuneef MA, Memish ZA, Balkhy HH, Alotaibi B, Algoda S, Abbas M, et al. Importance of screening household members of acute brucellosis cases in endemic areas; Epidemiol Infect. 2004;132:533-40.
5. Araj GF. Enzyme-linked immunosorbent assay, not agglutination, is the test of choice for the diagnosis of neurobrucellosis. Clin Infect Dis. 25:942.
6. Bayindir Y, Sonmez E, Aladag A, Buyukberber N. Comparison of five antimicrobial regimens for the treatment of brucellar spondylitis: a prospective, randomized study. J Chemother. 2003;15:466-71.
7. Chahota R, Sharma M, Katoch RC, Verma S, Singh MM, Kapoor V. Brucellosis outbreak in an organized dairy farm involving cows and in contact human beings, in Himachal Pradesh, India Vet Arh. 2003;73:95-102.

8. Ewals JA, [Brucellosis as an imported disease in a young man with arthritis]. [Case Reports, English Abstract, Journal Article]. Ned Tijdschr Geneeskd. 2005; 149(50):2810-4.
9. Giannacopoulos I, Eliopoulou MI, Ziambaras T, Papanastasiou DA. Transplacentally transmitted congenital brucellosis due to *Brucella* abortus. J Infect. 2002;45:209-10.
10. Gogia A, Dugga L, Dutta S, An unusual etiology of PUO [Case Reports, Journal Article J Assoc Physicians India. 2011. p. 47-9.
11. Gokhale YA, Ambardekar AG, Bhasin A, et al. *Brucella* spondylitis and sacroiliitis in the general population in Mumbai. [Journal Article, Research Support, Non-U.S. Gov't]. J Assoc Physicians India. 2003:659-66.
12. Gur A, Geyik MF, Dikici B, Nas K, Cevik R, Sarac J, et al. Complications of brucellosis in different age groups: a study of 283 cases in southeastern Anatolia of Turkey. Yonsei Med. J 2003;44:33-44.
13. Irmak H, Buzgan T, Evirgen O, Akdeniz H, Demiroz AP, Abdoel TH, et al. Use of the *Brucella* IgM and IgG flow assays in the serodiagnosis of human brucellosis in an area endemic for brucellosis. Am J Trop Med Hyg. 2004;70:688-94.
14. Kadri SM, Rukhsana A, Laharwal MA, et al. Seroprevalence of brucellosis in Kashmir (India) among patients with pyrexia of unknown origin. [Journal Article]. J Indian Med Assoc. 2000;98(4):170-1.
15. Kalla A, Chadda VS, Gauri LA, Gupta A, Jain S, Gupta BK, et al. Outbreak of polyarthritis with pyrexia in Western Rajasthan. J Assoc Physicians India. 2001; 49:9635.
16. Karabay O, Sencan I, Kayas D, Sahin I. Oxacin plus rifampicin versus doxycycline plus rifampicin in the treatment of brucellosis: a randomized clinical trial [ISRCTN11871179]; BMC Infect Dis. 2004;4:18.
17. Kochar DK, Gupta BK, Gupta A, Kalla A, Nayak KC, Purohit SK. Hospital-based case series of 175 cases of serologically confirmed brucellosis in Bikaner J Assoc Physicians India. 2007;55:271-75.
18. Kochar DK, Kumawat BL, Agarwal N, Shubharakaran N, Aseri S, Sharma BV, et al. Meningoencephalitis in brucellosis. Neurol India. 2000;48:170-3.
19. Kochar DK, Sharma BV, Gupta S, Jain R, Gauri LA, Srivastava T. Pulmonary manifestations in brucellosis: a report on seven cases from Bikaner (north-west India). J Assoc Physicians India. 2003;51:33-6.
20. Kumar S, Tuteja U, Sarika K, et al. Rapid multiplex PCR assay for the simultaneous detection of the *Brucella* Genus, B. abortus, B. melitensis, and B. suis. [Evaluation Studies, Journal Article] J Microbiol Biotechnol 2011;21(1):89-92.
21. Mangalgi S, Sajjan A, Mohite ST. Seroprevalence of brucellosis among Blood Donors of Satara District, Maharashtra (original article) Dept of Microbiology, Krishna Institute of Medical Sciences University, Karad, (Maharashtra), India JKIMSU. 2012;1(1):55-60.
22. Mantur B, Parande A, Amarnath S, et al. ELISA versus conventional methods of diagnosing endemic brucellosis. [Comparative Study, Journal Article, Research Support, Non-U.S. Gov't]. Am J Trop Med Hyg. 2010;83(2):314-8.
23. Mantur BG, Amarnath SK, Parande AM, et al. Comparison of a novel immunocapture assay with standard serological methods in the diagnosis of brucellosis. [Comparative Study, Controlled Clinical Trial, Journal Article. Clin Lab. 2011; 57(5-6):333-41.
24. Mantur BG, Mangalgi SS. Evaluation of conventional castaneda and lysis centrifugation blood culture techniques for diagnosis of human brucellosis. [Comparative Study, Journal Article]. J Clin Microbiol. 2004;42(9):4327-8.

25. Mathai E, Singhal A, Verghese S, D'Lima D, Mathai D, Ganesh A, et al. Evaluation of an ELISA for the diagnosis of brucellosis. Indian J Med Res. 1996;103:323-4.
26. Mirnejad R, Doust RH, Kachuei R, et al. Simultaneous detection and differentiates of *Brucella* abortus and *Brucella* melitensis by combinatorial PCR. [Evaluation Studies, Journal Article, Research Support, Non-U.S. Gov't]. Asian Pac J Trop Med. 2012; 5(1):24-8.
27. Pabuccuoglu O, Ecemis T, El S, et al. Evaluation of serological tests for diagnosis of brucellosis. [Comparative Study, Journal Article]. Jpn J Infect Dis. 2011; 64(4):272-6.
28. Palanduz A, Palanduz S, Guler K, Guler N. Brucellosis in a mother and her young infant: probable transmission by breast milk. Int J Infect Dis. 2000;4:55-6.
29. Purwar S, Metgud SC, Darshan A, et al. Infective endocarditis due to brucella. [Case Reports, Journal Article]. Indian J Med Microbiol. 2006; 24(4):286-8.
30. Rahman A, Dirk B, Fretin D, et al. Seroprevalence and Risk Factors for Brucellosis in a High-Risk Group of Individuals in Bangladesh. Food borne Pathogens and Disease. 2012;9(3):190-7.
31. Renukaradhya GJ, Isloor S, Rajasekhar M. Epidemiology, zoonotic aspects, vaccination and control/eradication of brucellosis in India. [Journal Article]. Vet Microbiol. 2002;90(1-4):183-95.
32. Renukaradhya GJ, Isloor S, Rajasekhar M. Epidemiology, zoonotic aspects, vaccination and control/eradication of brucellosis in India; Vet. Microbiol. 2002;90:183-95.
33. Roth F, Zinsstag J, Orkhon D, Chimed-Ochir G, Hutton G, Cosivi O, et al. Human health benefits from livestock vaccination for brucellosis: case study. Bull World Health Organ. 2003;81:867-76.
34. Roushan MR, Gangi SM, Ahmadi SA. Comparison of the efficacy of two months of treatment with co-trimoxazole plus doxycycline vs. co-trimoxazole plus rifampin in brucellosis. Swiss Med Wkly. 2004;134:564-8.
35. Ruiz-Mesa JD, Sanchez-Gonzalez J, Reguera JM, Martin L, Lopez-Palmero S, Colmenero JD. Rose Bengal test: diagnostic yield and use for the rapid diagnosis of human brucellosis in emergency departments in endemic areas. Clin Microbiol Infect. 2005;11:221-5.
36. Sen MR, Shukla BN, Goyal RK. Seroprevalence of brucellosis in and around Varanasi; J Commun Dis. 2002;34:226-7.
37. Sharma KD, Patil SD, Talib VH, Survey of brucellosis at Aurangabad. [Journal Article]. Indian J Med Sci. 1974;28(12):546-9.
38. Smits HL, Abdoel TH, Solera J, Clavijo E, Diaz R. Immunochromatographic Brucella-specific immunoglobulin M and G lateral flow assays for rapid serodiagnosis of human brucellosis. Clin Diagn Lab Immunol. 2008;10:1141-6.
39. Solera J, Geijo P, Largo J, Rodriguez-Zapata M, Gijon J, Martinez-Alfaro E, et al. A randomized, double-blind study to assess the optimal duration of doxycycline treatment for human brucellosis. Clin Infect Dis. 2004;39:1776-82.
40. Tikare NV, Mantur BG, Bidari LH. Brucellar meningitis in an infant—evidence for human breast milk transmission. [Case Reports, Journal Article]. J Trop Pediatr 2008;54(4):272-4.

8
Mycoplasma pneumoniae and Chlamydia

Baldev S Prajapati, Rajal B Prajapati

I. Mycoplasma pneumoniae

1. How common is mycoplasma infection in children? Is it worth to know for the practicing pediatrician?

Once considered to occur primarily among adolescents and young adults, *Mycoplasma pneumoniae (M. pneumoniae)* is increasingly being recognized as a cause of lower respiratory tract diseases in young children. The precise incidence of *mycoplasma* infections is unknown because surveillance is not conducted and laboratory confirmation is usually not obtained. However, prospective studies suggest that *M. pneumoniae* accounts for 7% to 30% of community-acquired lower respiratory infections in children between 3 to 15 years of age.

M. pneumoniae infection is no longer a benign condition as it was originally thought to be. Many atypical pulmonary and extrapulmonary manifestations affecting major organ systems like cardiovascular system (CVS), central nervous system (CNS), hematological system, gastrointestinal (GI) tract, renal and musculoskeletal system have been described.

Increasing reorganization of the condition has been reported from several centers of our country too. It is said that once a pediatrician becomes familiar with the condition, he starts to see more number of cases in his daily practice.

2. What type of organism is *Mycoplasma pneumoniae*? How does it causes disease in human being?

Mycoplasma are ubiquitous and are the smallest bacteria that can survive alone in nature. It was first isolated in cattle with pleuropneumonia.

Their size 150 to 350 nm is closer to that of viruses than of bacteria. Unlike viruses, however, *Mycoplasma* are able to grow in cell free media and possess both RNA and DNA. These organisms are unique in that they lack a cell wall, a feature largely responsible for their biologic properties such as their lack of reaction to Gram's stain and their lack of susceptibility to many commonly prescribed antimicrobial agents including beta-lactams. Mycoplasma organisms are usually associated with mucosa and rarely penetrate the submucosa, except in the case of immunosuppression or instrumentation.

M. pneumoniae is best known as the cause of walking or atypical pneumonia, but the most frequent clinical syndrome caused by this organism is tracheobronchitis or bronchiolitis, often accompanied by upper respiratory tract manifestations. Additionally, acute mycoplasmal respiratory tract infection may be associated with exacerbations of bronchial asthma. The role of *Mycoplasma* as a cofactor accelerating the progress of HIV infection has been speculated. Antibodies to the I antigen on erythrocytes, i.e. cold agglutinins are responsible for the anemia and are also an aid to the diagnosis. Extrapulmonary manifestations may be due to direct invasion or due to autoimmune mechanisms, as human antigens cross react with *Mycoplasma pneumoniae*.

3. **What are the clinical manifestations of *Mycoplasma pneumoniae* infections?**

Mycoplasma has a mild presentation and the severity is related to the patient underlying immune status and cardiopulmonary status.

Pulmonary manifestations

M. pneumoniae was first isolated during efforts to determine the cause of the clinical syndrome, referred as 'primary atypical pneumonia'. The failure of the patients with this infection to respond to penicillin or sulfonamide therapy—the standard therapy for pneumococcal pneumonia—was considered 'atypical'.

In young children, *M. pneumonia* may be indistinguishable from viral respiratory tract infections.
- In young children, the various respiratory tract infections are:
  - Croup
  - Bronchiolitis
  - Pneumonia
  - Lobar consolidation
  - Necrotizing pneumonia
  - Lung Abscess
  - Bronchiolitis obliterans
  - Acute respiratory distress syndrome (ARDS)
  - Respiratory Failure.

Extrapulmonary manifestations

It may be due to immune medicated mechanisms or direct invasion of the organ by dissemination.
- Central nervous system
  - Encephalitis or Meningoencephalitis
  - Transverse myelitis
  - Guillain Barre Syndrome
  - Bell's palsy
  - Cerebellar ataxia

- Cerebral infarction
- Psychosis
* Cardiac disease
  - Mycocarditis
  - Pericarditis
  - Myocardial infarction
  - Congestive cardiac failure (CCF)
  - Heart block
* Hematologic
  - Coomb's test positive hemolytis, anemia
  - Thrombosis
  - Thrombotic thrombocytopenic purpura
* Hepatic — Elevation of hepatic enzymes
* Occular
  - Conjunctivitis
  - Iritis
  - Optic disc edema
* Glomerulonephritis
* Acute pancreatitis
* Arthritis
* Rhabdomyolysis
* Dermatologic
  - Maculopapular rashes
  - Erythema multiforme
  - Stevens-Johnson Syndrome
  - Urticaria
  - Vesiclular-bullous
  - Erythema marginatum
  - Ulcerative stomatitis

4. What Investigations will be useful to diagnose *Mycoplasma* Infection?

* Complete blood cell (CBC)
  CBC is not likely to distinguish between respiratory tract infections caused by *M. pneumoniae* from infections caused by viruses or other bacteria. WBC may be normal or slightly elevated. Erythrocyte sedimentation rate (ESR) may be raised.
* Cold agglutinin test
  This may be performed at the bedside or in the laboratory and is positive in about 50 to 90% of the patients. Plasma from spun patient serum is combined with type O erythrocytes and incubated at 4° C for several minutes. The degree of agglutination is noted at this temperature and again after rewarming to 37° C to confirm resolution of the agglutination. The serum is diluted serially, and the test is repeated. The highest dilution resulting in agglutination at 4° C is reported as the cold agglutinin titer. A cold agglutinin titer of greater than or equal to 1:32 is

suggestive of *Mycoplasma* infections. Cold agglutinating antibodies are immunoglobulin M (IgM) autoantibodies directed against the I antigen on human erythrocytes. They appear within 7 to 10 days of initial symptoms and drop sharply after 2 to 3 weeks.

- Enzyme-linked immunosorbent assay (ELISA)
  ELISA or indirect immunoflourescence for IgM against *M. pneumonia* has specifity greater than 98% in all stages of infections, but the sensitivity varies depending on the stage of infection. The IgM result may be negative in early phase (7 to 10 days) and may not be helpful in guiding the initial therapy. These antibodies remain positive for few months after recovery. A fourfold increase in IgG *M. pneumonia* antibody titer by complement fixation or enzyme immunoassay (EIA) obtained 10 days to 3 weeks apart after the onset of infection is diagnostic.
- Polymerase chain reaction (PCR)
  PCR can be done rapidly and has a high specificity in all phases of infection, including early periods when the serum may be negative for antibody. PCR has a sensitivity of 92% and specificity of 98%. PCR can be performed on throat swabs, sputum, bronchoalveolar lavage fluid and nasopharyngeal aspirates. It can also be done on Cerebrospinal fluid (CSF), but it has a low diagnostic yield.
- Chest X-ray
  In the chest X-ray, there is no particular finding that is suggestive of mycoplasma.

5. What is the treatment of mycoplasma infections?

Antimicrobials are effective in reducing the length of illness due to *Mycoplasma pneumoniae*. Beta-lactams like penicillins and cephalosporins are ineffective because the organism lacks a cell wall.

The benefits of antimicrobial therapy for the treatment of upper respiratory tract symptoms caused by *M. pneumonia* have not been adequately studied in children. However, limited data in children suggest that a macrolide antibiotic or tetracycline (> 8 years of age) should be prescribed when a lower respiratory tract infection is likely to be caused by *M. pneumonia*.

Mycoplasma should be suspected under following circumstances:
- Prolonged mild presentation with unexplained radiological fluid in chest X-ray
- Multisystem or extrapulmonary manifestations along with pulmonary involvement
- Severe community acquired pneumonia or worsening of pneumonia despite appropriate therapy. Here, instead of escalating antimicrobials, consider atypical either as sole etiology or coinfection as the conventional beta-lactam antibiotics are not effective against them
- Pneumonia worsening wheeze
- Drugs and dosage for *Mycoplasma* infections

- Azithromycin —10 mg/kg OD on day 1 followed by 5 mg/kg OD for next 4 days
- Clarithromycin—5 mg/kg/day BID for 10 days.
- Erythromycin—30 to 40 mg/kg/day QID for 10 days
- Tetracycline (> 8 years of age)—20–50 mg/kg/day QID for 10 days
- Doxycycline (> 8 years of age)—2 to 4 mg/kg/day OD for 10 days

In hemolytic anemia and CNS involvement, antimicrobials may not have a major therapeutic role as these disorders are considered due to immune mediated mechanisms.

II. Chlamydia

6. What is *Chlamydia pneumoniae*? How is it common in children?

Chlamydiae are obligate intracellular pathogens. The first isolates of *C. pneumoniae* were obtained during studies on trachoma in the 1960s. Subsequent serologic studies demonstrated that the organism caused an outbreak of pneumonia among school children in Finland in 1978. In 1986, the organism was isolated from the respiratory tract of college students with acute respiratory disease. *C. pneumoniae* is primarily a human respiratory pathogen. The organism has also been isolated from non human species, including horse, reptiles, etc.

C. pneumoniae appears to affect individuals of all ages. The proportion of community-acquired pneumonia associated with *C. pneumoniae* infection is 2 to 19% varying with geographic location, the age group examined and the diagnostic methods used. Several studies on the role of *C. pneumoniae* in lower respiratory tract infection in pediatric population have found evidence of infection from none to more than 18%. Most of these studies have relied entirely on serology for diagnosis. A large multicenter study in 3 to 12 years of age found evidence of *C. pneumoniae* infection, based on culture in 14% and *Mycoplasma pneumoniae* in 22%.

Infections caused by *C. pneumoniae* cannot be readily differentiated from those caused by other respiratory pathogens especially *Mycoplasma pneumoniae*. The pneumonia usually presents as a classic atypical pneumonia characterized by mild to moderate constitutional symptoms including fever, malaise, headache, cough and frequently pharyngitis. However, severe pneumonia with pleural effusion and empyema has been reported.

C. pneumonia may serve as an infection trigger for asthma and can cause pulmonary exacerbations in patients with cystic fibrosis. It may cause otitis media. Asymptomatic respiratory infection has been documented in 2 to 5% adults and children and may persist for a year or more.

7. What are the laboratory diagnostic tests for *Chlamydia pneumoniae*?

It is not possible to differentiate *C. pneumonia* from other causes of atypical pneumonia on the basis of clinical findings. Rales and often wheezing are revealed on auscultation of chest. The chest X-ray often appears worse than patient's clinical status would indicate and may show mild, diffuse involvement or lobar infiltrates with small pleural effusions. The CBC may be unremarkable.

- Specific diagnosis of *C. pneumonia* is based on isolation of the organism in tissue culture. The optimum site for culture is the posterior nasopharynx. It can be isolated from sputum, throat cultures, bronchoalveolar lavage and pleural fluid. Few laboratories perform cultures because of technical problems
- PCR is the most promising technology
- Microimmunofluorescence (MIF) and complement Fixation (CF) tests have not been adequately validated.

8. What is the treatment of *Chlamydia Pneumonia*?

- Erythromycin 40 mg/kg/day BID for 10 days
- Clarithromycin 15 mg/kg/day BID for 10 days
- Azithroycin 10 mg/kg on day 1 and then 5 mg/kg/day on days 2–5.

Tetracyclines, ketolides and newer flluroquinolones (levofloxacin and moxifloxacin but not ciprofloxacin) are found effective in *Chlamydia* infections.

Clinical response to antibiotics therapy varies. Coughing often persists for several weeks even after the therapy.

Further Reading

1. Hammerschlag MR, Kohlhoff SA. *Chlamydophila pneumonia*. In: Kliegman RM, Stanton BF, Gemeler JWS, et al. editors, Nelson Text book of Pediatrics. 19th ed. New Delhi. Elsevier Saunders. 2011.p.1033-5.
2. Khosla 1. *Mycoplasma* Infections. In: Ghosh TK, Yewale V, Parthasarthy A, Shah NK, editors, IAP Speciality Series on Pediatric Infectious Diseases (Under IAP Action Plan 2006). 1st ed. Mumbai. Indian Academy of Pediatrics; 2006. p. 215-18.
3. Powell DA. *Mycoplasma pneumonia*. In: Kliegman RM, Stanton BF, Gemeler JWS, et al. editors, Nelson Textbook of Pediatrics 19th ed. New Delhi. Elsevier Saunders. 2011.p.1029-32.
4. Salaria M. Atypical pneumonia in children. Indian Pediatr. 2002; 39: 1061-2.
5. Shah SS. *Chlamydophila (Chlamydia) pneumoniae*. In: Long SS, Pickering LK, Prober CG, et al. editors. Principles and Practice of Pediatric Infectious Diseases. 3rd ed. Churchill Livingstone, 2008.p. 875-7.
6. Shah SS. *Mycoplasma pneumoniae*. In: Long SS, Pickering LK, Prober CG, et al. editors, Principles and Practice of Pediatric Infectious Diseases 3rd ed. Churchill Livingstone, 2008. p. 979-84.
7. Shivbalan SO. *Mycoplasma* infection. In: Parthasarathy A, Kundu R, Agrawal R et al. editors, Textbook of Pediatric Infectious Diseases. 1st ed. New Delhi. Jaypee Brothers Medical Publishers (P) Ltd; 2013.p.242-5.
8. Unadkat R, Gurav M, Parikh R. Unusual manifestations of *Mycoplamsa pneumonia* infection in children. Pediatric Infectious Disease, Journal of the Academy of Pediatrics, Infectious Disease Chapter. 2011;3:61-4.

9

Rickettsia

Atul Kulkarni

1. What are the rickettsial infections? What do we mean by spotted fever and typhus?

Rickettsiae comprise a group of microorganisms that phylogenetically occupy a position between bacteria and viruses. These are arthropod-borne bacteria belonging to the genus *Rickettsia* within the family *Rickettsia*. Most of these bacteria are associated with ticks, which are their vectors and reservoirs, but some are vectorized by lice, fleas or mites.

Rickettsia species were classically divided into "spotted fever" and "typhus" groups based on serologic reactions. The outer membrane protein A (OmpA) gene is present in spotted fever but not typhus group organisms. More than 19 types of spotted fever varieties are described depending upon the geographical area where these are prevalent, e.g. Rocky mountain spotted fever, meditarian spotted fever. Typhus group consist epidemic typhus, endemic typhus and scrub typhus.

2. What are the common features of various rickettsial infections?

Incubation period in children varies from 2 to 28 days. A history of exposure to tick or close contact with an infected pet animal may be forth coming. Often, history of travel from an endemic area or a similar illness in family members is available. Initially, the illness appears to be nonspecific and patients present with headache, fever, anorexia, myalgias and restlessness. Calf muscle pain and tenderness are common in children. Gastrointestinal symptoms include nausea, vomiting and diarrhea. Abdominal pain is a frequent complaint earlier in this disease. Skin rash is usually not present until after 2–4 days of illness. The typical triad of fever, headache and rash is observed in 44% of patients. Core body temperature may exceed 40ºC and can be remain high or it can fluctuate dramatically. Headache is severe, unremitting and usually unresponsive to analgesics.

Meningism, altered sensorium, seizures, coma, ataxia, auditory deficits and visual loss can be present when central nervous system is affected. Pulmonary involvement manifests as rales, infiltrates and non-cardiogenic pulmonary edema. Edema over the dorsum of hand or foot, periorbital edema, hepatomegaly and generalized lymphadenopathy are sometimes seen. Myocarditis, acute renal failure and vascular collapse can be seen in more severe form of disease.

3. **What is typical rash of rickettsial fever? Can we differentiate between various rickettsial diseases depending on type and distribution of rash?**

Rash is initially discrete. Pale rose red blanching macules or maculopapules appear characteristically on the extremities including the ankles, wrist, or lower limbs. Later, rash spreads rapidly to involve the entire body including palms and soles (Fig. 1). After several days, the rash becomes more petechial (Fig. 2) or hemorrhagic, sometimes with palpable purpura. In severe form of the disease, petechiae may enlarge into ecchymosis, which can become

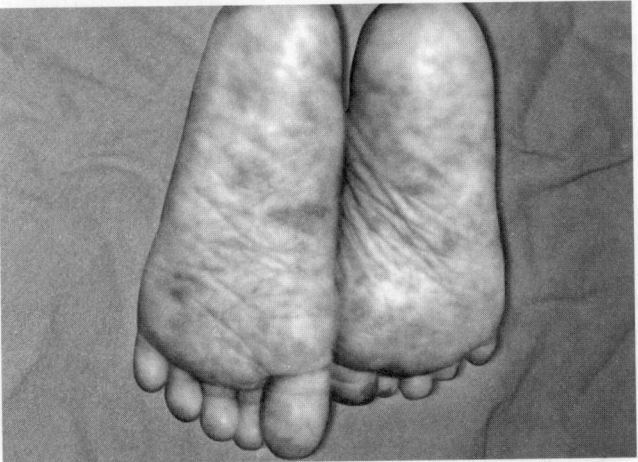

Figure 1: Rash on soles

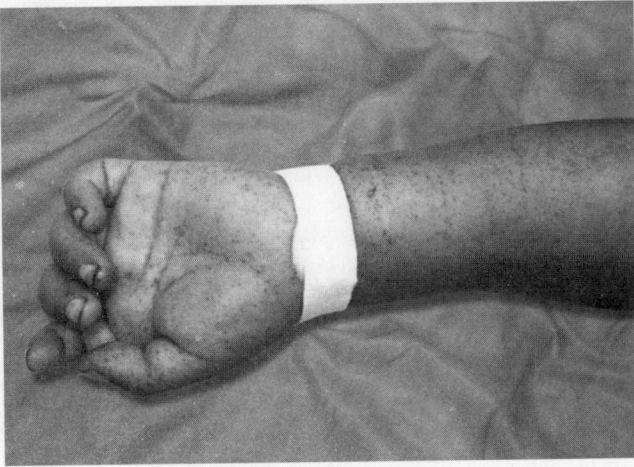

Figure 2: Petechial rash

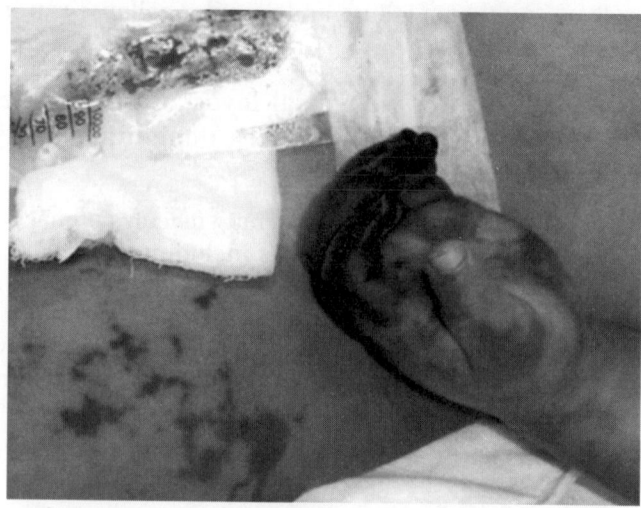

Figure 3: Gangrene of digits

necrotic. Severe vaso-occlusive disease secondary to rickettsial vasculitis and thrombosis is infrequent but can result in gangrene of the digits (Fig.3), toes, earlobes, scrotum, nose or entire limbs. Painless eschar, the tache noire, may be seen at the initial site of tick attachment and regional lymphadenopathy.

It is possible to differentiate between various rickettsial diseases depending on type and distribution of rash as shown in Table 1.

Table 1: Characteristic features of risckettsial diseases

Disease	Characteristic feature
Indian tick typhus	Rash on 3rd or 4th day as blanching macule on extremities and becomes petechial as it spreads later to the trunk. Eschar uncommon
Epidemic typhus	Rash and eschar first in axillary folds and on trunk. Later on spreads to palms and soles
Murine typhus	Rash is non-purpuric, non-confluent and less extensive
Scrub typhus	Frequently an eschar develops with satellite adenopathy
Rickettsial pox	Rash is in the form of vesicles and resembles varicella

4. What are the complications of rickettsial infection?

Complications include non-cardiogenic pulmonary edema from pulmonary microvascular leakage, cerebral edema from meningoencephalitis, and multi-organ damage (hepatitis, pancreatitis, cholecystitis, epidermal necrosis and gangrene) mediated either by rickettsial vasculitis or by accumulated effects of hypoperfusion and ischemia (acute renal failure). Hemophagocytics syndrome can rarely complicate the illness. Long-term neurologic sequelae are more likely to occur in patients who have been hospitalized for greater than or equal to 2 weeks and include paraparesis, motor dysfunction, hearing loss, peripheral neuropathy, and bladder and bowel incontinence. Language disorder and dysfunction of cerebellum and vestibule are also observed. Learning disabilities and behavioral problems are the most common neurologic sequelae among children who have survived severe disease.

Children with G6PD deficiency face an increased risk of developing a fulminant form of spotted fever disease.

5. What are the differential diagnoses of the rash?

Spotted fever can mimic a great number of febrile illnesses. Most important of these are meningococcemia, measles and enteroviral exanthemas. Other diseases included in differential diagnosis are typhoid fever, secondary syphilis, leptospirosis, toxic shock syndrome, scarlet fever, rubella, Kawasaki disease, parvo-viral infection, idiopathic thrombocytopenic purpura (ITP), thrombotic thrombocytopenic purpura (TTP), hemolytic uremic syndrome, Henoch-Schönlein purpura, dengue fever, infectious mononucleosis, drug reactions, malaria, tularemia and anthrax.

6. When to suspect rickettsial infection?

Rickettsial infection should be suspected in any febrile child with under mentioned clinical features.

Patient coming from endemic area. History of contact with pets like dogs and history of tick bite. Classical triad of fever, rash and headache (irritability in younger children). Rash without coryza. Rash extending over palms and soles, palpable purpura, necrotic rash, gangrene, eschar, lymphadenopathy. Edema over the body, pain in legs with hepatosplenomegaly, leukocytosis, anemia and thrombocytopenia. Children presenting with fever, rash with convulsion and altered sensorium. Pyrexia of unknown origin. Fever not responding to routine antibiotics.

7. How to diagnose rickettsial infection?

Laboratory findings are usually non-specific. Leukopenia in early stage and leukocystosis usually develops as the disease progresses. Anemia, thrombocytopenia, hyponatremia and elevated serum aminotransferase are other features. Roughly, 20% of the patients have elevated levels of proteins in CSF with mild pleocytosis.

Specific diagnosis

Diagnosis of rickettsial illness has most often been confirmed by serological testing. Serological evidence of Rickettsial infection occurs not earlier than two weeks after the onset of disease symptoms and hence a specific diagnosis may not be possible until after the patient has recovered or worsened.

- *Immunofloroscence assay:* It is the gold standard for serological diagnosis.
- *ELISA (Enzyme-linked immunosorbent assay):* It is sensitive and specific allowing for detection of IgM and IgG antibodies. It is now available in India and should be preferred for diagnosis.
- *Weil-Felix test:* It is a classical serological test, widely available but unacceptable for accurate diagnosis because of its low specificity and sensitivity. It should be interpreted in conjunction with history and clinical findings.
- *PCR (Polymerase chain reaction):* Confirmative test, costly not widely available.
- *Other tests*: Complement fixation, microagglutination test, indirect hemagglutination, latex agglutination, immunoperoxidase assay, western immunoblot assay.
- *Isolation of rickettsia*: Limited to research laboratory.

8. What is the treatment?

Delay in diagnosing and treating rickettsial disease may result in increased severity and at times may prove fatal. Since, no reliable diagnostic test is available to confirm rickettsial infection in the early stage, initial diagnosis and suitable treatment should be based on a high index of suspicion and appropriate clinical features.

Treatment should not be delayed until laboratory confirmation is obtained.

Tetracycline and chloramphenicol are the two time-tested drugs to effectively treat rickettsial infections in patients of all ages including children with spotted fever. Doxycycline is the drug of choice for all age groups. Chloramphenicol is reserved for patients with doxycycline allergy and for pregnant women.

Recommended treatment regimens

- *Doxycycline*: 2.2 mg/kg/dose Bid PO or IV, maximum 200 mg/day
- *Tetracycline*: 25–50 mg/kg/dose 6 hourly PO, maximum 2 g/day
- *Chlorampenicol*: 50–100 mg/kg/day 6 hourly, maximum 3 g/day

The therapy should be continued for a minimum of 5–7 days and for atleast 3 days until the patient is afebrile in order to avoid relapse. Patients treated with one of these regimens usually become afebrile within 48 hours and thus the entire therapy lasts for less than 10 days.

Other drugs

Mediterranean spotted fever has been effectively treated by azithromycin (10 mg/kg/day OD for 3 days), clarithromycin (15 mg/kg/day BID for 7 days) and fluoroquinolones besides doxycycline and chloramphenicol. However, doxycycline still remains the drug of choice. Specific fluoroquinolones regimens effective for children have not been established. Azithromycin or rifampicin may be used in doxycycline resistant scrub typhus.

Further Reading

1. Centre of Disease Control and Prevention (CDC). Rickettsial Diseases. [online] Available from http://www.cdc.gov/ncidod/ diseases/sunmenus/sub_rickettsial.htm. [Accessed May, 2009].
2. Kulkarni A. Childhood rickettsiosis. Indian J Pediatr. 2011; 78(1):81-7.
3. Raoult D, Parola P. Rickettsial Diseases. New York: Informa Healthcare; 2007.
4. Reller ME, Dumler JS. Rickettsial Infections. Nelson's Textbook of Paediatrics, 19th edition. 1038-53.
5. Scola B, Raoult D. Laboratory diagnosis of rickettsioses. J Clinical Microbiology. 1997;33:2715-27.

10

Leptospira

Janani Sankar

1. What is the epidemiology of leptospirosis, especially in urban areas?

Leptospirosis is presumed to be the most widespread zoonosis in the world. The source of infection in humans is usually either direct or indirect contact with the urine of an infected animal. The incidence is significantly higher in warm-climate countries than in temperate regions, this is due mainly to longer survival of leptospires in the environment of warm and humid conditions. The disease is seasonal, with peak incidence occurring in summer or spring in temperate regions, where temperature is the limiting factor in survival of leptospires, and during rainy seasons in warm-climate regions, where rapid desiccation would otherwise prevent survival.

Generally, veterinarians, farmers, soldiers, abattoir, sewer and rodent-control workers are considered as high-risk group. But rapid urbanization has nullified this concept. In present scenario, urban population, especially those who are involved in recreational activities like swimming, canoeing, surfing, fishing are also at risk.

Transmission

1. Cuts and abrasions in the skin.
2. Intact mucous membranes—Mouth, nose, eyes.
3. Through waterlogged skin.
4. Inhalation of droplets of urine or via water.
5. Human to human—Rarely sexual, transplacental, breast milk.
6. Urine and blood from a patient may be infectious.

2. What are the various manifestations of leptospirosis?

Anicteric form

The clinical presentation of leptospirosis varies widely. It can range from an acute febrile illness to a severe syndrome of multiorgan dysfunction. The more common, mild, anicteric form of the disease is characterized by nonspecific symptoms, such as fever, headache, chills and severe myalgia restricting mobility. It may closely mimic acute infectious polyradiculomyelitis. CPK levels are usually very high. It may present with lymphadenopathy and generalized maculopapular rash mimicking mucocutaneous lymphnode syndrome. Other manifestations include meningoencephalitis, where children have severe headache and neck stiffness.

Similar to any enteroviral infections it can cause myocarditis, which is more common in infants and toddlers. A short febrile illness with disproportionate tachycardia, muffled heart sounds and cardiomegaly with or without raised creatine phosphokinase-MB (CPK-MB) is usually the clinical picture. Polyserositis is usually seen in the form of pleural and pericardial effusion, ascites and gallbladder wall edema. This is usually associated with reduced serum albumin and occasionally these fluids may test positive for dark field microscopy (DFM). Transient glomerular dysfunction, which closely mimics nephrotic syndrome is seen in some children. Hepatorenal syndrome is a more serious condition, which may require peritoneal or hemodialysis. It can involve the eyes and cause severe conjunctival congestion and uveitis.

Icteric form (Weil's syndrome)

This closely mimics acute viral hepatitis and the probable differentiating features may be the presence of polyserositis and cholecystitis. This is a severe form of the infection and occurs less commonly in children and can sometimes coexist with hepatitis A infection. When it coexists with Hepatitis A infection, the severity and the duration of illness is longer. Renal manifestations are common, with abnormal urine analysis (hematuria, proteinuria, hyaline and granular casts) and azotemia, which is often associated with oliguria or anuria. Acute renal failure occurs in a few cases and is the commonest cause of mortality. Both acute renal failure and jaundice are less common in children than in adults.

3. What are modified Faine's criteria for diagnosis of leptospirosis?

This criteria is found to be very useful in a presumptive case of leptospirosis while awaiting the lab reports. It applies clinical criteria, epidemiological criteria and lab criteria with individual scores. It is more useful in older children.

Part A: Clinical data	
Question	Score
Headache	2
Fever	2
Temprature > 39° C	2
Conjunctival suffusion	4
Meningism	4
Muscle pain	2
Conjunctival suffusion + Meningism + Muscle pain	10
Jaundice	1
Albuminuria/nitrogen retention	2
Total score	

| Part B: Epidemiological Factors ||
Question	Score
Rainfall	5
Contact with contaminated environment	4
Animal contact	1
Total score	
Part C: Bacteriological and Lab Findings	
Isolation of leptospira in culture—Diagnosis certain	
Positive Serology	Score
ELISA IgM positive+	15
SAT–positive	15
MAT–Single high titer+	15
Rising titer (paired sera)	25
Total score	

- Current leptospirosis should be considered when score is 26 or more using Parts A + B alternatively 25 or more using Parts A + B + C.

4. What are the various laboratory tests for diagnosis of leptospirosis?

Serological tests

serologic testing is mostly used for diagnosis. Enzyme-linked immunosorbent assay (ELISA) for detection of IgM antibodies (which is positive from the fifth day of illness onwards) and IgM-specific dot-ELISA tests are now recommended in clinical practice; these tests have a sensitivity > 80–90% and are done at many regular pathological and microbiological laboratories. Two to four fold rise in titer is suggestive of leptospirosis. Single high titer is usually seen during the 2nd or 3rd week of illness.

The slide agglutination method, Dri-Dot assay, LEPTO Dipstick, latex agglutination, complement fixation assay, indirect immunofluorescent test, and indirect hemagglutination test are also available; these tests too have good sensitivity of up to 85%.

The microscopic agglutination test (MAT) (serogroup-specific assay) using live antigen suspension of leptospiral serovars is the reference method. This test is available only in a few research institutes and is not helpful for diagnosing leptospirosis during the acute illness; however, it remains important for epidemiological research purposes. The test is read by dark-field microscopy for agglutination and the titers are determined; a four-fold or greater increase in titer in paired sera is confirmative. Agglutinins usually appear by the 12th day of illness and reach the maximum titer by the 3rd week. Due to lack of specific live serovars MAT is not regularly done. MAT titer of 1:100 is usually seen in the general population in endemic area and does not suggest active infection. High titers are usually required to make a diagnosis of active disease. The limitations of MAT are:

1. Antibody titers rise and peak only in 2nd or 3rd week making it a less sensitive test.
2. High titers of past infection persist for long time and therefore interfere with diagnosis of current infection.
3. The cut off titer for diagnosis of current infection depends on whether the area is endemic or nonendemic the cut off titers varies from 1/100 – 1/800. Therefore, a second sample is usually required to diagnose current infection. Seroepidemiological studies are required for determining the cut off values.
4. The test is complicated requiring dark field microscopy and cultures of live serovars.

Demonstration of organism in cultures

Though not commonly employed in routine practice, demonstration of the organisms in the patient's blood and culture of the organism can be used for diagnosis before the 10th day of the illness. Spirochetes can be demonstrated by phase-contrast or dark-field microscopy but these are not very sensitive tests. The definitive method for laboratory diagnosis of leptospirosis is to culture the *Leptospira* from blood, CSF or urine. *Leptospira* are easily cultured on media containing rabbit serum or bovine serum albumin and long-chain fatty acids. All cultures are incubated at room temperature in the dark for up to 6 to 8 weeks. *Leptospira* can be recovered from the blood or CSF during the first 10 days of illness and from the urine after 14 days up to 30 days after the onset of symptoms.

Detection of DNA

DNA hybridization techniques or nucleic acid amplification procedures, including polymerase chain reaction (PCR), can be used to detect the presence of *Leptospira* in body fluids or culture supernatants.

5. What is the gold standard for diagnosis of leptospirosis?

The microscopic agglutination test (MAT) is considered the "gold standard" or cornerstone of serodiagnosis because of its unsurpassed diagnostic (serovar/serogroup) specificity in comparison with other currently available tests.

6. What is the treatment of leptospirosis?

Leptospirosis usually responds to oral amoxycillin (50–100 mg/kg/day for 7 days), azithromycin (10 mg/kg/day for 3 days), cefixime (10 mg/kg/day for 7days) and doxycycline (5–10 mg/kg/day for 7 days).

Antibiotic administration especially before the 7th day of illness reduces length of hospitalization and leptospiruria. In children, even late institution of antibiotic treatment has been shown to prevent complications. Treatment with parenteral penicillin 50,000–1,00,000 U/kg/day is usually reserved for very sick children with meningoencephalitis, myocarditis and renal involvement.

Adequate attention to supportive care, including maintenance of the fluid-electrolyte balance, treatment of cardiovascular collapse and provision of dialysis for renal failure are equally important. Frequent monitoring of vital parameters and hemodynamic assessment, careful charting of fluid input and output and prompt use of ionotropes in patients with hypotension refractory to fluid therapy are important considerations in the management of the disease.

7. How leptospirosis can be prevented?

Important measures for prevention are rodent control and avoidance of contact with contaminated water and soil. Parents should instruct children not to wade through flood waters or play in puddles or stagnant water. Participation in water sports should also be monitored. Immunization of livestock (cattle, sheep, pigs, and horses) and family pets (cats and dogs) has been recommended as a means of eliminating some of the animal reservoirs. Awareness of importance of environmental hygiene should be stressed and propagated.

8. What is the differential diagnosis in early stage of leptospirosis?

   i. Influenza
  ii. Dengue
 iii. Malaria
  iv. Aseptic meningitis
   v. Typhoid
  vi. Viral hepatitis
 vii. Rickettsial infections
viii. Acute polyradiculomyelitis
  ix. Infectious mononucleosis
   x. Viral myocarditis
  xi. Meningencephalitis
 xii. Pyrexia of unknown origin (PUO).

Further Reading

1. Azim P. Nelson Text book of Pediatrics, 19th edition. Philadelphia:Saunders;2011. pp. 984-5.
2. Stoddard R, Shadomy SV. CDC Health information for international travel 2012; The Yellow Book.
3. Terpstra WJ. Human leptospirosis: Guidance for diagnosis, surveillance and control world health organization, International Leptospirosis Society;2003.

PART B: VIRAL INFECTIONS

11

Measles

Ketan H Shah

1. How measles is transmitted?

Measles is highly contagious disease. Virus enters through the respiratory tract or conjunctivae following contact with large droplets or small droplet aerosols in which virus is suspended. Patients are infectious 3 days before to upto 4-6 days after the onset of rash. Approximately, 90% of exposed susceptible individuals experience measles. Face to face contact is not necessary. Viable virus may be suspended in air for as long as one hour after the patient with the source case leaves a room. In physician's office and also in hospitals' secondary cases do occur.

2. What is the risk to the pregnant woman in the household where a child is suffering from measles?

If mother develops measles, child is at risk of having prematurity and low-birth weight. Pregnant woman have chance of miscarriage.

3. How to diagnose measles, especially in early stage, and what are the differential diagnoses?

In case of measles outbreak, high index of suspicion is most important. Clinical diagnosis is usually recommended. The profile of clinical presentation gives clue to diagnosis. It starts with fever, coryza, conjunctival redness, and Koplik's spot. These are initial findings. After 3-4 days, macular rash starts from face, spreading on trunk. Fever increases with appearance of rash. After 2-3 days, rash disappears in same order as it has appeared. Coughing increases with appearance of rash. Serological diagnosis is not routinely recommended. Virus isolation can be done. Molecular detection by Polymerase chain reaction (PCR) is the research tool.

Complete hemogram shows decreased white blood cells. Lymphocytes, decreased more than neutrophils. C-Reaction protein (CRP) and erythrocyte sedimentation rate (ESR) in uncomplicated measles are normal. Absolute neutropenia is known to occur.

Differential diagnosis in typical case is unlikely to mimic the diagnosis. Koplik's spot is diagnostic of measles. In later stage of disease, many exanthematous disease can confuse measles. Rubella, adenovirus, enterovirus, Epstein-Barr virus, exanthema subitum, erythema infectiosum may be confused with measles. *Mycoplasma pneumonia* and group A Streptococci may also produce similar rash. Drug rash and Kawasaki's disease can also have same findings as measles. Meningococcemia has fever, rash and very fast progress of disease. Table 1 shows the differential diagnosis.

4. Which children are likely to have severe measles?

Immunocompromised child are likely to have fatal measles. Children under 5 years of age and adults over 20 years are likely to have complications. Malnutrition and poor healthcare system also make children vulnerable.

5. What are the common complications in a child with measles?

Complications range from relatively mild to severe. Mild diarrhea, measles related pneumonia, otitis media, acute encephalitis and corneal ulceration leading to corneal scarring can occur. Gangrene appears to be secondary to purpura fulminans or disseminated intravascular coagulation. Measles may cause interstitial pneumonia. In HIV patients, it is fatal. Post measles bronchopneumonia and pneumonia due to secondary bacterial infection is common. They are associated with Pneumococci, Streptococci, Staphylococci and *Haemophilus influenzae*. Exacerbation of tubercular lesions and temporary loss of hypersensitivity to tuberculin test are quite common. Encephalitis can occur in one out of every 1000 children having measles. Other neurological complications are Gullian Barre syndrome, retrobulbar neuritis, hemiplegia, and cerebral thrombophiltis, but they are rare.

6. What is the relation between measles and SSPE and how to recognize it?

SSPE (Subacute sclerosing panencephalitis) is neurodegenerative disorder caused by measles virus. There is a persistent infection in CNS by altered measles virus. Virus is harbored intracellular in CNS for several years. After 7-10 years, virus regain virulence and attacks CNS causing cell death. This is nearly fatal disease. Measles at early age favors SSPE.

Clinical manifestation appears after 7-10 years of the disease. Subtle changes in behavior or school performance appears, including irritability, temper outburst, reduced attention span. This is phase one. This stage may be often missed.

Phase two starts with sudden onset of myoclonus; that coincide with inflammation in deep CNS structure. Myoclonus affects axial and appendicular muscles. Consciousness is maintained. In phase three, involuntary movements are replaced by choreoathetosis, immobility, dystonia, and lead pipe rigidity. Sensorium deteriorates, gradually stupor; dementia and coma occurs. Fourth phase is characterized by loss of critical centers that support respiration, heart rate and blood pressure. Death soon ensues. These stages may have acute, sub-acute, or chronic progressive course.

Table 1: Differential diagnosis of measles

Disease	Etiology	Important Clinical features	Laboratory findings	Remark
Measles	Viral infection Paramyxoviridae family	• Koplik's spot • Typical rash • Coryza, cough • Age group <5 years	• Low WBC • Normal ESR • Normal CRP	Epidemiology outbreak helps in diagnosis
Rubella	Viral infection Togaviridae family	• Lymphadenopathy • Rash—not distinctive • With onset of rash, oropharynx may reveal tiny, rose colored lesions (Forchheimer spots), or petechial lesions on soft palate • Rash fades as it progresses. Whole body may or may not be involved. No desquamation. Rash fades within 3 days.	• Low WBC • May have mild thrombocytopenia.	Congenital rubella syndrome is a serious disease
Enterovirus (coxsackie and HFM disease)	Belongs to Picornaviridae family and enterovirus genus	• Maculo-papular lesions on hand, foot, mouth. They are tender. Occasionally vesicular eruptions may be seen • Constitutional symptoms may present.	• Variable hemogram • Non specific	Epidemiology gives clue

Contd...

Contd...

Erythema infectiosum (fifth disease)	Parvovirus	• Slapped check rash • Lacy reticulated appearance of rash • Arthropathy • Transient aplastic crisis • Gloves and socks syndrome	Serological test for B-19 specific IgM	In immunocompromised patient serious sequel can occur
Exanthema subitum (sixth disease) or (Roseola Linfantum)	Human herpes virus 6 and 7	• High grade fever • Appears with crisis and disappears with lysis. • Rash is faint pink, non-pruritic, morbilliform on trunk. Rash may last for few hours. • Ulcers at uvulopalatal glossal junction (Nagayama spots)	• Low WBC • Occasionally thrombocytopenia, • Elevated liver enzymes, • Atypical lymphocytes	Specific diagnosis may not be needed in classical case
Adenovirus	Different group of presentation	• Pharyngo-conjunctival fever • Conjunctivitis, pharyngitis • Bronchitis	No specific findings in hemogram	Preauricular and cervical lymphadenopathy may be seen
Mononucleosis like disease	Epstein Barr virus	• Exudative tonsillitis, • Cervical lymphadenopathy • Hepatosplenomegaly • Palatal catarrh, macular rash on trunk	May have high WBC count, atypical lymphocytes are seen Raised liver transaminase	Splenic rupture Neurological complication can occur Hematological malignancy can occur

Contd...

Contd...

			Classical features
Kawasaki disease	Of unknown etiology	• Strawberry tongue • Cervical lymhnodes • Cracked lips • Mucus membrane involvement • Edema of foot, palm	May have high WBC count, High platelet in 2nd week Raised CRP, ESR	Cardiac complications
Mycoplasma	Mycoplasma pneumoniae	• Respiratory findings are predominant • No rash	IgM level study	CNS and Hematological complication can occur
Streptococcal disease (scarlet fever)	Group A beta hemolytic streptococci	• High fever, strawberry tongue • Sand paper rash • Pruritis, toxic child • Rash in neck, elbow	High count	May have desquamation after fever subsides
Drug eruption	Due to any drug	• Fever may occur • Macular rash • No catarrh	May see eosinophilia	After withdrawing the drug rash may disappear

7. What is the role of vitamin A in measles?

Vitamin A deficiency in developing countries is associated with increased morbidity with measles. Low level of retinol is associated with high mortality and complications with measles. Vitamin A supplementation is recommended as a treatment for children with measles by WHO regardless of their Vitamin A status. It is given for 2 days, at the following dose:
- 200000 IU for children of 12 months of age or older;
- 100000 IU for infants 6 through 11 months of age;
- 50,000 IU for infants younger than 6 months of age.
- An additional (i.e. a third) age specific dose should be given 2 through 4 weeks later to children with clinical sign and symptoms of Vitamin A deficiency.

8. What are the key strategies of measles elimination and measles control program?

WHO's expanded program on immunization has significantly helped to reduce global morbidity and mortality from measles. Measles can be controlled if 100% of the population is immunized with a vaccine which is 100% effective. There are chances of good control. Identification of the distribution of cases, ages of susceptible children and reduction of their concentration throughout the community should be considered. Priority should be given to urban and densely populated rural areas. In large urban areas, high coverage of infants must be achieved soon after the age at which they lose their maternal antibodies and become susceptible. This will be facilitated by the introduction of high-dose measles vaccines, which can be given at 6 months of age. Where measles incidence is increasing among children aged over 2 years, immunization of older children may be considered during contacts with the health care system, or at primary school entry, if this does not divert resources from immunization of younger children. Health workers should be informed of the predicted changes in measles epidemiology following immunization. The collection, analysis and use of data on measles (vaccine coverage, morbidity and mortality) should be improved at all levels of the health care system in order to monitor the immunization program's overall impact, identify pockets of low coverage, and allow early detection of and response to measles outbreaks.

The current global goal for measles control, as stated in the Global Immunization Vision and Strategy (GIVS), 2006–2015 of the World Health Organization and United Nations Children's Fund, is to reduce measles deaths by 90% by 2010 compared to the estimated number in 2000.

World Health Assembly (WHA) has also endorsed the same after the review by WHO's Strategic Advisory Group of Experts (SAGE) on immunization. The key strategies being followed globally are:
- High coverage of measles first dose: Coverage for first dose measles vaccine must be ≥90% at national level and ≥80% for each district in routine immunization

- Sensitive laboratory supported surveillance: Outbreak and case based surveillance is fully supported by laboratories for serological and virological classification. An outbreak is considered confirmed if measles immunoglobulin M (IgM) is detected in serum from at least two suspected cases
- Appropriate measles case management: Includes administration of vitamin A to reduce mortality and complications
- Providing second dose of measles vaccine:
  (a) Single dose in routine immunization—In India, states with ≥80% evaluated coverage for 1st dose of measles vaccine in Routine Immunization (RI) will have the second dose of measles vaccine in RI with Diphtheria, tetanus and pertussis (DPT) booster.
  (b) Supplementary immunization activity (SIA) for measles through catch up immunization campaigns and/or follow up immunization campaigns: States with <80% evaluated coverage of first dose of measles vaccine in routine immunization are conducting measles catch up campaigns since 2010 in a phased manner.

India's decision to introduce MCV2 (measles containing vaccine)

Building on global experience and recognizing that measles represents a significant source of preventable child mortality, the Government of India announced in May 2010, its decision to implement the National Technical Advisory Group on Immunization (NTAGI) recommendation to introduce MCV2. As recommended by the NTAGI, the implementation strategy of MCV2 at the state level is determined by the underlying performance of the routine immunization (RI) program. In total, 14 states with measles vaccine coverage <80% (Arunachal Pradesh, Assam, Bihar, Chhattisgarh, Gujarat, Haryana, Jharkhand, Madhya Pradesh, Manipur, Meghalaya, Nagaland, Rajasthan, Tripura and Uttar Pradesh) will introduce MCV2 through catch up vaccination campaigns. In the remaining 21 states with better performing routine immunization systems (i.e. ≥ 80% routine measles coverage), 17 will introduce MCV2 for children aged 16-24 months through the routine program. The remaining four States and Union Territories (Delhi, Goa, Pondicherry and Sikkim) have already used a second dose of measles vaccine in their RI program (as mumps measles-rubella vaccine) financed with state resources. After the campaigns in the districts of 14 states, these districts will start the MCV2 in routine immunization at 16-24 months old children after 6 months of completing the campaigns.

Supplementary immunization activities and measles catch-up campaigns

Measles catch-up campaigns are indeed SIAs just like polio Sub/National immunization days (SNIDs/NIDs). Supplementary Immunization activities are mass campaigns targeting all children in a defined age group, with the objective of reaching a high proportion of susceptible individuals. Each campaign is conducted over a wide geographical area (e.g. province or country) in order to achieve a rapid reduction in the number of susceptible children. This is a one-time effort to vaccinate all children in a defined age group (based on the epidemiology of the country), irrespective of their prior immunization status (history or record). The goal is to rapidly reduce the susceptible proportion in a population and to rapidly enhance population immunity, i.e. the 'herd immunity'. It is not usual to conduct screening for vaccination status and prior disease history (i.e. the campaigns are usually 'non selective'). Hence anyone who has already received measles vaccine (or MCV) or has history of measles disease in the past is also vaccinated. During SIAs, many established principles of vaccination practices are not adhered to. For example, if a child has received a dose of measles or MCV just a day before the campaign, is also targeted for a campaign dose. Even being a live vaccine, extra doses of measles vaccine do not harm, and in fact, may benefit few children with primary vaccine failure even after second dose. This campaign in fact will increase awareness amongst community for vaccination. With this campaign, 100% coverage is targeted. This will increase immunity of community.

Further Reading

1. Mason WH. Measles. In: Kliegman RM, Stanton BF, St. Geme JW, Schor NF, Behrman RE, editors. Nelson textbook of pediatrics, 19th edition: Elsevier Saunders 2011. pp. 1069-75.
2. Measles. In: Red book. 2012 Report of the committee on Infectious diseases. American academy of Pediatrics, 29th edition; 2012.pp. 489-99.
3. Measles Catch Up Immunization Campaign–Guidelines for Planning and Implementation. New Delhi: Ministry of Health and Family Welfare, Government of India; 2010.
4. Minutes and Recommendations of National Technical Advisory Group on Immunization (NTAGI), 16th June 2008, Ministry of Health and Family Welfare, Government of India. Available at http://mohfw.nic.in. Accessed on June 6, 2013.
5. Principle of measles control .Bull world Health organ. 1991;69(1):1-7. URL: http://www.ncbi.nlm.nih.gov/pmc/articles/PMC2393212/. Accessed on June 6, 2013.
6. Shah AK. Measles. In: Parthsarthy A, Agarwal R, Kundu R, editors. Text book of Pediatric infectious diseases. Jaypee Brothers Medical Publishers (P) limited; 2013. pp. 263-7.
7. Vashishtha VM, P Choudhury P, BansalCP, Gupta SG. Measles Control Strategies in India: Position Paper of Indian Academy of Pediatrics. Indian Peditr. 2013; 50:561-4.

12

Mumps

Ashok Rai

1. How to clinically diagnose mumps and what are the differential diagnosis?

Mumps is an acute systemic viral infection characterized by swelling of one or more of the salivary glands, usually the parotid glands. This illness presents with a prodrome of fever, headache, malaise, neck pain and sore throat.

Parotitis is the most common manifestation and occurs in 30-40% of children. It usually starts unilaterally, but involves the other side in about 70-75% cases.

Swollen glands are tender on palpation and painful. Ingestion of sour or acidic foods usually increases the pain in parotid area.

Approximately, one third of infections do not cause clinically apparent salivary gland swelling and may manifest primarily as respiratory tract infections.

Other salivary glands namely submandibular and sublingual glands may also become inflamed, but in 10% cases, these glands are involved in isolation. Edema over the manubrium and upper chest may also occur due to lymphatic obstruction in severe cases.

Differential diagnosis

Variety of illnesses may simulate mumps but can be easily differentiated on the basis of clinical features. Parotitis may be caused by other viruses namely cytomegalovirus, parainfluenza virus type 1 and 3, influenza A virus, coxsackie virus and other enteroviruses, lymphocytic chorio meningitis virus, human immuno deficiency virus (HIV).

Purulent parotitis is usually caused by *Staphylococcus aureus* and other gram negative organisms, mainly occurs in debilitated patients, premature newborns and during postoperative period. Recurrent parotitis is not rare in children and usually caused by salivary duct calculi. Collagen vascular disease, SLE and certain drug reactions (e.g. phenylbutazone thiouracil) are the other causes of parotid swelling.

2. What are the common complications in a child with mumps?

The most common complications of mumps are aseptic meningitis, encephalitis, orchitis or oophoritis and pancreatitis.

Aseptic meningitis is second to enterovirus as a common cause of viral meningitis and may be the presenting syndrome while only half have clinical evidence of parotitis. Symptomatic involvement (headache, vomiting, neck rigidity) occurs in 10-30% of children suffering from meningitis and it may resolve without sequelae in 3-10 days. This complication is more common in boys than girls (3:1 ratio) and adults are more at risk than children.

Meningo-encephalitis usually develops 5 days after parotitis. It usually occurs due to primary infection of neurons by the viruses or may be post infectious encephalitis with demyelination. Recovery is usually complete with rare fatalities. Occasionally meningitis or encephalitis may occur without parotitis.

Other less common neurological complications are transverse myelitis, facial palsy, aqueductal stenosis, ascending polyradiculitis and cerebellar ataxia.

Orchitis with or without epididymitis is less common in prepubertal males. Orchitis was noted in 30-40% males after puberty. It is bilateral in approximately 30% of affected males. It is usually associated with high grade fever, chills, malaise, rapid painful swelling of the testes and reddening of overlying scrotal skin. It may be associated with atrophy of testes but sterility is very rare even with bilateral involvement.

Oophoritis is rare in childhood and estimated to occur in 7% of female patients. It manifests with lower abdominal pain and tenderness.

Pancreatitis is usually subclinical or mild infections are seen in cases of mumps; however, severe infections are rarely reported. It usually presents with fever, vomiting, epigastric pain and increased serum amylase levels are suggestive of the disease.

Deafness occurs in approximately 1 per 20,000 reported cases. It occurs due to neuritis of the auditory nerve and is usually unilateral.

3. How to approach a child with recurrent parotid swelling?

Recurrent Parotitis is characterized by intermittent swelling of unilateral or bilateral parotid glands, often associated with fever, malaise, pain with mastication and swallowing.

The disease usually manifests between 3 and 6 years of age, but earlier and later occurrence has been observed.

The number of attacks varies individually, with attacks every three to four months being the commonest pattern. The swelling lasts from several days to two weeks and resolves spontaneously, independent of any treatment.

Ultrasound is the appropriate initial investigation and is usually supplemented by sialography. Sialographic examination reveals numerous scattered punctate/globular pools of contrast medium which usually measure 1-2 mm in diameter.

Ultrasonography of the parotid gland reveals enlarged parotid gland in majority of patients with multiple small hypoechoic areas measuring 2-3 mm in diameter.

Flow chart 1: Investigations in a case of recurrent parotitis

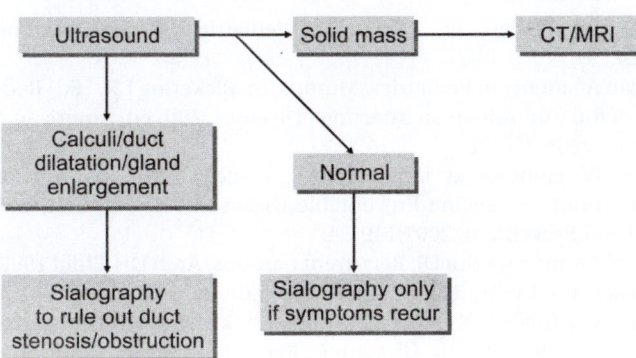

Following investigations should be performed, if there is a clinical suspicion of recurrent parotitis as shown in Flow chart 1.

The recurrent attacks are usually treated conservatively with antibiotics and analgesics. Other treatment options include sialogogic agents to increase salivary fluid, warmth, massage, duct probing and good oral hygiene. More aggressive treatment is justified only for those patients with persistent problems. This may be parotid duct ligation, parotidectomy or tympanic neurectomy, depending upon preference and experience of the treating physician.

4. What is the vaccination strategy against mumps?

Prophylactic immunization is necessary to protect children against mumps and its complications.

Mumps vaccine is a live attenuated vaccine, available in India as MMR vaccine. Though mumps vaccine is also available as single antigen preparation, combined with rubella vaccine, combined with measles and rubella vaccine or combined with measles, rubella and Varicella vaccine (MMRV).

Seroconversion rates against Mumps are more than 90% but clinical efficacy and long-term protection is 60-90% with single dose; outbreaks have been reported in previously vaccinated population. Hence, two dosages are needed for proper protection.

Mumps vaccine should be given as MMR vaccine routinely to children at 12-15 months of age, with a second dose of MMR at 4 to 6 years of age or any time 8 weeks after the first dose. The second dose of mumps vaccine provides an additional safeguard against primary and secondary vaccine failure. The recommended dose of MMR vaccine is 0.5 mL to be given subcutaneously.

Mumps vaccine is generally safe and adverse reactions are very rare. Orchitis, parotitis and low-grade fever have been reported after immunization. This vaccine is contraindicated in pregnancy, severe immunodeficiency and patients with severe allergy to vaccine or its components.

Further Reading

1. Agrawal KN. Mumps. In: Textbook of Pediatrics. 1st Ed. Ana Book Pvt Ltd; 2010;124.
2. American Academy of Pediatrics. Mumps. In: Pickering LK, (Ed) Red book 2009: Report of the Committee on Infectious Diseases. 28th ed. American Academy of Pediatrics. 2009;468-71.
3. Atkinson W, Homborsky J, McIntyre L, Wolfe. C. Mumps. In: Epidemiology and Prevention of Vaccine-Preventable Diseases. 10th Ed. Centres for Disease Control and Prevention, 2007;149-54.
4. Chitre VV, Premachandra DJ, Recurrent parotitis. Arch Dis Child 1997;77:359-63.
5. Committee on Immunization, Indian Academy of Pediatrics. In: Yewale V, Chaudhary P, Thacker N (Eds). IAP Guide Book on Immunization; 2011:73-4.
6. Ericson S, Zetterlund B, Ohman J. Recurrent parotitis and sialectasis in childhood. Clinical, radiologic, immunologic, bacteriologic, and histologic study. Ann Otol Rhinol Laryngol. 1991;100:527-35.
7. Galili D, Marmary Y. Juvenile recurrent parotitis: clinicoradiologic follow-up study and beneficial effect of sialography. Oral Surg Oral Med Oral Pathol 1986; 61:550-6.
8. Jain V, Mani NBS, Singh M, Kumar L. Juvenile Recurrent Parotitis. Indian Pediatrics. 2000;37:1126-9.
9. Knlov LR, Swenson P. Acute parotitis associated with influenza A infection. J infect Dis. 1985;152:853.
10. Li NW, Chan WM, Kwan YW, Leung CW. Recurrent parotitis in children. HKJ Pediatric (New series) 2011;16:36-40.
11. Mandal BK, Wilkins EG, Dunbar EM, Mayon-white RT Mumps. In: Lecture notes on infectious diseases. 5th ed. Blackwell Science Ltd. 1996;58-9.
12. Mandel L, Kaynar A. Recurrent parotitis in children. N Y State Dent J 1995;61:22-5.
13. Murrat ME, Buckenham TM, Joseph AE. The role of ultrasound in screening patients referred for sialography: a possible protocol. Clin Otolaryngol. 1996; 21:21-3.
14. Nozaki H, Harasawa A, Hara H, Kohno A, Shigeta A. Ultrasonographic features of recurrent parotitis in childhood. Pediatr Radiol 1994;24:98-100.
15. Parthasarathy A. Mumps. In: IAP Text Book of Pediatrics. 3rd Ed. Jaypee Brothers Medical Publishers (P) Ltd. 2006:242-3.
16. Robinson MJ, Roberton DM. Infectious diseases of childhood. In: Practical pediatrics. 3rd Ed. B.I. Churchill Livingstone Pvt Ltd. 1995; 277-8.
17. Som PM, Shugar MA, Train JS, Biller HFG. Manifestations of parotid gland enlargement. Radiographic, pathologic and clinical correlations. Radiology 1981;141:415-9.

13

Rubella

P Ramachandran

1. How to clinically diagnose rubella?

Rubella can manifest as postnatal infection and congenital rubella syndrome. Postnatal rubella is generally a mild exanthematous infection in children and adults with minimal morbidity and mortality.

Postnatal rubella

Clinical features

Prodromal symptoms are more in adolescents and adults characterized by sore throat, eye pain, headache, fever, diarrhea and nausea. These symptoms precede the onset of rash by 1 to 5 days and may not be seen in many. Lymphadenopathy is a major clinical manifestation, characteristically involving suboccipital, retroauricular and posterior cervical lymph nodes but generalized lymphadenopathy can also occur. Lymphadenopathy starts at least 24 hours before rash and remains for 1 week or more.

Discrete maculopapular rash starts over face and spreads over the whole body in about 24 hours. Rash may become confluent over face. Large areas of flushing over body are seen. Rash normally disappears by third day. Rubella infection without rash is seen in upto 50%.

An enanthem in the form of discrete rose colored spots (Forchheimer spots) may be seen in the soft palate in 20% cases. They may coalesce and extend over the fauces.

Polyarthritis or arthralgia is seen more commonly in adults, especially in women. Small joints of the hands are frequently involved, often knees and wrists are also involved, but practically any joint may be involved. The joint involvement lasts for several days to two weeks and rarely up to 3 months.

In some, rubella infection is totally asymptomatic.

Diagnosis

Mild forms of measles, scarlet fever, roseola infantum, enteroviral infections and drug fever are to be considered in the differential diagnosis, A combination of exanthem and suboccipital lymphadenopathy can also occur in entero- or adenoviral infection, infectious mononucleosis and *mycoplasma pneumoniae* infection in adolescents.

To bring about uniform diagnostic criteria, WHO has defined probable rubella infection as fever, maculopopular rash and cervical, suboccipital or posterior cervical lymphadenopathy or arthralgia/arthritis. Confirmed rubella is a probable case with IgM seropositivity within 28 days of onset of rash.

2. **What is the risk to the fetus of a nonimmune pregnant woman getting infected in different trimesters of pregnancy?**

Risk can be classified as: a) fetal infection; and b) congenital defects.

Risk for fetal infection

One of the most critical factors determining the frequency of fetal infection and severity of disease in neonate is the time during which rubella infection occurs. The risk for fetal infection after serologically confirmed maternal rubella is as follows:

In first trimester, the risk is quite high, 81%. Out of those, it is 90% for fetuses exposed in first 11 weeks and 67% for fetuses exposed between 11 and 12 weeks. The infection risk comes down to 39% when exposure occurs in second trimester. It increases to 53% in third trimester. The risk is 35%, 60% and 100% in the last 3 months of pregnancy respectively.

Fetal infection is less between 12 and 28 weeks. The placental barrier becomes relatively ineffective in the last month, almost to the same extent as in the first trimester. Anyhow, the fetus is at risk throughout pregnancy to varying degrees.

Risk for congenital infections

The estimates of risk of defects depend on serologic status and age at evaluation of the child. Congenital defect rate is 100% in first 11 weeks, 30% in 11-20 weeks and none thereafter.

Maternal infection after the 16th week of pregnancy poses a low risk for congenital defects, although infection of the fetus may occur.

Cataract and glaucoma occur when maternal rubella occurs in first 2 months of gestation. Congenital heart disease can result when maternal rubella occurs in the first 3 months, deafness during the first 4 months and retinopathy during the first 5 months.

3. **What are the salient features of congenital rubella syndrome (CRS) and how to diagnose it?**

CRS is the result of in utero fetal infection which usually occurs during the first 12 weeks of pregnancy. Classical congenital rubella syndrome comprises of triad of cataract, sensorineural hearing loss and congenital heart disease. It was later expanded to include many other clinical manifestations. Many infants have only one or a few of these manifestations.

Clinical manifestations of congenital rubella

General
  i. Fetal loss (spontaneous abortion and stillbirths)
  ii. Low birth weight
  iii. Micrognathia.

Ears and central nervous system

Sensorineural deafness is the most common manifestation of CRS, seen in 80% to 90% of cases and it is generally bilateral. Frequently, this is the only manifestation. In many cases, it may not be apparent in infancy or early childhood. 10-20% babies suffer from active meningoencephalitis at birth. Mental retardation, behavioral disturbances and speech defects may occur later.

Cardiovascular system
  i. Patent ductus arteriosus
  ii. Pulmonary artery stenosis
  iii. Ventricular septal defects
  iv. In severe CRS with multisystem involvement, myocarditis may occur and often is the cause of death.

Eyes
  i. Retinopathy, pigmentary changes of "salt-and-pepper" appearance can be seen
  ii. Cataracts: pearly, dense, nuclear; 50% bilateral
  iii. Microphthalmia.

Transient neonatal manifestations
  i. Thrombocytopenia, with or without purpura
  ii. Hepatitis
  iii. Dermal erythropoiesis (Blue berry muffin lesions)
  iv. Meningoencephalitis
  v. Bony radiolucencies
  vi. Adenopathies.

Late-emerging or developmental

Late-onset interstitial pneumonitis can occur at age 3-12 months. These are depicted in Table 1.

The clinical manifestations of CRS can be classified under three groups.

Diagnosis of congenital rubella syndrome

1. Viral isolation or identification by PCR from nasopharyngeal, urine or CSF specimen of infant is the best method. Virus isolation may be possible upto 6-12 months and occasionally for longer period.

Table 1: Congenital rubella syndrome—manifestations	
Time of manifestation	Features
Manifestations of active infection seen at birth	• Hepatitis • Dermal erythropoiesis (Blue berry muffin lesions) • Thrombocytopenic purpura • Anemia • Hepatosplenomegaly • Meningoencephalitis • Myocarditis
Permanent manifestations at birth through the first year	Deafness, cataract, structural cardiac lesions, microcephaly, mental and motor retardation
Delayed manifestations (not manifest in early life)	Deafness, endocrinopathies (thyroid deficiency, hyperthyroidism, insulin deficiency), vascular effects.

2. Rubella-specific IgM is readily detected in first 6 months of life in infected infants and to a lesser extent upto 1 year of age. Its detection usually indicates prenatal rather than postnatal infection.
3. Persistence of rubella-specific IgG beyond 6 months can be seen in 95% of infants with CRS. It may also indicate a postnatal infection. Identification of low avidity IgG may indicate a prenatal infection.
4. Prenatal diagnosis of fetal rubella infection can be confirmed by viral isolation or RT-PCR positivity from amniotic fluid or identification of rubella-specific IgM in cord blood.

WHO case definitions for CRS:

Compatible CRS (when laboratory data not sufficient for confirmation):
Any two complications listed below in (a) or one from (a) and one from (b):
a. Cataract or congenital glaucoma, congenital heart disease, hearing loss, pigmentary retinopathy.
b. Purpura, splenomegaly, microcephaly, mental retardation, meningo-encephalitis, radiolucent bone lesions, jaundice with onset within 24 hours of birth.

Confirmed CRS
Congenital defects and laboratory confirmation.

4. What is the vaccine strategy against rubella?

The rubella vaccine is available in the form of MMR vaccine. As per IAP recommendations, the first dose is given after 1 year of age and the second dose is recommended at 4–6 years of age. The second dose can be given before 4 years also, provided an interval of minimum 4 weeks is maintained from the first dose.

MMR vaccine can be administered for unimmunized older children in the age group of 7–18 years as 2-dose vaccine with a minimum interval of 4 weeks between the doses. A single dose will suffice if the child has received MMR vaccine in the past.

Postpubertal females without previous rubella immunization can be immunized unless they are known to be pregnant. If immunized, they should be recommended not to become pregnant for 28 days after vaccination.

Further Reading

1. Cherry JD. Rubella virus. In: Feigin RD, Cherry JD, Demmler-Harrison GJ, Kaplan SL. Feigin and Cherry's Textbook of Pediatric Infectious Diseases. 6th Edn. Saunders Elsevier, Philadelphia, USA. 2009;2271-300.
2. Cooper LZ. The history and medical consequences of rubella. Reviews of infectious diseases, 1985,7(suppl. 1):S2-10.
3. Cutts FT, Robertson SE, Diaz-Ortega JL, Samuel R. Control of rubella and congenital rubella syndrome in developing countries, Part 1: Burden of disease from congenital rubella syndrome. Bull WHO 1997;75:55-68.
4. Dudgeon JA. Congenital rubella. Journal of Pediatrics, 1975;87:1078-86.
5. Indian Academy of Pediatrics Committee On Immunization (IAPCOI). Consensus Recommendations on Immunization and IAP Immunization Timetable 2012. Indian Pediatr 2012;49:549-64.
6. Miller E, Cradock-Watson JE, Pollock TM. Consequences of confirmed maternal rubella at successive stages of pregnancy. Lancet 1982;320:781-4.
7. Veda K, Nishida Y, Oshima K, et al. Congenital rubella syndrome. Correlation of gestational age at the time of maternal rubella with type of defect. J Pediatr 1979; 94:763.

14 Non-polio Enteroviruses

Dhanya Dharmapalan

1. What are the common non-polio enteroviruses affecting children and what diseases do they cause?

Enteroviruses are small RNA viruses which have been classified into polioviruses and four alphabetically designated HEV species (HEV-A, B, C and D). These viruses have four structural proteins VP1, VP2, VP3 and VP4, of which VP1 is the major capsid protein used for molecular typing of the enteroviruses.

Coxsackie and echoviruses are the common non-polio enteroviruses affecting children and generally cause benign illnesses in children. They have a wide spectrum of diseases in children from common cold to fatal conditions like myocarditis and meningitis.

Diseases caused by non-polio enteroviruses

Their most common manifestation is nonspecific febrile illness, accounting for 47% to 63% of cases requiring hospitalization to rule out bacterial sepsis in a young infant.

Respiratory manifestations range from common cold (Coxsackie A21), pharyngitis, herpangina (Coxsackie A10), stomatitis (Coxsackie A16), parotitis, croup and pneumonia. Gastrointestinal manifestations include vomiting, diarrhea and abdominal pain. Other diseases caused by viruses of this group are acute hemorrhagic conjunctivitis (EV 70), myocarditis (Coxsackie B5), orchitis (group B Coxsackie), Hand, foot and mouth disease (entero virus 71, Coxsackie virus A16) and exanthemas (echoviruses).

Among the neurological manifestations, aseptic meningitis is the commonest with a good prognosis if seen in isolation but with significant mortality when accompanied by multisystem disease. Encephalitis, GBS and acute paralysis are other neurological complications which can occur.

Just as we are marching towards the global eradication of polio, the fact that the non-polio viruses are associated with acute flaccid paralysis is a growing concern. In a recent study from South-Western India, of the 422 non-polio enteroviruses isolated from the stool samples of 2186 AFP cases, it was found that NPEV positive AFP cases were significantly higher in children aged below 2 years with residual paralysis. Echoviruses (81.9%) and Coxsackie viruses (57.3%) constituted the major component of NPEV positive samples.

2. What is hand, foot and mouth disease, how to recognize it and what are the differential diagnoses?

Clinical manifestations

As the name implies, hand, foot and mouth disease (HFMD) is characterized by sudden appearance in crops of erythematous papulovesicular lesions over specific locations like the hand, feet, knees, buttocks and perioral or intraoral areas. It may be preceded or accompanied by constitutional symptoms like fever and malaise.

HFMD is seen mostly in young children below 10 years and is caused commonly by Coxsackie virus A16 (CA16) and human enterovirus 71 (HEV71). It may also be caused by other serotypes of HEV-A like CA serotypes 2-8, 10, 12 and 14. The disease may occur sporadically or in epidemics and is transmitted through droplet infection or direct contact with the vesicular fluid.

The vesicles may initially contain clear fluid but can become turbid. There is characteristic perilesional erythema. Children are infectious until the blisters have disappeared. The disease usually resolves spontaneously in 7-10 days.

Recurrences have been reported presuming an absence of protective immunity or the possibility of infection by a different strain.

HFMD outbreak associated with Coxsackie virus A6 (CA6) in Japan unlike the typical HFMD was distributed over trunk and extremities and less frequently on soles and hands and was associated with onychomadesis (shedding of nails). Healing took place by crust formation.

The most common problem seen in HFMD is dehydration due to inadequate intake of fluids resulting from mouth ulcers causing odynophagia. Recently, there have been severe fatalities associated with HEV71 from South Asian Countries like Taiwan and China with the development of neurogenic pulmonary edema.

Differential diagnoses

HFMD is mainly a clinical diagnosis. Though the lesions may resemble varicella zoster, papular urticaria, impetigo and herpetic gingivostomatitis, aphthous stomatitis, insect bite allergy, the classical distribution of the lesions helps in clinching the diagnosis.

The varicellar lesions heal by crusting while HFMD vesicles heal when the vesicular fluid gets reabsorbed, except in the recent outbreak with CA6 witnessed in Japan, where healing took place by crusting.

Scabies also causes pustules and vesicles over hands and feet but is associated with predilection for the interdigital space and associated with severe pruritus.

The aphthous stomatitis is associated with larger and very painful ulcerative lesions in the oral mucosa and is not associated with constitutional symptoms. Children with herpetic gingivostomatitis are toxic with high fever, gingival erythema/bleeding and cervical lymphadenopathy. Insect bite allergy may present as urticarial maculopapular lesions, but have absence of constitutional symptoms and oral lesions.

Laboratory diagnosis by real-time PCR, viral neutralization tests, and viral isolation from nasopharyngeal or stool specimens are possible but rarely indicated since this is a clinical diagnosis. The management is largely supportive as it is usually a self-limiting illness which resolves in about seven days.

3. What are the life-threatening infections of non-polio enteroviruses?

In neonates, enteroviruses are responsible for nonspecific febrile illness and meningitis but can also cause multiorgan involvement with hepatic necrosis and coagulopathy (HNC) and/or myocarditis, which can be fatal. Factors such as an elevated bilirubin level and concurrent myocarditis were significantly associated with death in HNC syndrome.

Myocarditis caused by Coxsackie B enterovirus can lead to fulminant cardiogenic shock with acute cardiovascular collapse, or even sudden death.

Meningitis/encephalitis, especially when associated with multisystem involvement, can be life-threatening.

Recently, there have been several deaths reported with the development of neurogenic pulmonary oedema during HFMD outbreak associated with HEV71 from South Asian Countries like Taiwan and China. Postmortem specimens of brainstem of the deceased in HFMD outbreak primarily caused by E71 in Malaysia showed extensive neuronal degeneration, inflammation, and necrosis, suggesting that a central nervous system infection was responsible for the disease, with the cardiopulmonary dysfunction being neurogenic in origin.

Further Reading

1. Chan LG, Parashar UD, Lye MS, et al. Deaths of Children during an Outbreak of Hand, Foot and Mouth Disease in Sarawak, Malaysia: Clinical and Pathological Characteristics of the Disease. Clin Infect Dis. 2000;31(3):678-83.
2. Dias E, Dias M. Recurring hand, foot and mouth disease in a child. 2012;5(1): 40-41.
3. Enteroviruses and Paechoviruses. In: Feigin RD, Cherry JD, editors. 2009. Textbook of Pediatric Infectious Diseases, 6th edition. Philadelphia: W.B. Saunders Co. 2110-70.

4. Hawkes MT and Vaudry W. Nonpolio enterovirus infection in the neonate and young infant. Paediatr Child Health. 2005 September; 10(7): 383-8.
5. Kobayashi M, Makino T, Hanaoka N, et al. Clinical manifestations of Coxsackievirus A6 infection associated with a major outbreak of hand, foot and mouth disease in Japan. Jpn J Infect Dis. 2013;66(3):260-1.
6. Laxmivandana R, Yergolkar P, Gopalkrishna V, Chitambar SD. Characterization of the non-polio enterovirus infections associated with acute flaccid paralysis in South-Western India. PLoS One. 2013 Apr 22;8(4):e61650.
7. Liao HT, Hung KL. Neurologic involvement in an outbreak of enterovirus 71 infection: a hospital-based study. Acta Pediatr Taiwan. 2001 Jan-Feb; 42(1):27-32.
8. Nilendu Sarma. Relapse of Hand, Foot and Mouth Disease: Are We at More Risk? Indian J Dermatol. 2013 Jan-Feb; 58(1):78-9.

15

Herpes Simplex

Niranjan Mohanty

1. What are the type of infections caused by human Herpes simplex virus (HSV) 1 and 2?

The type of infection depends upon the age and immune status of the patient. In childhood, the primary HSV infection beyond neonatal period is asymptomatic. The most common clinical manifestation causes by HSV is gingiovostomatitis with or without perioral vesicular lesion, fever, irritability tender submandibular lymphadenopathy.

In adolescent, the primary HSV infection is mainly caused by HSV2 and is characterized by vesicular or ulcerative lesions of the male or female genitalia and perineum.

In immunocompromised patients, it causes severe local lesions and disseminated HSV infection with visceral involvement.

HSV Encephalitis (HSE) can result from primary or recurrent HSV1 infection.

HSE usually involves the temporal lobe. Temporal lobe abnormalities on imaging and Electroencephalography (EEG) are highly probable of HSE. HSV can also cause meningitis and is usually associated with HSV2 infection. A number of unusual CNS manifestations including Bell's palsy, trigeminal neuralgia, ascending myelitis post infection encephalomyelitis. Conjunctivitis and keratitis can result from primary or recurrent HSV infection.

Reactivation of latent virus leads to recurrent herpes labialis (HSV1) and recurrent genital herpes (HSV2), characterized by less severe vesicular lesion on lips and genital area including buttocks, respectively.

2. What are the clinical characteristics of neonatal herpes?

- HSV2 is most common infecting agent
- Neonatal herpes is never asymptomatic and is always more severe in nature
- Presentation depends on timing of infection, portal of entry and extent of spread.

Intrauterine infection

Presents as skin vesicles, scarring of skin, chorioretinitis, keratoconjunctivitis and microcephaly. Infection during delivery or postpartum period is the most common mode of transmission. It presents as localized SEM disease (Skin, eye and mouth disease), encephalitis with/without SEM disease and disseminated HSV infection.

Localized SEM disease

Presents within 5-11 days of life, and is present in approximately 40-45% cases.

Encephalitis with/without SEM disease

Presents within 8-17 days of life, and causes mortality of about 50% cases.

Disseminated HSV infection

Presents within 5-11 days of life with sepsis syndrome and severe liver dysfunction and 90% mortality.

3. **What is the management of neonatal herpes?**

All patients of proven or suspected HSV infection should be treated. Acyclovir 20 mg/kg, 8 hourly should be given intravenously. In SEM disease, the treatment duration is 14 days. In encephalitis or disseminated disease the duration is 21 days. Treatment can be discontinued, if the laboratory testing shows no infection in suspected cases.

4. **What is the epidemiology and clinical features of childhood and adolescent herpes. How to manage them?**

HSV 1 is more common in this age group. Prevalence is more in those who belong to low socio-economic status.

Clinical features

Mainly asymptomatic. Typical lesions are small to large vesicles surrounded by erythematous base.

Orolabial herpes

a. Primary—High fever, irritability, drooling of saliva, pain, submandibular lymphadenopathy, vesicoulcerative lesion, pharyngitis in older children. Most lesions heal without scar formation.
b. Reactivation—Usually asymptomatic.

Cutaneous

Severe pain, burning, itching before eruption of lesion. Lesions are vesicles with erythematous base which progresses to ulcer and heal without scarring.

Genital

a. Primary—Fever, headache, myalgia, backache. Lesions evolve from vesicles and pustules to wet ulcers and then healing occurs with crusting. Distributed over penis in males and over labia, mons pubis, vagina and cervix in females.

b. Reactivation—Mostly asymptomatic. Tender lymphadenopathy, dysuria, vaginal discharge may occur.

Ocular

Follicular conjunctivitis with pain, photophobia, tearing, chemosis, periorbital edema, pre auricular tender lymphadenopathy.

CNS

Usual features are fever, headache, vomiting, nuchal rigidity, seizure and altered sensorium. Other uncommon features are anosmia, memory loss, aphasia and hallucination.

Immunocompromised patients

Skin lesion is deep and necrotic. Mucositis and esophagitis may be present. Other uncommon features are pneumonia, tracheobronchitis, Disseminated intravascular coagulation (DIC), shock, adrenal involvement and retinal lesions.

Treatment

i. Mucocutaneous HSV infection
   Oral ayclovir 15 mg/kg/dose (maximum-1 g/day), 5 times a day for 7 days, better if started within 72 hours.
ii. Herpes labialis
   Oral treatment is superior to topical. In primary cases, no treatment is necessary.
   In recurrent cases, 200–400 mg/dose 5 times a day for 5 days is given. Long term acyclovir/valacyclovir is given to individuals with frequent relapse.
iii. Genital-
   a. Primary
      In adolescents, acyclovir 400 mg PO TID for 7–10 days
      Famciclovir 750 mg PO TID for 7–10 days
      Valacyclovir 100 mg PO TID for 7–10 days
      In Children, acyclovir 10mg/kg/dose PO QID for 7–10 days.
   b. Recurrent
      Episodic therapy—Acyclovir 800mg PO TID for 2 days
      Famciclovir 100 mg PO BID for 1 day
      Valacyclovir 500 mg PO BID for 3 days
      Long term therapy—Acyclovir 400 mg PO BID
      Famciclovir 250 mg PO BID
      Valacyclovir 500 mg PO QID is given for 1 year duration.
iv. CNS
   IV Acyclovir 10 mg/kg/dose is given 8 hourly for 14–21 days.
v. Ocular
   Topical therapy—1% trifluridine, 0.1% iodo-deoxyuridine or 3% vidarabine is used.
      For recurrent ocular infection, additional treatment with oral acyclovir 80 mg/kg/day TID is given.

5. **How to prevent the transmission during pregnancy and delivery?**

   i. During pregnancy
      a. If the mother is infected, daily oral acyclovir/valacyclovir/famciclovir can be given during the last 4 weeks of gestation.
      b. If vaginal delivery is being done in case of a woman with first episode of genital herpes—anticipatory acyclovir therapy for atleast 2 weeks.
      c. In case of a recurrent genital herpes with vaginal delivery, caregivers are explained the signs and symptoms of the disease and told to seek help when signs and symptoms develop.
   ii. During delivery—Cesarean section to be done within 4-6 hour of rupture of membrane to minimize the transmission.

Further Reading

1. Cook GC, Zumla AI. Cutaneous Viral Diseases. In: Cook GC, Zumla AI, editors. Manson's Tropical Diseases. 22nd edition: Saunders Elseviers; 2009 .p. 845-6.
2. Gutierrez KM, Arvin AM. Herpes Simplex Virus 1 & 2. In: Feigin R, Cherry J, Demmler-Harisson G, Kaplan S, editors. Text Book of Pediatric Infectious Diseases; 6th edition. Philadelphia: Saunders Elsevier; 2009.p.1993-2021.
3. Pickering LK, Becker CJ, Long SS, McMillan JA. Herpes Simplex. In: Pickering LK, Becker CJ, Long SS, McMillan JA, editors. RED BOOK, 27th edition. New Delhi: CBS Publishers and distributers; 2008.p.361-70.
4. Stanberry LR. Herpes Simplex Virus. In: Stanton B, Schor N, St Geme J, Berhman R, editors. Nelson's Text Book of Pediatrics. 19th edition. Philadelphia: Saunders Elsevier; 2012.p.1097-1103.

16 Varicella

Parang Mehta

1. How varicella is transmitted in various settings?

Varicella is transmitted mainly person to person, by droplet infection. The incidence of infection among nonimmune people exposed to the disease varies with the type of contact. Casual contact for a short time carries a low risk. Close contact, as in the home, class room, or day care center, is associated with secondary attack rates approaching 100%. Varicella is a highly infectious disease.

Other modes of transmission include congenital varicella, if the mother develops varicella during pregnancy. Incidence of congenital varicella is highest, if maternal chicken pox occurs during week thirteen to twenty of pregnancy.

2. How long a child is contagious following varicella infection?

A child with varicella is infectious a day or two before the skin lesions appear. This is the dangerous period. The child continues to be infectious till all the lesions have crusted.

3. What are the clinical manifestations in immunocompetent and immunocompromised children?

The incubation period of varicella is 10-21 days. After this, children have prodromal symptoms before the appearance of the skin lesions. These consist of:
  i. Low-grade fever.
  ii. Abdominal pain in some children.
  iii. Headache, malaise, and loss of appetite.
  iv. Cough, cold and sore throat.

The rash usually starts on the head and trunk. It later spreads to the rest of the body. Most children have significant itching. The skin lesions start as papules, then become fluid filled vesicles and pustules, and finally dry up with crust formation. The lesions do not affect the eyes, unlike small pox. A few lesions may appear in the oropharynx.

New lesions appear for 3-5 days. Most children have 250-500 lesions, but normal children may have as many as 1500. Different stages of the rash are often seen in the same child (pleomorphic rash). This is the hallmark of chicken pox. Lesions usually crust by 6 days, but may be quicker or slower (2-12 days). Complete healing takes about 16 days, but may take as long as a month.

Immunocompromised children have similar but more severe manifestations. New lesions continue to erupt for a longer time, the number of lesions is higher, and fever is prolonged. In normal children, fever subsides in four days. Prolonged fever should raise suspicion of immunocompromise, or a secondary infection. Complications are also more frequent in this population.

4. What is breakthrough varicella? Is it contagious?

Chicken pox occurring in people who have received the varicella vaccine at least 42 days earlier is called breakthrough varicella. In general, it is a milder disease than varicella in unvaccinated people.

It is contagious, and outbreaks can be spread by people who develop breakthrough varicella. There is some evidence that the number of skin lesions have a direct relation to infectiousness in breakthrough varicella.

5. What are shingles?

Shingles is derived from the Latin word '*cingulum*', which means girdle. It is a late complication of infection with the varicella zoster virus. Following an episode of chicken pox, the virus persists in the sensory ganglia of the cranial nerves and the spinal dorsal root ganglia. This residual virus reactivates when immunity diminishes, usually in old age.

The lesions consist of small papular vesicular lesions spread in one dermatome (the distribution of the spinal nerve that harbors the virus). The lesions are painful, sometimes intensely so, that the disease can occur repeatedly in the elderly.

6. What are the consequences if a pregnant mother develops varicella?

Varicella is a viral disease, and can affect the fetus in utero. Some babies develop the fetal varicella syndrome, consisting of intrauterine growth restriction (IUGR), low birgh weight (LBW), cicatricial skin lesions, limb hypoplasia or paresis, microcephaly and ophthalmic lesions (microphthalmia, chorioretinitis, and cataracts). The incidence depends on the timing of infection—it is highest in the second trimester (about 2%). Beyond 20 weeks, it is rare, but does occur. Among children exposed to varicella during pregnancy but born normal, about one percent develop herpes zoster during childhood.

7. How do we protect a newborn who is exposed to a case of varicella?

Varicella can be severe and even fatal during the newborn period. The mortality can be as high as 30%. The risk to the newborn depends on the timing of diagnosis of varicella in the mother.

If the mother developed chicken pox seven days or more before delivery, the baby gets the virus, but also the neutralizing antibodies made by the mother. Such babies develop mild disease.

If the mother developed chicken pox less than seven days before delivery or two days after delivery, the baby gets the virus only, and usually, a large inoculums. Such babies are at risk for severe disease.

The vaccine is not recommended at this young age, and the recommended protection is VZIG (varicella zoster immune globulin). This should be given as soon as possible after birth, or after the mother develops chicken pox. The protection is best when VZIG is given within four days. It may be given upto ten days later, as it has been shown to attenuate the disease. The dose varies from product to product, but generally, 125 mg per 10 Kg is recommended.

If VZIG is not available, acyclovir is another option. It is given intravenously in a dose of 20 mg/Kg/8 hourly for 5-7 days. Oral therapy is not considered reliable.

8. How do we treat varicella in newborn, infants, children, adolescents and immunocompromised children?

Varicella can be a serious disease in newborns. It requires hospitalization, close monitoring, and intravenous acyclovir therapy.

In children, varicella is usually a benign and self limited disease. Treatment is generally not recommended. If acyclovir is started within 24 hours of the disease onset, it may slightly reduce the duration of fever and number of lesions.

Adolescents are more likely to have severe varicella, including varicella pneumonitis, which has a significant mortality. They should be treated with oral acyclovir (20 mg/kg, 6 hourly), monitored closely, and hospitalized if indicated.

Varicella in immunocompromised children is a high risk situation. These children are likely to have prolonged high fever, extensive rashes lasting for more than 1 week, disseminated varicella, hepatitis, and primary viral pneumonia. The mortality is significant. These children should be hospitalized, and given intravenous acyclovir (500 mg/square meter, 8 hourly).

9. How to prevent infection following exposure to varicella zoster virus?

If the child has received the varicella vaccine, or has suffered chicken pox in the past, nothing needs to be done. Susceptible children are at risk of developing the disease, and should be offered prophylaxis.

The best way is to use the varicella vaccine, and this option should be used in all children above one year of age who are exposed to chicken pox. Post exposure vaccination is effective at preventing or attenuating varicella, and provides long term protection also. It should be given as soon as possible, as it is maximally effective when given within three days of exposure.

In children below the age of one year, the vaccine cannot be used. VZIG is the next best option, followed by acyclovir.

10. What are the indications and contraindications of varicella vaccine?

The varicella vaccine is recommended for all children as a part of childhood immunization. It is specially recommended for:
  i. Children with humoral immunodeficiencies.
  ii. Children with HIV infection but with CD4 counts 15% and above the age related cut off.
  iii. Leukemia but in remission and off chemotherapy for at least 3–6 months.
  iv. Children on long term salicylates. Salicylates should be avoided for at least 6 weeks after vaccination.
  v. Children likely to be on long term steroid therapy.
  vi. In household contacts of immunocompromised children.
  vii. Adolescents who have not had varicella in past and are known to be varicella IgG negative, especially if they are leaving home for studies in a residential school/college.
  viii. Children with chronic lung or heart disease.
  ix. Seronegative adolescents and adults, if they are inmates of or working in the institutional set up, e.g. school teachers, day care center workers, military personnel and health care professionals.
  x. For post-exposure prophylaxis in susceptible healthy non pregnant contacts preferably within 3 days of exposure (efficacy 90%), and potentially upto 5 days of exposure (efficacy 70%, against severe disease 100%).

Contraindications

  i. Severe reaction to an earlier dose.
  ii. Immunosuppression due to leukemia, lymphoma, generalized malignancy, immune deficiency disease, or immunosuppressive therapy.
  iii. Systemic steroid therapy at a dose of 2 mg/kg/day of prednisolone or higher.
  iv. Pregnancy.

11. What is the indication of varicella zoster immunoglobulin?

Varicella zoster immunoglobulin provides immediate but passive immunity to varicella. It is recommended for protection after exposure in:
  i. Immunocompromised patients.
  ii. Neonates whose mothers develop varicella 5 days before to 2 days after delivery.
  iii. Preterm infants born at 28 weeks gestation or later who are exposed during the neonatal period and whose mothers do not have evidence of immunity to varicella.

iv. Preterm infants born earlier than 28 weeks' gestation or who weigh 1,000 g or less at birth and were exposed during the neonatal period.
v. Pregnant women.
vi. Normal children exposed to varicella who cannot be vaccinated because of the age or other contraindication.

12. When should a child be vaccinated following varicella zoster immunoglobulin administration?

Varicella vaccine is a live vaccine, and it needs to replicate in the body to generate a robust immune response. Circulating antibodies to the virus will prevent the vaccine from being effective.

The persistence of the antibodies varies from product to product, and can be from three to eleven months. The vaccine should be given at least after 5 months.

Further Reading

1. Aronson J, Mc Sherry G, et al. Varicella in children with HIV infection. Pediatric Infectious Diseases J 1992;11:1004.
2. Choo P W, Donahue J G, Mausen J, et al. The Epidemiology of varicella and its complications. J Infect Dis 1995;172:706.
3. Fegin, Cherry, Demlee, Kaplan. The Textbook of Pediatric Infectious Diseases 5th edition, Philadelphia: WB Sunders, 2004.
4. Gresham M N, Russap LA, et al. Varicella zoster virus infections in children with underlying HIV infections. J Infectious Diseases 1997;176:1496.
5. Markin GM, Lawrence R, Jane FS. In: Behrman RS, Kleigman, Jenson FS, editors. Nelson Textbook of Pediatrics, 17th edition. Philadelphia: WB Saunders, 2004.
6. Prevention of varicella: update recommendations. Advisory Committee Immunization Practices (ACIP). Pediatrics, 2004.

17

Epstein-Barr Virus

S Balasubramanian, Sumanth Amperayani, K Dhanalakshmi

1. Epstein-Barr Virus (EBV) is implicated in which disease?

EBV in implicated in Infectious mononucleosis, characterized by systemic somatic complaints consisting primarily of fatigue, malaise, fever, sore throat, and generalized lymphadenopathy. It was originally described as glandular fever. It may also cause Hodgkin's disease, hematological neoplasias and nasopharyngeal carcinoma. EBV infection may result in a spectrum of proliferative disorders ranging from self-limited, usually benign disease such as infectious mononucleosis to aggressive, non-malignant proliferations such as the virus associated hemophagocytic syndrome to lymphoid and epithelial cell malignancies. Benign EBV-associated proliferations include oral hairy leukoplakia, primarily in adults with AIDS, and lymphoid interstitial pneumonitis, primarily in children with AIDS. Malignant EBV-associated proliferations include nasopharyngeal carcinoma, Burkitt's lymphoma, Hodgkin's disease, lymphoproliferative disorders, and leiomyosarcoma in immunodeficient states, including AIDS. X-linked lymphoproliferative syndrome (Duncan's syndrome), an X chromosome–linked recessive disorder of the immune system associated with severe, persistent, and sometimes fatal EBV infection. EBV is also associated with carcinoma of the salivary glands.

2. How does EB Virus spread?

Among children, transmission may occur by exchange of saliva from child to child, such as occurs between children in out-of-home child care or by sharing water bottles at school. Non intimate contact, environmental sources, and fomites do not contribute to spread of EBV. EBV can spread through close interpersonal contact and primitive personal hygiene like overcrowding and roommates in hostels. The role of the oropharynx as a dominant route of transmission had been suggested earlier by Hoagland's observations which raised the possibility of actively infectious saliva, even after a long incubation period of 34–49 days.

Demonstration of the presence of EBV-DNA in exfoliated buccal mucosa cells by in situ nucleic acid hybridization techniques suggests that epithelial cells of the buccal mucosa may also be a source of EBV. Iatrogenic sources, like transfusion of fresh whole blood, plasma, or packed red blood cells and transplantation of bone marrow entail risk of infection to the susceptible recipient.

3. What are the hallmarks of infectious mononucleosis? What are the other causes or pathogens responsible for similar illness?

Hallmarks of infectious mononucleosis include—fever, generalized lymphadenopathy, hepatosplenomegaly, tonsillar enlargement and exudates, cough and rhinorrhea, epitrochlear lymphadenopathy and atypical lymphocytosis.

A growing number of pathogens have been reported to cause heterophile negative mononucleosis—like illnesses, including cytomegalovirus (CMV), human herpesvirus 6 (HHV-6), human immunodeficiency virus (HIV), adenovirus, herpes simplex virus (HSV), *Streptococcus pyogenes* and *Toxoplasma gondii*.

4. How to diagnose infectious mononucleosis?

Leukocytosis with atypical lymphocytosis is characteristic of EBV infections in majority of cases. Mild thrombocytopenia and anicteric hepatitis is frequently seen.

Heterophile antibody tests (Paul Bunnel Test) were the only tests available till recently for diagnosis. Titers >1:28 or >1:40 are considered positive. Positivity may remain for upto 2 years. If the heterophile test result is negative and an EBV infection is suspected, EBV-specific antibody testing is indicated.

Testing for specific Epstein-Barr Virus antibodies is useful to confirm acute EBV infection, especially in heterophile negative cases, or to confirm past infection and determine susceptibility to future infection. The antibodies tested are Early Antigen (EA), Viral Capsid Antigen(VCA) and Nuclear Antigen (NA). The IgM response to VCA is transient and is considered as the diagnostic serological test for acute infection, but can be detected for at least 4 weeks and occasionally for upto 3 months. Antibodies to the cytoplasmic-restricted component of EA, early antigen-restricted (EA-R), emerge transiently in the convalescence from infectious mononucleosis and often attain high titers in patients with EBV-associated Burkitt, lymphoma. Anti-EBNA antibodies are the last to develop in infectious mononucleosis, gradually appearing 3–4 months after the onset of illness and remaining at low levels for life.

5. How to treat infectious mononucleosis?

There is no specific treatment for infectious mononucleosis. Antibiotics have no role in prevention of secondary infections. Therapy with high doses of acyclovir, with or without corticosteroids, decreases viral replication and oropharyngeal shedding during the period of administration but does not reduce the severity or duration of symptoms or alter the eventual outcome. Rest and symptomatic treatments are the mainstays of management. Bed rest is necessary only when the patient has debilitating fatigue. As soon as there is definite symptomatic improvement, the patient should be allowed to begin to resume normal activities. Because blunt abdominal trauma may predispose patients to splenic rupture, it is customary and prudent to advise against participation in contact sports and strenuous athletic activities during the first 2–3 weeks of illness or while splenomegaly is present. Not all sore throats are caused by bacteria.'Ampicillin rash', a phenomenon unique to patients with Epstein-Barr virus acute infectious mononucleosis (AIM) treated with ampicillin, was first reported in the 1960s. But the incidence of rash in pediatric patients with AIM after treatment with the current oral amino-penicillin (amoxycillin) is much lower than originally reported.

Acyclovir is known for its antiviral activity against some pathogenic viruses such as the Epstein-Barr virus (EBV) that causes infectious mononucleosis (IM) and IM-like illness. Acyclovir is a potential therapeutic agent for both EBV-IM and IM like-illnesses. Future studies should further examine its mechanism of action.

6. What are the indications of steroids in infectious mononucleosis?

Some appropriate indications for steroid use in infectious mononucleosis include incipient airway obstruction, thrombocytopenia with hemorrhage, autoimmune hemolytic anemia, seizures, and meningitis. A recommended regimen is prednisone 1 mg/kg/day (maximum 60 mg/day) or equivalent for 7 days followed by a dosage taper over another 7 days. Corticosteroids should not be used in uncomplicated cases of infectious mononucleosis.

Further Reading

1. Balasubramanian S, Ganesh R, Kumar JR. Profile of EBV associated infectious mononucleosis. Indian Pediatr. 2012;49:837-8.
2. Blacklow NR, Watson BK, Miller G, et al: Mononucleosis with heterophile antibodies and EB virus infection acquired by an elderly patient in the hospital. Am J Med; 1971; 51:549-52.
3. Căinap S, Răchişan A, Fetică B, Cosnarovici R, Mihuţ E, Popa G, et al. EBV in pediatricneoplasia—intensity of infection as independent prognostic factor. J Med Life; 2012;5:283-7.
4. Chovel-Sella A, Ben Tov A, Lahav E, Mor O, Rudich H, Paret G et al. Incidence of rash after amoxicillin treatment in children with infectious mononucleosis. Pediatrics. 2013;131:e1424-7.
5. Hal. B. Jenson. Epstein-Barr Virus. In: Robert M. Kliegman, MD, Bonita M.D. Stanton, MD, Joseph St. Geme, Nina Schor, MD, PhD and Richard E. Behrman, MD editors. Nelson Textbook of Pediatrics, 19th ed. Philadelphia: Elsevier Saunders; 2011. Chapter 246.
6. Herling M, Rassidakis GZ, Vassilakopoulos TP. Impact of LMP-1 expression on clinical outcome in age-defined subgroups of patients with classical Hodgkin's lymphoma. Blood; 2006;107:1240.
7. Hoagland RJ: The transmission of infectious mononucleosis. Amer J Med Sci. 1955; 229:262-72.
8. Hurt C, Tammaro D. Diagnostic evaluation of mononucleosis-like illnesses. Am J Med. 2007;120:911.e1-8.
9. Kwon JM, Park YH, Kang JH. The effect of Epstein-Barr virus status on clinical outcome in Hodgkin's lymphoma. Ann Hematol. 2006;85:463-68.
10. Lemon SM, Hutt LM, Shaw JE, et al: Replication of EBV in epithelial cells during infectious mononucleosis. Nature. 1977; 268:268-70.

11. Luzuriaga K, Sullivan JL: Infectious mononucleosis. N Engl J Med 2010; 362:1993-2000.
12. Montalban C, Abraira V, Morente M. Epstein-Barr virus latent membrane protein 1 expression has a favorable influence in the outcome of patients with Hodgkin's disease treated with chemotherapy. Leuk Lymphoma. 2000;39:563-72.
13. Niederman JC. Infectious mononucleosis: observations on transmission. Yale J Biol Med; 1982;55:259-64.
14. Sullivan JL, Wallen WC, Johnson FL. Epstein-Barr virus infection following bone marrow transplantation. Int J Cancer. 1978;22:132-5.
15. Turner AR, MacDonald RN, Cooper BA: Transmission of infectious mononucleosis by transfusion of pre-illness plasma. Ann Int Med; 1972;77:751-53.
16. Usami O, Saitoh H, Ashino Y, Hattori T. Acyclovir reduces the duration of fever in patients with infectious mononucleosis-like illness. Tohoku J Exp Med. 2013; 229:137-42.
17. Vouloumanou EK, Rafailidis PI, Falagas ME. Current diagnosis and management of infectious mononucleosis. CurrOpinHematol. 2012;19:14-20.
18. Wising PJ: A study of infectious mononucleosis (Pfeiffer's disease) from the etiological point of view. Acta Med Scand; 1942; 1:507-12.

18
Influenza and Parainfluenza

A K Prasad

1. What are the types and subtypes of influenza virus and what is the basis of the classification?

Influenza viruses belong to the Orthomyxoviridae family and are divided into types A, B and C. Influenza types A and B are responsible for epidemics of respiratory illness that are often associated with increased rates of hospitalization and death. Influenza type C causes a subclinical to a mild infection of insignificant illness. It does not cause epidemics, like influenza types A and B viruses.

All influenza viruses have negative strand RNA with a segmented genome. Influenza type A and B viruses have 8 genes that code for 10 proteins, including the surface proteins hemagglutinin (HA) and neuraminidase (NA). In the case of influenza type A viruses, further subdivision can be made into different subtypes according to differences in these two surface proteins.

Till date, 16 HA subtype and 9 NA subtypes have been identified. However, during the last century, the human influenza A subtypes that circulated extensively were A (H1N1), A (H1N2), A (H2N2), and A (H3N2). All other known subtypes of influenza type A viruses have been isolated from birds and can affect a range of mammal species. As with humans, the number of influenza A subtypes that have been isolated from other mammalian species is limited. Influenza type B viruses almost exclusively infect humans.

2. What are "Antigenic Drift" and "Antigenic Shift" and what are the implications as regards to disease?

The characteristics of influenza viruses are their ability to undergo antigenic change, which occurs as the following:

Antigenic drift—A gradual process and is continuous change in the viral HA and NA proteins. This results in outbreaks and small epidemics. This also necessitates the use of influenza preventive seasonal vaccine as an annual event to update the protective capability for the drifted strain.

It results from the accumulation of point mutations in the HA and NA genes during viral replication. Both influenza type A and B viruses undergo antigenic drift, leading to new virus strains. The emergence of these new strains necessitate the frequent updating of influenza vaccine virus strains. As antibodies to previous influenza infections may not provide full protection against the new strains resulting from antigenic drift, individuals can have many influenza infections over a lifetime.

Outbreaks and influenza epidemic generally occur each year or every alternate year due to drift in the surface H & N antigen. The severity depends upon the amount of drift but, when there is a shift in the surface H & N antigen, the infection spreads globally in absence of any protective antibody in the world population. There is no vaccine as the change is unpredictable and the pandemic strain is not available.

Antigenic shift—It is a total change in either H or N or both influenza surface proteins from the existing in virus in circulation.
   i. A virus bearing new HA and NA proteins can arise through the genetic reassortment of nonhuman and human influenza viruses
   ii. An influenza virus from other animals (e.g. birds or pigs) can infect a human directly without undergoing genetic reassortment or
   iii. A nonhuman virus may be passed from one type of animal (e.g. birds) through an intermediate animal host (such as a pig) to humans.

3. What is the period of contagiousness?

The disease has a short incubation period of 1–2 days and normally recedes in 5–7 days as self limiting infection. A person recovers in 2–4 weeks time in uncomplicated cases. The sick person is infectious from a day before the onset of symptoms and till 1–2 weeks post infection.

4. What are the characteristic features of influenza infection?

Sudden symptoms characterized by fever, headache, myalgia, and sore throat, followed by dry or running nose, feeling of weakness in legs, pressure in eyes and anorexia occurs. One observes a sudden increase in similar cases in the OPD. In case of school going children, there will be large absentees with similar symptoms.

5. What is pandemic influenza?

During the last 20th century, the only influenza A subtypes that circulated extensively in humans were A(H1N1), A(H1N2), A(H2N2), and A(H3N2). The hallmark of human influenza viruses is their ability to undergo antigenic change:

1919—The "Spanish flu" A (H1N1) pandemic led to more than 40 million deaths worldwide (Palese, 2004). Nearly half of these deaths were among people of 20–40 years of age, and case of fatality rates of 30% were reported among pregnant women.

1957-1958—The "Asian flu" A (H2N2) pandemic was associated with a total excess mortality of more than 1 million deaths globally (Lipatov, et al, 2004).

1968-1969—Despite the lack of well-established estimates, the global excess mortality caused by the "Hong Kong flu" A(H3N2) pandemic has been calculated at around 1 million (Lipatov et al, 2004).

Influenza and Parainfluenza **113**

In all cases, the pandemic spread throughout the world within a year of its initial detection. Outbreaks of the 'Asian flu' were first reported in late February 1957 in China and spread to other parts of Asia by April–May. Quarantine efforts were not helpful in curtailing the spread.

Although the highest rates of seasonal influenza-related illness occur among school-age children, the highest rates of associated hospitalizations occur among: children under 2 years of age, people of any age with certain chronic medical conditions (including chronic heart disease, lung disease such as asthma, diabetes, renal failure or immunocompromising conditions); those aged 65 years or older, and pregnant women.

For example, one study from the United States (Izurieta et al, 2000) estimated that healthy children under 2 years of age have 12 times the risk of influenza-related hospitalization as healthy children aged 5–17 years. Influenza-associated hospitalization rates are also higher among those with chronic medical conditions than among otherwise healthy people of the same age group.

6. **What is typical about influenza virus circulation, especially with respect to climate of that region?**

The timing of influenza activity around the world varies depending upon the climate of each region. In temperate climate zones, the onset and peak of influenza activity may vary substantially from one influenza season to the next but activity generally begins to increase in late autumn. In temperate regions of the northern hemisphere, influenza viruses are frequently isolated in the autumn, winter and spring. Periods of peak influenza activity typically occur between December and March and last for 6–8 weeks. In temperate regions of the southern hemisphere, influenza activity typically peaks in May to September. Although temperate regions of the world experience such seasonal peaks in influenza activity, influenza viruses can be isolated sporadically throughout the year, usually associated with outbreaks in closed environments such as nursing homes and summer camps.

The timing of seasonal peaks in influenza activity in tropical and subtropical countries also varies by region, and in some areas more than one peak of activity may occur in the same year. Such variability in influenza seasonal peaks in tropical and subtropical countries illustrate the importance of country-specific and regional epidemiological and virological data including decisions on timing of vaccination programs. Influenza viruses in tropical and subtropical regions can circulate at low levels at any time of the year and can cause isolated cases of influenza as well as outbreaks outside the peak periods of activity.

The Pandemic influenza in addition to the annual seasonal epidemics of influenza seen in some regions, pandemics of influenza have occurred infrequently and at irregular intervals.

In all age groups, influenza infection rates are generally higher during pandemics than during annual epidemics. As with epidemics, school-age children play an important role in the spread of pandemic influenza in the community.

The Pandemic (H1N1) 2009 was even more rapid due to the high mobility and interconnectedness of 21st century societies. Within 6 weeks of first being described, it had affected all regions resulting in the declaration of a pandemic. Once again schools appeared to play an important role in the amplification of virus transmission.

The overall rates of severe disease, however, were considerably lower than those recorded for the pandemic of 1918. The rapidity with which the pandemic (H1N1) 2009 virus spread, highlighted the need for timely and effective surveillance systems to detect emerging viruses with pandemic potential, and the need for standard platforms for data sharing and dissemination.

7. What are the vaccines for influenza?

Annual vaccination is the primary means of reducing the impact of seasonal influenza. Vaccination is associated with reductions in: Influenza-related respiratory illness and physician visits among all age groups, hospitalizations and deaths among people at high risk, otitis media among children, and work absenteeism levels among adults.

Currently, seasonal influenza vaccines contain a mixture of four inactivated strains of the influenza viruses (two type influenza A and two influenza B viruses), likely to circulate during the next influenza season. Because influenza viruses are constantly changing, the seasonal influenza vaccines are updated and administered annually to provide the necessary protection.

Live attenuated and inactivated seasonal influenza vaccines

Live attenuated seasonal influenza vaccines have been advised for healthy people aged 2–49 years to avoid influenza infection themselves or if they are in close contact with people at high risk of developing serious complications from influenza infection.

Inactivated seasonal influenza vaccines are similar in many respects to live attenuated influenza vaccines. They both contain similar strains of influenza viruses representative of the recommended strains. The virus strains for both types of vaccine are selected annually, and one or more of these may be changed based on the results of global influenza surveillance and the emergence of new strains.

8. What is the role of antiviral drugs?

Amantadine and rimantadine are chemically related drugs that specifically inhibit the replication of Influenza types A viruses—but not influenza type B viruses.

The mechanism of action of adamantine derivatives is not completely understood, but it is believed that they interfere with the function of the transmembrane domain of the M2 protein of influenza type A viruses. They also interfere with influenza type A virus assembly during viral replication. As a result, they prevent the release of infectious influenza A viral particles from the host cell.

Effectiveness—Controlled studies have found that when administered within 48 hours of the onset of illness, both drugs are effective in decreasing viral shedding and in reducing the duration of illness of influenza type A infections by approximately one day compared with placebo administration. The recommended duration of treatment is usually 5 days. When used for chemoprophylaxis, both drugs are approximately 70–90% effective in preventing the symptoms of illness resulting from influenza type A infection. When used for treatment, neither appears to affect the ability of the body to develop antibodies to influenza A, and antibodies can also be produced during prophylaxis should viral exposure occur while taking the drug. The efficacy and effectiveness of both drugs in preventing the complications of influenza type A are unknown.

Side-effects—Adverse gastrointestinal and central nervous system effects have been reported during controlled chemoprophylaxis studies in healthy adults and elderly nursing-home residents. The chemoprophylactic use of both drugs has been associated with central nervous system toxicity effects such as light-headedness, difficulty in concentrating, nervousness, insomnia and seizures in patients with pre-existing seizure disorders. Rimantadine use has been associated with fewer central nervous system side-effects than amantadine. Amantadine is teratogenic and embryo toxic in animals. Rimantadine has not been found to be mutagenic. The safety of amantadine and rimantadine use during pregnancy has not, however, been established.

Neuraminidase (NA) inhibitors

Zanamivir and oseltamivir are chemically related members of a new class of antiviral drugs active against both influenza type A and B viruses. Zanamivir is an orally inhaled powder, whereas oseltamivir is given as an orally administered capsule or oral suspension. Other forms of delivery of these drugs (e.g. intravenous) and additional NA-inhibitors are currently being developed.

Antiviral activity—the mechanism of action of both drugs involve blocking the active site of the viral enzyme neuroaminidase, which is common to both influenza type A and B viruses. It results in viral aggregation at the infected host cell surface and the prevention of progeny virus release from the cell. The recommended duration of treatment is 5 days. Oseltamivir is indicated for the treatment and chemoprophylaxis of influenza type A and B in adults and children aged one year and older. Zanamivir is indicated for the treatment and chemoprophylaxis of influenza type A and B in adults and children aged >5 years.

Side-effects—Oseltamivir use has been associated with nausea and vomiting during controlled treatment studies compared with placebo administration.

Nausea, diarrhoea, dizziness, headache and cough have been reported during zanamivir treatment but the frequencies of adverse events were similar to those seen with orally inhaled powder placebo. Besides, few serious central nervous system adverse effects have been reported for these drugs. Zanamivir is not generally recommended for use in people with underlying respiratory disease because of the risk of precipitating bronchospasm. Serious respiratory adverse events resulting from zanamivir use have been reported in people with chronic pulmonary disease and in healthy adults. Data are limited regarding the potential use of these drugs to treat influenza during pregnancy.

Antiviral resistance —In 2008, a high proportion of seasonal H1N1 viruses were found to have resistance to Oseltamivir but were still sensitive to zanamivir. Influenza types A (H3N2) and B viruses remain sensitive to both NA inhibitors. The majority of pandemic (H1N1) influenza viruses characterized in 2009 were sensitive to oseltamivir but a small number of resistant viruses were detected. All pandemic (H1N1) 2009 viruses analyzed in 2009 were sensitive to zanamivir. In vitro studies have found that resistance to NA inhibitors does not affect the susceptibility of viruses to adamantane derivatives.

9. Who are at increased risk for developing influenza related complications?

At both extremes of the age spectrum, however, rates of influenza-related hospitalization are elevated, even among those without chronic medical conditions. Rates of seasonal influenza-associated hospitalization are highest for people aged 85 years or older. The rates are lower for children and young adults, but children younger than 5 years old have hospitalization rates similar to people aged 50-64 years. Pregnant women also appear to be at increased risk of complications from influenza.

Further Reading

1. Arden A, et al. Vaccine Use and the Risk of Outbreaks in a Sample of Nursing Homes during an Influenza. American Journal of Public Health, 1995; 85(3):399-401.
2. Aymard-Henry MT, et al. Influenza virus neuraminidase and neuraminidase inhibition test procedures. Bulletin of the World Health Organization. 1973; 48:199-202.
3. Barker WH, Mullooly JP. Pneumonia and influenza deaths during epidemics: implications for prevention. Archives of Internal Medicine. 1982; 142(1):85-9.
4. Barr IG, et al. Epidemiological, antigenic and genetic characteristics of seasonal influenza A(H1N1), A(H3N2) and B influenza viruses: Basis for the WHO recommendation on the composition of influenza vaccines for use in the 2009-2010 Northern Hemisphere season. Vaccine; 2010; 28:1156-67.
5. Burch J, et al. Prescription of anti-influenza drugs for healthy adults: A systematic review and meta-analysis. The Lancet Infectious Diseases; 2009; 9(9):537-45.
6. Colman PM. Neuraminidase inhibitors as antivirals. Vaccine, 2002; 20 (Suppl. 2):S55-S58.

7. Couch RB (2000). Prevention and treatment of influenza. New England Journal of Medicine, 343:1778-87.
8. Dawood FS, et al. Emergence of a Novel Swine-Origin Influenza A (H1N1) Virus in Humans: Novel Swine-Origin Influenza A (H1N1) Virus Investigation Team. New England Journal of Medicine, 2009; 360(25):2605-15.
9. Fiore AE, et al. Prevention and control of seasonal influenza with vaccines. Recommendations of the Advisory Committee on Immunization Practices (ACIP), 2009. Recommendations and Reports, Centers for Disease Control and Prevention. Morbidity and Mortality Weekly Report, 2009; 58(RR-8):1-52.
10. Glezen WP. Emerging infections: pandemic influenza. Epidemiologic Reviews, 18:64-76. Antigenic and genetic characteristics of influenza A(H5N1) and influenza A(H9N2) viruses and candidate vaccine viruses developed for potential use in human vaccines-February 2010. Weekly Epidemiological Record, 1996; 11(85):100-8.
11. Hayden FG. Antivirals for pandemic influenza. The Journal of Infectious Diseases, 1997; 176 (Suppl. 1):S56-S61.
12. Lackenby A, et al. Rapid quantitation of neuraminidase inhibitor drug resistance in influenza virus quasispecies. Antiviral Therapy, 2008; 13(6):809-20.

19
Respiratory Syncytial Virus

M Govindraj

1. What is the epidemiology of respiratory syncytial virus infection?

Outbreaks of RSV infections occur in temperate climates with striking regularity during winter and early spring. In other parts of the world, epidemics occur during the rainy season, which corresponds to "winter" in temperate climates. Although, no clear link between climate and the onset of epidemics has been established, it has been suggested that the weather conditions themselves predispose to outbreaks. More likely is the fact that poor weather, regardless of the climate, forces humans to stay indoors and in closer contact. Initial infection with RSV usually occurs during the first year of life, and most infants are infected by 24 months of age. Repeated infections are common in childhood and can also occur in adult life despite the presence of specific local and systemic neutralizing antibodies. Most infections are symptomatic; about one third of initial infections involve the lower respiratory tract, and reinfections are largely limited to the upper respiratory tract. Most hospitalizations occur in 2-to 6-month-old children. Rates of hospitalization for bronchiolitis and pneumonia exceed 24 per 1000 young infants experiencing primary RSV infection. Severe RSV disease is more common in males, in infants from industrialized areas, and in infants exposed to passive parental cigarette smoke.

Humans are the only source of infection. Transmission usually is by direct or close contact with contaminated secretions, which may involve droplets or fomites. Respiratory syncytial virus can persist on environmental surfaces for many hours and for a half-hour or more on hands. Infection among hospital personnel and others can occur by self-inoculation with contaminated secretions. Enforcement of infection control policies is important to decrease the risk of health care-related transmission of RSV. Health care-related spread of RSV to organ transplant recipients or patients with cardiopulmonary abnormalities or immunocompromised conditions has been associated with severe and fatal disease in children and adults. The period of viral shedding usually is 3 to 8 days, but shedding may last longer, especially in young infants and in immunosuppressed individuals, in whom shedding may continue for as long as 3 to 4 weeks. The incubation period ranges from 2 to 8 days; 4 to 6 days is most common.

2. What are the clinical characteristics of bronchiolitis and what other organisms cause bronchiolitis?

- Nasal obstruction ± rhinorrhea and an irritating cough are noticed first.
- After 1–3 days there follows increasing tachypnea and respiratory distress. The chest is often over-expanded.
- Auscultatory signs are very variable: Fine inspiratory crackles are often heard early, becoming coarser during recovery; expiratory wheeze is often present, initially high-pitched, with prolonged expiration.
- Respiratory distress may be mild, moderate or severe.
- Fever of 38.5°C or greater is seen in about 50% of infants with bronchiolitis.
- Apnea may be the presenting feature, especially in very young, premature or low-birth weight infants. It often disappears, to be replaced by severe respiratory distress.
- The radiographic manifestations of bronchiolitis are nonspecific and include diffuse hyperinflation of the lungs, flattening of the diaphragm, prominence of the retrosternal space, and bulging of the intercostal spaces. Patchy or peribronchial infiltrates suggestive of interstitial pneumonia occur in the majority of infants. Atelectasis is observed in most infants, but consolidation is observed in only 24% of patients. Pleural fluid is rarely observed and, when present, is minimal. Some (13%) infants with illness severe enough to require hospitalization have normal chest roentgenograms.

Organisms causing bronchiolitis

RSV is the most common pathogen (85%), but other organisms occasionally produce a similar clinical picture:
- Adenovirus (11%) occasionally causes a similar syndrome with a more virulent course.
- Epidemics of bronchiolitis due to parainfluenza virus usually begin earlier in the year and tend to occur every other year.
- Other less common etiologic agents include the following:
  - *Mycoplasma pneumoniae*
  - Enterovirus
  - Influenza virus
  - Rhinovirus
  - *Chlamydia pneumoniae*.

3. How do you treat RSV infection?

Most previously healthy infants infected with RSV do not require hospitalization, and many who are hospitalized improve with supportive care and are discharged in fewer than 5 days. Characteristics that increase the risk of severe or fatal RSV infection are preterm birth; cyanotic or complicated congenital heart disease, especially conditions causing pulmonary hypertension; underlying pulmonary disease, especially chronic lung disease of prematurity; and immunodeficiency disease or therapy causing immunosuppression at any age.

Most infants with RSV bronchiolitis or pneumonia can be managed at home with supportive care. Infants unable to feed because of respiratory distress or those who require supplemental oxygen should be hospitalized. A small percentage of infants will need intubation and respiratory support with a mechanical ventilator because of respiratory compromise. A trial of aerosolized bronchodilators is reasonable but should not be continued unless a favorable clinical response is noted. Corticosteroids are not useful in RSV bronchiolitis and should not be used.

At present, the only antiviral drug with in vitro efficacy against RSV is ribavirin. Early trials of ribavirin in RSV bronchiolitis suggested a reduction in the severity of illness with a decrease in viral shedding and improved oxygenation. However, concern about the efficacy of ribavirin, its safety in exposed health care workers and its high cost has dampened enthusiasm for this therapy. The American Academy of Pediatrics Committee on Infectious Diseases recommends that "decision about ribavirin administration should be based on the particular clinical circumstances and physicians' experience."

Prevention of RSV Infections

Palivizumab, a humanized mouse monoclonal antibody that is administered intramuscularly, is available to reduce the risk of RSV hospitalization in high-risk children.

4. What relation it has with asthma?

There is now sufficient evidence supporting the notion that severe infantile RSV infection is associated with recurrent wheezing and asthma later in childhood. However, the underlying mechanisms are not fully defined, perhaps suggesting genetic and environmental risk factors playing role in dictating final outcome. In early life Th2 biased responses is likely an important in hosts that are atopic or predisposed to become atopic. RSV infection in neonates may bias both the systemic immune response and the response in lung. This Th2 biased setting seen with RSV reinfection and development of IgE specific antibodies may induce cross sensitization or lower threshold to allergen induced responses. This combination may manifest as increased asthma susceptibility.

Further Reading

1. Chernick V, Boat TF, Wilmott RW, Bush A. Kendig's disorders of the respiratory tract in children. Elsevier Inc. 7th edition, 2006.
2. Fitzgerald DA, Kilham HA. Bronchiolitis: assessment and evidence-based management. MJA 2004; 180 (8): 399-404.
3. Han J, Takeda K, Gelfand EW. The role of RSV infection in asthma and progression. Pulmonary medicine vol. 2011(2011).
4. Javed Akhter, Sameera Al Johani. Epidemiology and diagnosis of human respiratory syncytial virus infections. Book on Human Respiratory Syncytial Virus Infection. 2011. ISBN 978-953-307-718-5.
5. Larry K, Pickering CJ, Baker SS, Long JA. McMillan. Red book; Report of the committee on infectious diseases 27th edition. Publisher: American Academy of Pediatrics. 2006.
6. Louden M. Pediatrics, Bronchiolitis. 2007. eMedicine Specialties. Website: www.emedicine.com.

20

Dengue

Jaydeep Choudhury

1. What is the epidemiology of dengue including transmission and disease burden?

Dengue fever was reported for the first time in India in 1956 from Vellore town of Tamil Nadu. During the two decades from 1991 to 2010, out of 35 states and Union Territories, 31 have reported dengue cases.

The case fatality rate (deaths per 100 cases) due to dengue was 3.3% in 1996. Though it declined thereafter but consistently had been above 1.0% till 2007. After the National Guidelines on clinical management of DF/DHF/DSS were developed and circulated in 2007, the case fatality rate started declining.

Dengue virus has four serologically distinct serotypes DEN-1, DEN-2, DEN-3 and DEN-4. Infection with one dengue virus serotype confers long-term immunity only to that serotype, and does not offer cross-protection to other serotypes. So, one may be infected by dengue up to four times by four different dengue serotypes. Humans are the main reservoir for dengue virus.

Mosquitoes of the genus aedes, such as *Aedes aegypti* and *A. albopictus*, transmit dengue virus. *A. aegypti* is the principal vector found worldwide in the tropics and subtropics. The mosquito is well adapted to life in urban settings and typically breeds in clean, stagnant water in containers that collect rainwater, such as tin cans, pots and buckets. It feeds preferentially on human blood, has an almost imperceptible bite. Characteristically, it is a daytime feeder and is capable of biting several people in a short period for one blood meal. Peak dengue transmission occurs about six to eight weeks after the peak rainfall. DHF cases usually start to rise after about 4 weeks of the peak rainfall and within the next 4 weeks, the peak dengue transmission is recorded. Vertical transmission in newborns has also been reported.

2. What are the recent classifications of dengue and how to recognize them?

The clinical presentation of dengue is a large spectrum, which extends from asymptomatic infection to dengue shock syndrome. Dengue is endemic in most parts of the country. Any child presenting with fever with or without rash and thrombocytopenia should be suspected to suffer from dengue infection. The following features, if present, should alert the clinician that it could probably be a case of dengue and these children should be closely monitored. These children may develop the warning signs and they are at risk to progress to severe dengue. The recent WHO classification of dengue is as follows:

Criteria for probable dengue
  i. Live in/travel to dengue endemic area
  ii. Fever and two of the following criteria:
     a. Nausea, vomiting
     b. Rash
     c. Aches and pains
     d. Positive tourniquet test
     e. Leukopenia
     f. Any warning sign.

Dengue with warning signs
  i. Abdominal pain and tenderness
  ii. Persistent vomiting
  iii. Clinical fluid accumulation
  iv. Mucosal bleeds
  v. Lethargy, restlessness
  vi. Liver enlarged more than 2 cm
  vii. Laboratory—Rise in hematocrit with rapid fall in platelets.

Criteria for severe dengue
Severe dengue is characterized by severe plasma leakage, severe hemorrhage and severe organ impairment.
A. Severe plasma leakage:
   i. Shock (Dengue Shock Syndrome—DSS)
   ii. Fluid accumulation with respiratory distress
B. Severe bleeding:
   As evaluated by the clinician
C. Severe organ involvement:
   i. Liver enzymes—AST/ALT more than 1000
   ii. CNS—Impaired consciousness
   iii. Heart and other organ dysfunctions

The previous WHO classification of dengue along with clinical and laboratory criteria are shown in Table 1.

Unusual manifestations of dengue infection
1. Encephalopathy and, less often, encephalitis
2. Hepatic failure
3. Cardiomyopathy
4. Dengue fever with severe hemorrhage
5. Acute respiratory distress syndrome
6. Acalculous cholecystitis

Table 1: WHO classification of dengue

Dengue Fever (DF) grade	Clinical criteria	Laboratory criteria
Dengue Fever (DF)	Fever with 2 or more of following signs: Headache, retro-orbital pain, myalgia, arthralgia	Leukopenia, occasionally thrombocytopenia with no plasma leakage
Dengue Hemorrhagic Fever (DHF) I	Above signs plus positive tourniquet test	Hematocrit rise > 20% platelets < 100,000
Dengue Hemorrhagic Fever (DHF) II	Above signs plus spontaneous bleeding	Hematocrit rise > 20% platelets < 100,000
DHF III (Dengue Shock Syndrome—DSS)	Above signs plus circulatory failure	Hematocrit rise > 20% platelets < 100,000
DHF IV (DSS)	Profound shock with undetectable BP and pulse	Hematocrit rise > 20% platelets < 100,000

Role of tourniquet test

The tourniquet test is performed by inflating a blood pressure cuff to a point midway between the systolic and diastolic pressures for five minutes. The test is considered positive when 10 or more petechiae per 2.5 square cm (1 square inch) are observed. In severe dengue with hemorrhagic manifestation, the test usually gives a definite positive result with 20 petechiae or more. The test may be negative or only mildly positive during the phase of profound shock. It usually becomes positive, sometimes strongly positive, if it is conducted after recovery from shock.

3. What are the laboratory diagnoses of dengue?

Dengue-specific tests

Virus isolation

Although this is the most definitive method for the diagnosis of dengue infection, it is only performed in very few research laboratories.

Detection of dengue ribonucleic acid (RNA)

The use of polymerase chain reaction to detect dengue RNA is not a routine procedure and should be considered more of a research tool. It is indicated when there is a diagnostic problem.

Serology

The serologic tests that have been used for the diagnosis of dengue infections include hemagglutination inhibition (HI) test, complement fixation test (CFT), neutralization tests (NT), IgM capture ELISA, IgG capture ELISA, immunofluorescence assays, dot blot immunoassays, dipstick enzyme immunoassays and the rapid immunochromatographic card tests. The HI test, CFT and NT are performed only in reference laboratories. The ELISA and the rapid card tests are most commonly used for dengue diagnosis in current clinical practice.

In the primary dengue infection, 80% of the individuals demonstrate IgM ELISA antibodies by day 5, 93% by day 6-10 and 99% by day 10-20. IgM antibodies peak at 2 weeks and then decline over the next 2-3 months. IgG antibodies rise later and to lower levels as compared to IgM, then decline gradually but may persist at low levels for life.

In secondary dengue infections, there is a brisk and rapid IgG response much higher than that seen in primary dengue infections, which peaks at 2 weeks and then declines slowly over the next 3-6 months. The IgM response in secondary dengue infections is slower and lower than IgG with some individuals showing no detectable IgM.

In early infection, serology may be negative and, hence, impart a false sense of security. In most cases, by the time serology is positive and is able to differentiate primary from secondary infections, the diagnosis is fairly clinically evident. Dengue serology, though is useful in diagnosis of dengue illnesses, it is ineffectual in differentiating these clinical syndromes. While these tests are capable of differentiating primary from secondary responses, it is worth knowing that secondary serological responses are not synonymous with DHF, only six to eight percent of secondary infections culminate to dengue hemorrhagic fever. One of the shortcomings of dengue serology is the time interval of six days, when they become clinically meaningful. In DF, the mild variety of illness, by the time serological tests become positive, disease might have already been over in good number of cases. Contrarily, in majority of DHF, disease may lend into a serious stage, by the time tests results become positive. Therefore, repeated physical assessment and serial blood counts are the basis for the clinical diagnosis and management of various dengue illnesses.

NS1 antigen

NS1 is a highly conserved glycoprotein of dengue virus. It is secreted in the circulation and disappears as antibodies appear. So, NSI antigen can be detected upto twelve days. It declines as the illness advances. NS1 antigen presents with lower levels in secondary dengue infections.

The specificity of NS1 antigen is nearly 100%. The sensitivity of NS1 antigen for primary dengue fever in the first 4 days is 90% and for secondary dengue, it is 70%. Interpretation of NS1 and dengue serology is shown in Table 2.

Table 2: Interpretation of NS1 and dengue serology

NS1 antigen	IgM	IgG	Interpretation
Positive	Negative	Negative	Early (< 4 dys)
Negative/Positive	Positive	Negative	Primary
Negative	Positive	Positive low titers	Current/Recent
Negative/Positive	Positive	Positive high titers	Secondary
Negative	Positive	Positive high titers	Secondary
Negative	Negative	Positive low titers	Past infection

Supportive tests

Complete blood cell count

i. Leucopenia is common initially, but WBC may also be normal. Neutrophils usually predominate. Towards the end of the febrile phase, there is a drop in the total number of white cells as well as in the number of polymorphonuclear cells. A relative lymphocytosis with more than 15% atypical lymphocytes is commonly observed towards the end of the febrile phase and at the early stage of shock.

Absence of leucopenia and a relatively low percentage of typical lymphocytes predict severe dengue illness.

ii. A rise in hematocrit greater than 20% is a sign of hemoconcentration and precedes shock. An initial hematocrit of > 40% warrants close monitoring. The hematocrit level should be monitored at least every 24 hours to facilitate early recognition of dengue hemorrhagic fever (DHF) and every 3-4 hours in severe cases of DHF or dengue shock syndrome (DSS).

iii. Thrombocytopenia and hemoconcentration are constant findings in DHF. A drop in platelet count to below $100,000/mm^3$ is usually found between the third and eighth days of illness. A rise in hematocrit occurs in all DHF cases, particularly in shock cases. Hemoconcentration with hematocrit increased by 20% or more is considered objective evidence of increased vascular permeability and leakage of plasma. It should be noted that the level of hematocrit may be affected by early volume replacement and by bleeding. Platelet counts of less than 100,000 are seen in DHF or DSS and occur before defervescence and the onset of shock.

Like hematocrit, the platelet count should be monitored at least every 24 hours to facilitate early recognition of DHF.

Metabolic tests

i. *Hyponatremia*—It is the most common electrolyte abnormality observed in patients with DHF or DSS.
ii. *Metabolic acidosis*—It is observed in those with shock, and it must be corrected rapidly.
iii. *BUN*—Elevated in those with shock.

Liver function tests

Mild elevations in transaminase levels may be seen. Low albumin is a sign of hemoconcentration.

Coagulation studies

It may help guide therapy in patients with severe hemorrhagic manifestations.

i. Partial thromboplastin time (PTT) and prothrombin time (PT)—Prolonged in about one-half and one-third of DHF cases respectively.

Thrombin time is also prolonged in severe cases. Deranged prothrombin time (PT) is a significant risk factor for DSS.
ii. Low fibrinogen and elevated fibrin degradation product levels are signs of disseminated intravascular coagulation. Assays of coagulation and fibrinolytic factors show reductions in fibrinogen, prothrombin, factor VIII, factor XII, and antithrombin III. A reduction in antiplasmin (plasmin inhibitor) has been noted in some cases. In severe cases with marked liver dysfunction, reduction is observed in the vitamin K-dependent prothrombin family, such as factors V, VII, IX and X. Serum complement levels are reduced.

Imaging studies

Chest radiograph—Right-sided pleural effusion is typical. Bilateral pleural effusions are common in patients with DSS.

Ultrasound—Ultrasound examination detects plasma leakage in multiple body compartments around the time of defervescence. Ultrasonographic signs of plasma leakage are detectable before changes in hematocrits. Ultrasound is a useful tool for detecting plasma leakage in dengue infection. Gallbladder wall thickening measured by ultrasound is significantly associated with severe dengue.

Other tests

Arterial blood gas determinations should be performed in severe cases to assess pH, oxygenations and ventilation. A transient mild albuminuria is sometimes observed. Occult blood is often found in the stool.

4. When to admit a child with dengue?

Criteria for Hospitalization
1. Lethargy or restlessness.
2. Cold extremities.
3. Rapid weak pulse.
4. Capillary refill time >2 seconds.
5. Hypotension or pulse pressure <20 mm of Hg.
6. Oliguria.
7. Bleeding in any form.
8. Hematocrit 40 or rising hematocrit.
9. Platelet count less than 100,000/mm^3.
10. Acute abdominal pain.
11. Evidence of plasma leakage—pleural effusion, ascites.
12. Condition where proper monitoring at home is not possible.

5. What are the aspects of monitoring and fluid therapy in various stages of dengue?

Monitoring a child with dengue is of utmost importance as a child suffering from probable dengue may quickly turn to be a severe dengue. A careful monitoring may help in early detection and controlling progression.

Monitoring in a child with dengue

1. Every 30 minutes—Pulse, BP and respiration.
2. Hematocrit and hemoglobin every 2 hours for first 6 hours and then every 4 hours until the patient is stable.
3. Fluid balance sheet—Type, volume and rate.
4. Urine output—Frequency and volume.

Parents must bring the child back immediately to the nearest hospital in the presence of any one of the following situations:

 i. Not drinking/feeding poorly.
 ii. Passing less urine than usual.
 iii. Abdominal pain.
 iv. Bleeding in any form.
 v. In older children, inability to sit up and giddiness.
 vi. Irritability, drowsiness and restlessness.
 vii. Child continues to be unwell.

Management

Management of shock in dengue infection encompasses the following:

1. Airway, breathing and circulation and administration of 100% oxygen.
2. If vascular access is not available, then intraosseous route may be established.
3. Intravenous fluids—20 mL/kg of 0.9% NS over 10–15 minutes. If no improvement, the cycle may be repeated. If no response to fluids, colloid can be used (5% albumin, or blood products).
4. Consider central venous pressure (CVP). If CVP < 10 mm Hg, continue fluid therapy CVP > 10 mm Hg with poor perfusion, give vasoactive agents.
5. Place urinary catheter and maintain urine output 1–2 mL/kg/hour.

Treatment is planned according to Groups A–C as shown in Figure 1.

Group A

These patients may be managed at home. They tolerate adequate volumes of oral fluids, pass urine at least once every six hours and do not have any of the warning signs (particularly when fever subsides).

The parents should be given clear, definitive advice on the care of the patient at home, i.e. bed rest and frequent oral fluids. Patients with 3 days or more of illness should be reviewed daily for disease progression (indicated by decreasing white blood cell and platelet counts and increasing hematocrit, defervescence and warning signs) until they are out of the critical period. Those with stable hematocrit can be sent home but should be advised to return to the hospital immediately if they develop any of the warning signs and to adhere to the following action plan:

 i. The choice of fluids should be based on the local culture. Coconut water, rice water or barley water may be given. Oral rehydration solution or soup and fruit juices may be given to prevent electrolyte imbalance. Sufficient oral fluid intake should result in a urinary frequency of at

128 FAQs in Pediatric Infectious Diseases

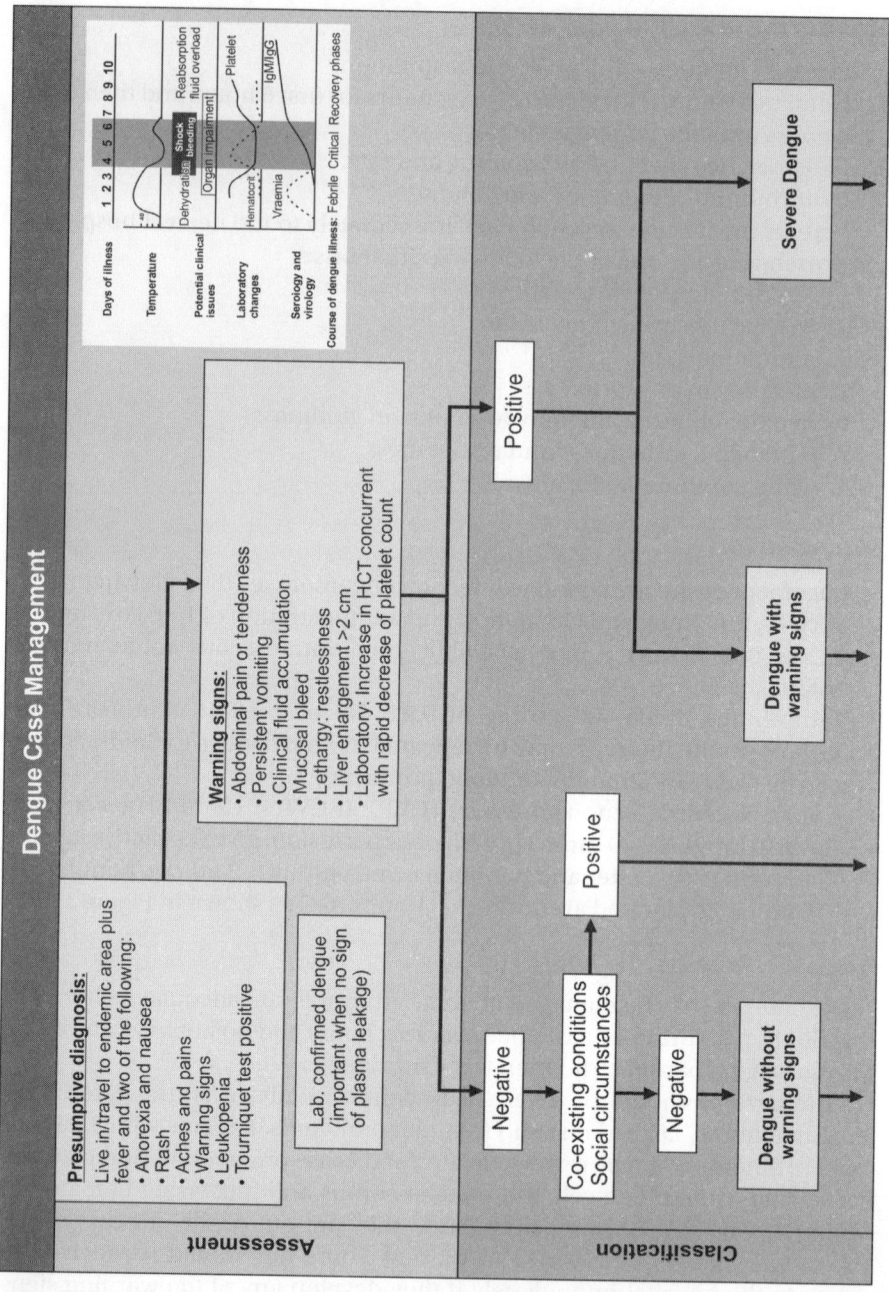

Contd...

Dengue

	Group A May be sent home	Group B Referred for in-hospital care	Group C Requires emergency treatment
Management	**Group criteria** Patients who do not have warning signs, **And** Who are able: • To tolerate adequate volumes of oral fluids • To pass urine at least once every 6 hours **Laboratory tests** • Full blood count (FBC) • Hematocrit (Hct) **Treatment** Advice for: • Adequate bed rest • Adequate fluid intake • Paracetamol, 4 grams max. per day in adults and accordingly in children Patients with stable Hct can be sent home **Monitoring** • Daily review for disease progression • Decreasing WBC • Defervescence • Warning signs (until out of critical period) • Advice for immediate return to hospital if development of any warning signs • Written advice of management (e.g. home care card for dengue)	**Group criteria** Patients with any of the following features: • Co-existing conditions such as pregnancy, infancy, old age, diabetes mellitus • Social circumstances such as living alone or living far from the hospital **Or** Existing warning signs: • Abdominal pain or tenderness • Persistent vomiting • Clinical fluid accumulation • Mucosal bleeding • Lethargy/restlessness • Liver enlargement >2 cm • Laboratory: increase in Hct **Laboratory tests** • Full blood count (FBC) • Hematocrit (Hct) **Treatment** • Encouragement for oral fluids • If not tolerated, start intravenous fluid therapy 0.9% saline or Ringer Lactate at maintenance rate **Treatment** • Obtain reference Hct before fluid therapy • Give isotonic solutions such as 0.9% saline, Ringer lactate, start with 5–7 mL/kg/hr for 1–2 hrs, then reduce to 3–5 mL/kg/hr for 2–4 hrs, and then reduce to 2–3 mL/kg/hr or less according to clinical response **Reassess clinical status and repeat Hct** • If Hct remains the same or rises only minimally → continue with 2–3 mL/kg/hr for another 2–4 hours • If worsening of vital signs and rapidly rising Hct → increase rate to 5–10 mL/kg/hr for 1–2 hours **Reassess clinical status, repeat Hct and review fluid infusion rates accordingly** • Reduce intravenous fluids gradually when the end of the critical phase **This is indicated by:** • Adequate urine output and/or fluid intake • Hct decreases below the baseline value in a stable patient **Monitoring** • Vital signs and peripheral perfusion (1–4 hourly until the patient is out of critical phase) • Urine output (4–6 hourly) • Hct (before and after fluid replacement, then 6–12 hourly) • Blood glucose • Other organ functions (renal profile, liver profile, coagulation profile, as indicated)	Patients with any of the following features: • Severe plasma leakage with shock and/or fluid accumulation with respiratory distress • Severe bleeding • Severe organ impairment **Laboratory tests** • Full blood count (FBC) • Hematocrit (Hct) • Other organ function tests, as indicated **Treatment of compensated shock** Start IV fluid resuscitation with isotonic crystalloid solutions at 5–10 mL/kg/hr over 1 hr • Reassess the patient's condition **If the patient improves:** • IV fluids be reduced gradually to 5–7 mL/kg/hr for 1–2 hrs; then to 3–5 mL/kg/hr for 2–4 hrs, then to 2–3 mL/kg/hr for 2–4 hrs and then reduced further depending on hemodynamic status • IV fluids can be maintained for up to 24–48 hrs. **If the patient is still unstable:** • Check Hct after first bolus • If Hct increases/is still high (>50%), repeat a second bolus of crystalloid solution at 10–20 mL/kg/hr for 1 hr • If there is improvement after bolus, reduce rate to 7–10 mL/kg/hr for 1–2 hrs, continue to reduce as above • If Hct decreases, this indicates bleeding and one needs to crossmatch and transfuse blood as soon as possible **Treatment of hypotensive shock** Initiate IV fluid resuscitation with crystalloid or colloid solution at 20 mL/kg as a bolus for 15 mins. **If the patient improves:** Give a crystalloid/colloid solution of 10 mL/kg/hr for 1 hr, then reduce gradually as above **If the patient is still unstable** • Review the Hct taken before the first bolus • If Hct was low (<40% in children and adult females, <45% in adult males), this indicates bleeding, the need to crossmatch and transfuse (see above) • If Hct was high compared to the baseline value, change to IV colloids at 10–20 mL/kg as a second bolus over 1 hr, reassess after second bolus • If improving, reduce the rate to 7–10 mL/kg/hr for 1–2 hrs, then back to IV crystalloids and reduce rates as above • If the condition is still unstable, repeat Hct after second bolus • If Hct decreases, this indicates bleeding as above • If Hct increases/remains high (>50%), continue colloid infusion at 10–20 mL/kg as a third bolus over 1 hr. Then reduce to 7–10 mL/kg/hr for 1–2 hrs, then change back to crystalloid solution and reduce rates as above **Treatment of haemorrhagic complications** Give 5–10 mL/kg of fresh-packed red cells of 10–20 mL/kg fresh whole blood
	Discharge criteria: → All of the following criteria must be present	• No fever for 48 hours • Improvement in clinical picture	• Increasing trend of platelet count • No respiratory distress	• Stable hematocrit without intravenous fluids

Figure 1: Treatment plan for dengue case management

least 4 to 6 times per day. A record of oral fluid and urine output could be maintained and reviewed daily in the ambulatory setting.
  ii. Paracetamol for high fever if the patient is uncomfortable, recommended dose is 10 mg/kg/dose, not more than 3–4 times in 24 hours in children (and not more than 3 g/day in adults). Sponge with tepid water if the patient still has a high fever. Acetylsalicylic acid (aspirin), ibuprofen or other non-steroidal anti-inflammatory agents (NSAIDs) or intramuscular injections should not be given, as these aggravate gastritis or bleeding.
 iii. Patient should be brought to hospital immediately if there is no clinical improvement, deterioration around the time of defervescence, severe abdominal pain, persistent vomiting, cold and clammy extremities, lethargy or irritability/restlessness, bleeding (e.g. black stools or coffee ground vomiting), shortness of breath, not passing urine for more than 4–6 hours.

Group B

These patients should be admitted for in-hospital management. These include patients with warning signs, those with co-existing conditions that may make dengue or its management more complicated (such as infancy, hypertension, heart failure, renal failure, chronic hemolytic diseases and autoimmune diseases), and those with certain social circumstances (such as living far from a health facility without reliable means of transport). Rapid fluid replacement in patients with warning signs is the key to prevent progression to the shock state.

The action plan should be as follows and applies to infants and children:
   i. Obtain a reference hematocrit before intravenous fluid therapy begins. Only isotonic solutions such as 0.9% saline or Ringer's lactate. Start with 5–7 mL/kg/hour for 1–2 hours, then reduce to 3–5 mL/kg/hour for 2–4 hours, and then reduce to 2–3 mL/kg/hour or less according to the clinical response.
  ii. Reassess the clinical status and repeat the hematocrit. If the hematocrit remains the same or rises only minimally, continue at the same rate (2–3 mL/kg/hour) for another 2–4 hours. If the vital signs are worsening and the hematocrit is rising rapidly, increase the rate to 5–10 mL/kg/hour for 1–2 hours. Reassess the clinical status, repeat the hematocrit and review fluid infusion rates accordingly.
 iii. Give the minimum intravenous fluid volume required to maintain good perfusion and a urine output of about 0.5 mL/kg/hour. Intravenous fluids are usually needed for only 24–48 hours. Reduce intravenous fluids gradually when the rate of plasma leakage decreases towards the end of the critical phase. This is indicated by urine output and/or oral fluid intake improving, or the hematocrit decreasing below the baseline value in a stable patient.
 iv. Patients with warning signs should be monitored by healthcare providers until the period of risk is over. Parameters that should be

monitored include vital signs and peripheral perfusion (1–4 hourly until the patient is out of the critical phase), urine output (4–6 hourly), hematocrit (before and after fluid replacement, then 6–12 hourly), blood glucose and other organ functions (such as renal profile, liver profile and coagulation profile as indicated).

v. If the patient has dengue with co-existing conditions but without warning signs, the action plan should be to encourage oral fluids. If not tolerated, start intravenous fluid therapy of 0.9% saline or Ringer's lactate with or without glucose at the appropriate maintenance rate. Give the minimum volume required to maintain good perfusion and urine output. Intravenous fluids are usually needed only for 24–48 hours.

Group C

These patients with severe dengue require emergency treatment and urgent referral because they are in the critical phase of the disease. They have:
  i. Severe plasma leakage leading to dengue shock and/or fluid accumulation with respiratory distress;
  ii. Severe hemorrhages;
  iii. Severe organ impairment (hepatic damage, renal impairment, cardiomyopathy, encephalopathy or encephalitis).

Patients with severe dengue should be admitted to a hospital with access to blood transfusion facilities. Judicious intravenous fluid resuscitation is essential and usually sole intervention required. Plasma losses should be replaced immediately and rapidly with isotonic crystalloid solution. In case of hypotensive shock, colloid solution is preferred. If possible, obtain hematocrit levels before and after fluid resuscitation.

Blood transfusion should be given only in cases with established severe bleeding, or suspected severe bleeding in combination with otherwise unexplained hypotension. Here larger volumes of fluids (e.g. 10–20 ml/kg boluses) are administered for a limited period of time under close supervision, to evaluate the patient's response and to avoid the development of pulmonary edema.

The goals of fluid resuscitation include:
  i. Improving central and peripheral circulation, i.e. decreasing tachycardia, improving BP and pulse volume, warm and pink extremities, a capillary refill time < 2 seconds;
  ii. Improving end-organ perfusion, i.e. achieving a stable conscious level (more alert or less restless), and urine output ≥ 0.5 mL/kg/hour or decreasing metabolic acidosis.

Treatment of shock

The action plan for treating patients with shock is as shown in Figures 2 and 3. Consider reducing intravenous fluid earlier if oral fluid intake improves. The total duration of intravenous fluid therapy should not exceed 48 hours.

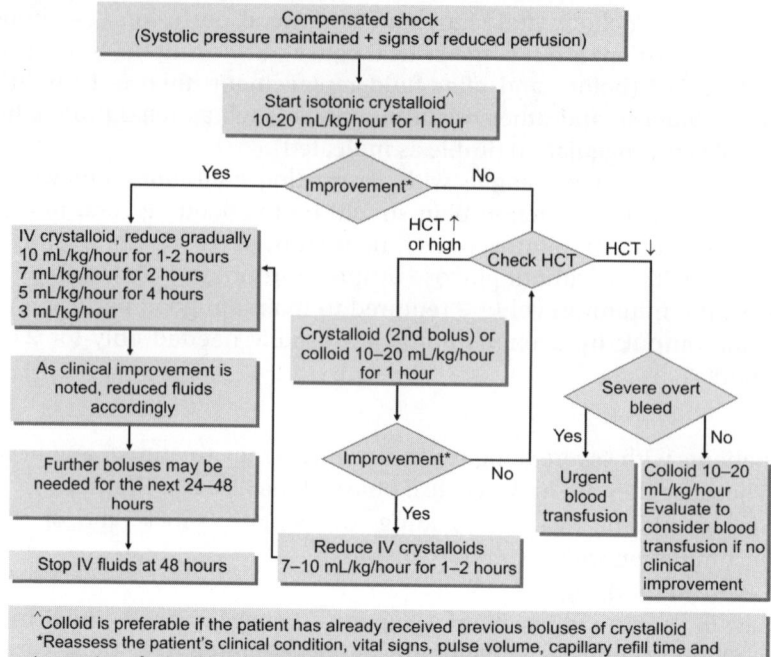

Figure 2: Fluid management of compensated shock: in infants and children

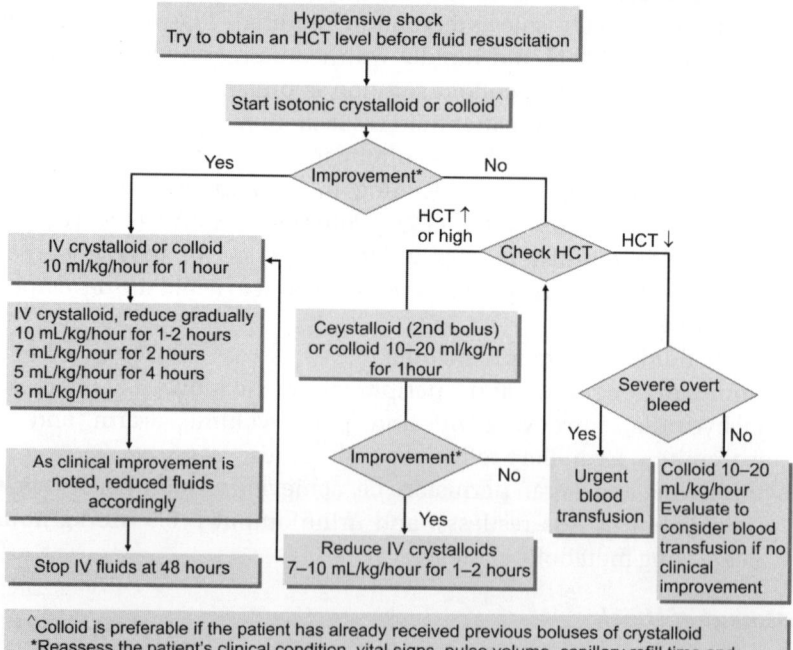

Figure 3: Management in hypotensive shock—infants, children and adults

When to stop intravenous fluid therapy

Recognizing when to decrease or stop intravenous fluid as part of the treatment of severe dengue is crucial to prevent fluid overload. When any of the following signs are present, intravenous fluids should be reduced or discontinued:
  i. Signs of cessation of plasma leakage;
  ii. Stable BP, pulse and peripheral perfusion;
  iii. Hematocrit decreases in the presence of a good pulse volume;
  iv. Apyrexia (without the use of antipyretics) for more than 24–48 hours;
  v. Resolving bowel/abdominal symptoms;
  vi. Improving urine output.

Further Reading

1. Guzman MG, Kouri G. Dengue: an update. Lancet Infect Dis. 2002;2:33-42.
2. Halstead SB. Dengue and dengue hemorrhagic fever. In: Feigin, Cherry, Demmler, Kaplan, editors. Textbook of Pediatric Infectious Diseases, 5th edition. 2004;2178-200.
3. Handbook for Clinical Management of Dengue. World Health Organization. Geneva: WHO, 2012.
4. Kabra SK, Jain Y, Singhal T, Ratageri VH. Dengue hemorrhagic fever: clinical manifestations and management. Indian J Pediatr. 1999;55:93-101.
5. Lall R, Dhandha V. Dengue hemorrhagic fever and dengue shock syndrome in India. Natl Med J India. 1996;9:20-3.
6. Rigau-Perez JG. Severe dengue: the need for new case definitions. Lancet Infect Dis. 2006;6:297-302.

21

Rabies

Jaydeep Choudhury

1. Why children are more vulnerable to animal bites and rabies?

Children are more vulnerable to animal bites and consequent rabies due to the following reasons:
   i. Children are curious and love to play with animals, particularly dogs and cats.
  ii. They often play provocatively with animals which results into bites.
 iii. Their relative short height makes them more vulnerable to bites to head, face, neck and hands.
  iv. They do not have any knowledge about danger of animal scratches and bites, and also possible outcome. Also they often fail to report animal bites to their parents.
   v. Traversing time of virus from periphery to central nervous system is short.

2. How rabies is transmitted to man and which animals are usually responsible?

All warm-blooded animals can be infected by rabies virus. Human rabies is acquired by bites, licks or scratches of rabid animals. Dogs account for 90–96% of animal bites in India.

Apart from dogs, which are the main culprits other warm-blooded animals like cat, fox, jackals, etc. transmit rabies. The domestic animals like cow, buffalo, goat, pig and sheep can also transmit rabies when they are bitten and get infected by rabid animals. Monkey can also transmit rabies if they are infected. Man to man transmission is rare except in cases of cornea transplant from donors with undiagnosed rabies.

Common modes of transmission

   i. Bite and scratch from infected animals
  ii. Lick—on broken skin and intact mucus membranes.

Rare modes of transmission

   i. Aerosol transmission
  ii. Organ transplantation

Bites by insectivorous bats can also transmit rabies and rabies can also spread by aerosol infection in bat infested caves but these are not problems of India.

3. What are the various categories of exposure?

The following Table 1 shows the WHO classification of animal bites.

Table 1: WHO classification of animal bites, type of contact, exposure and recommended post-exposure prophylaxis

Category	Type of contact	Type of exposure	Recommended post-exposure prophylaxis
I	Touching or feeding of animals Licks on intact skin	None	None, if reliable case history is available
II	Nibbling of uncovered skin Minor scratches or abrasions without bleeding	Minor	Wound management Anti-rabies vaccine
III	Single or multiple transdermal bites or scratches, licks on broken skin Contamination of mucous membrane with saliva (i.e. licks)	Severe	Wound management Rabies immunoglobulin Antirabies vaccine

Note: After carefully assessing the category of exposure, the treating doctor should evaluate the course of action to be taken, based on the following general considerations. He should also keep in the mind that with the presently available safe cell culture rabies vaccines (CCRV), it is always safe to offer treatment rather than withhold in doubtful situations

4. How to manage animal bite wound?

Treatment following an exposure to potentially rabid animal (bite, scratch or lick on broken wounds in skin or directly on mucous membrane, i.e. on oral cavity or on anus by suspected rabid animal) will consist of the following stages:

   i. Proper wound management.
   ii. Infiltration of rabies immunoglobulin (RIG) in all category III exposures rabies.
   iii. Antirabies vaccination with modern cell culture rabies vaccine (CCRV).
   iv. Antitetanus prophylaxis if required.
   v. Supportive treatment with antipyretic/analgesics, local and/or systemic antibiotic as required.

The initial and the most important step is proper wound management. Rabies infection can be prevented to a large extent if the wound is managed properly.

Wound management

In wound management, the most important steps are the following:
  i. Thorough washing of wounds under running tap water for at least 10 minutes with the aim of physical elimination/shedding of the viral loads and application of soap/detergent for chemical treatment and changing the pH of the wounds.
  ii. Application of disinfectants like povidone-iodine, spirit, household antiseptics, etc. to remove the remaining virus particles and prevention of secondary infection.

It is to be noted that in wound management application of irritants, cauterization and suturing, i.e., closing of wounds are to be avoided. If suturing is needed for the purpose of hemostasis, it can be done only after administration of RIG.

Do's of wound management	
Wash with running tap water for up to 15 minutes.	Mechanical removal of virus from the wound
Washing the wound with soap and water, dry and apply antiseptic	Inactivation of the virus
Infiltration of rabies immuno-globulins in the depth and around the wound in Category III exposures	Neutralization of the virus
Don'ts of wound management	
• Touch the wound with bare hand	
• Apply irritants like soil, chillies, turmeric, oil, herbs, chalk, betel leaves, etc.	

5. **What is the recommendation for exposure to small mammals like rats, rabbits and guinea pigs?**

Domestic rats do not transmit rabies virus but wild rodents do transmit. Bites by house rats, squirrels and rabbits ordinarily do not require post-exposure prophylaxis (PEP) but when exposures occur in strange or peculiar situation and when in doubt, the treating physician may consider providing rabies PEP. The bites by snakes, lizards, birds and insects do not require rabies PEP.

6. **Does the management differ depending on whether it was provoked or unprovoked bites?**

Whether a dog bite was provoked or unprovoked should not be considered a guarantee that the animal is not rabid as it can be difficult to understand what a dog considers provocation for an attack.

7. What is post-exposure prophylaxis (PEP)?

India being a rabies endemic country, every animal bite is suspected as a potentially rabid bite, the treatment should be started immediately. Because of long and variable incubation period of rabies, which is typical of most cases of human rabies, it is possible to institute rabies prophylaxis following a rabies exposure. PEP should be started at the earliest to ensure that the individual will be effectively protected before the rabies virus reaches the nervous system. The risk of infection occurring in children depends on severity of bite; the amount of virus inoculated at the site of wound, virulence of the virus and some as yet unknown host factors. The PEP depends on the severity of exposure. To ensure standardization and uniformity globally, the classification of animal bites/rabies exposures for post-exposure prophylaxis has been based on these WHO recommendations Table 1.

Rabies immunoglobulin (RIG)

The antirabies serum/rabies immunoglobulin provides passive immunity to counter the initial phase of infection. RIG has the property of binding to rabies virus, thereby resulting in neutralization of the virus.

Two types of RIGs available are the following:

Equine rabies immunoglobulin (ERIG): ERIG is of heterologous origin raised by hyperimmunization of horses. The currently manufactured ERIGs are highly purified and enzyme refined. The occurrence of adverse events is also significantly less.

Human rabies immunoglobulin (HRIG): These are prepared from the serum of healthy people hyperimmunized with modern rabies vaccines. As it is homologous, HRIG is free from the side effects that are encountered in a serum of heterologous origin. It has longer half life, thus it can be given in half the dose of equine antirabies serum. The antirabies sera which are stored in the refrigerator between 2 to 8 degree centigrade should always be brought to room temperature (20–25°C) before injection.

Dose of rabies immunoglobulin: The dose of ERIG is 40 IU per kg body weight of patient and is given after testing for sensitivity. Its dosage is up to a maximum of 3000 IU. The ERIG produced in India contains 300 IU per mL. The dose of the human rabies immunoglobulin (HRIG) is 20 IU per kg body weight (maximum 1500 IU). The HRIG does not require any prior sensitivity testing. HRIG preparation is available in concentration of 150 IU per mL.

Out of the calculated dose of RIG, the maximum quantity that is anatomically feasible should be infiltrated into and around the wounds. Multiple needle injections into the wound should be avoided. Any RIG remaining after all wounds have been infiltrated, should be administered by deep intramuscular injection at an injection site distant from the site of vaccine injection. Animal bite wounds inflicted can be severe and multiple, especially in small children. In such cases, the calculated dose of the rabies immunoglobulin may not be sufficient to infiltrate all wounds. In such situations, it is advisable to dilute the RIG in sterile normal saline to a volume sufficient for infiltration of all wounds.

If RIG was not administered when antirabies vaccination was begun, it can be administered up to seventh day after the administration of the first dose of vaccine. Beyond the seventh day, RIG is not indicated since an antibody response to antirabies vaccine is presumed to have occurred. The RIG should never be administered in the same syringe or at the same anatomical site as rabies vaccine.

Skin test: Inject 0.1 mL ERIG diluted 1:10 in sterile physiological saline intradermally into the flexor surface of the forearm to raise a bleb of about 3–4 mm diameter. Inject an equal amount of sterile normal saline as a negative control on the flexor surface of the other forearm. After 15 minutes an increase in diameter to >10 mm of induration surrounded by flare, swelling, pseudopodia, etc. is taken as positive skin test, provided the reaction on the saline test is negative. An increase or abrupt fall in blood pressure, syncope, hurried breathing, palpitations and any other systemic manifestations should be taken as positive test. A negative skin test must never reassure the physician that no anaphylactic reaction will occur.

WHO has recently recommended abolishing the skin sensitivity test as it is considered not predictive of adverse events/reactions to occur. But in India, it is obligatory on the part of physician to do it as mentioned in the product insert due to prevailing drug laws and until it is withdrawn.

8. What is to be done if a patient requires rabies immunoglobulin but none is available?

Greater emphasis should be given to proper wound management followed by regular schedule of modern rabies vaccine with double dose of vaccine on day 0 at 2 different sites intramuscularly (one dose each on left and right deltoid) followed by one dose each by IM on day 3, 7, 14 and 28. It is emphasized that doubling the first dose of CCV is not a replacement to RIG. However, all efforts should be made to refer the patient to the nearest facility providing RIG to receive the same within seven days of starting rabies vaccine.

9. What is the recommendation for exposure to immunized pet animals?

Although unvaccinated animals are more likely to transmit rabies, vaccinated animals can also do so, if the vaccination of the biting animal was ineffective for any reason. A history of antirabies vaccination in an animal is not always a guarantee that the biting animal has seroconverted adequately and is not rabid. Animal vaccine failures may occur because of improper administration or poor quality of the vaccine, poor health status of the animal, and the fact that one dose of vaccine does not provide long-lasting protection against rabies infection in dogs.

PEP may be deferred only if the pet is more than a year old and has a vaccination certificate indicating that it has received at least 2 doses of a potent vaccine, the first not earlier than 3 months of age and the second within 6 to 12 months of the first dose and in the past 1 year. If vaccination is deferred, the pet should be observed for 10 days. Patient should receive full rabies PEP if the animal shows any signs of illness during this period.

Another option is pre-exposure conversion of post-exposure schedule. After an exposure, antirabies vaccine is given on day 0 and day 3. Then the patient comes back for 3rd dose on day 7 (which is the day 8th day of the bite). If the biting animal under observation is living healthy, then the vaccine is not administered and advised to wait for 2 more days and to again report to the doctor. If on day 10, the same patient reports that the dog is still living healthy; the 3rd dose is postponed to day 28. Thus, a postexposure schedule is converted to pre-exposure schedule skipping the 3rd and 4th dose. This is applicable only for pet dogs and cats under observation.

11. What is the recommendation for drinking milk of rabid animal?

Raw milk from an infected cow can transmit rabies virus as rabies virus can penetrate intact mucus membrane. Rabies virus is killed by proper boiling of infected milk, hence boiled milk is safe for consumption.

12. What is the management of re-exposure following completed pre and post-exposure prophylaxis?

Patient who has been previously vaccinated with rabies vaccine, either pre-exposure or post-exposure schedule with documented evidence, the treatment protocol is as follows:
  i. Local treatment of wound
  ii. Vaccination schedule—One dose immediately (day 0) and second on day 3. The dose is either 1 standard intramuscular dose (which may be 1 ml or 0.5 ml depending on vaccine type) or one intradermal dose of 0.1 ml per site
  iii. No RIG should be applied
  iv. However full treatment should be given to persons—
   - Who have received pre- or post-exposure treatment with vaccines of unproven potency.
   - Person who have not demonstrated acceptable rabies neutralizing antibody titer.

13. What are the different rabies vaccines and their merits and demerits?

Active immunization is achieved by administration of antirabies vaccines, either cell culture vaccine (CCV) or purified duck embryo vaccine (PDEV). The dosage schedule is same irrespective of the body weight or age of the children. It is recommended that these vaccines should be kept and transported at a temperature range of 2-8°C. Freezing does not damage the lyophilized vaccine but there are chances of breakage of ampoule containing the diluent. The lyophilized vaccine should be reconstituted just prior to use with the diluent provided with the vaccine. After reconstitution, if there is delay, it should be used within 6–8 hours.

Vaccines

Cell culture vaccines (CCV):
  i. Human diploid cell vaccine (HDCV)—produced locally in private sector. It is an adsorbed (liquid) vaccine.
  ii. Purified chick embryo cell vaccine (PCECV)—produced locally in private sector.
  iii. Purified vero cell rabies vaccine (PVRV)—imported and produced locally in public and private sectors.
  iv. Purified duck embryo vaccine (PDEV)—produced locally in private sector.

All CCVs and PDEV used for PEP should have potency (antigen content) greater than 2.5 IU per intramuscular dose irrespective of whether it is 0.5 mL or 1.0 mL vaccine by volume.

The cell culture vaccines/PDEV presently in the market are safe and generally do not produce any side effects. Occasional local or systemic side effects may be seen. Commonly seen local side effects are pain and tenderness at the injection site. Systemic side effect may include fever, malaise, urticaria and rarely lymphadenopathy. Generally these side effects are self-limiting and occasionally require medication.

Currently available CCVs and PDEV are administered by Essen Intramuscular (IM) regimen. Some CCVs which are also approved for ID use can be administered by cost effective intradermal regimens.

Intramuscular (IM) regimen

The currently available vaccines and regimens in India for IM administration are described below:

Essen schedule: Five dose intramuscular schedules is recommended for post-exposure prophylaxis. It consists of intramuscular administration of five injections on days 0, 3, 7, 14 and 28. Day 0 indicates the date of first injection and may not be the day/date of bite/exposure.

Site of injection: Anterolateral thigh is ideal for injection of these vaccines. Gluteal region is not recommended because the fat present in this region retards the absorption of antigen and hence, impairs the generation of optimal immune response.

Intradermal (ID) regimen

Intradermal regimen consists of administration of a fraction of intramuscular dose of CCVs at multiple sites in the layers of dermis of skin. The use of intradermal route leads to considerable savings in terms of total amount of vaccine needed for full pre- or post-exposure vaccination, thereby reducing the cost of active immunization. Single dose (0.5 mL/1 mL) of rabies vaccine/antigen when given by IM route gets deposited in the muscles. Thereafter the antigen is absorbed by the blood vessels and is presented to antigen presenting cells which triggers immune response. Whereas in ID route, small amount (0.1mL) of rabies vaccine/antigen is deposited in the layers of the skin at 2 or more sites. The antigen is directly taken up by the antigen presenting cells (Langerhans cells) within the layers of the skin, which then migrate to regional lymph nodes generating a stronger and quicker antibody response.

Updated Thai Red Cross (updated TRC-ID) schedule (2-2-2-0-2) is the ideal ID schedule. This involves injection of 0.1 mL of reconstituted vaccine per ID site and on two such ID sites per visit (one on each deltoid area, an inch above the insertion of deltoid muscle) on days 0, 3, 7 and 28. The day 0 is the day of first dose administration of IDRV and may not be the day of rabies exposure/animal bite. No vaccine is given on day 14.

14. Can the vaccines be used interchangeably?

Switch over from one brand of CCV/PDEV to other brand/type should not be encouraged as literature supports that good immunity is best achieved with same brand. However, under unavoidable circumstances, available brand/type of rabies vaccine may be used to complete PEP.

15. If a child is brought to you 2 months after a dog-bite and the fate of the dog is not known, should you start a course of rabies vaccination?

Definitely rabies vaccination has to be started, since the incubation period for rabies is anything between 4 days to 4 years and beyond, although the majority of human rabies cases occur within 3 months of exposure.

16. Under which circumstances should we consider pre-exposure prophylaxis in children?

Since 40–60% of all animal bite cases occur in children less than 15 years of age, the WHO considers them to be a vulnerable group and has recommended pre-exposure vaccination for children in "canine rabies endemic" countries.

It may be unrealistic and unnecessary, to consider all children for pre-exposure prophylaxis but one can perhaps focus on the "at-risk" group of children, such as:
  i. Where there is a pet dog in the house, even if immunized, since animals with a history of prior rabies vaccination, have also been known to transmit rabies.
  ii. A pet dog at a neighbor's house which the child visits, or if the dog comes to the child's house.
  iii. Where there are "community pets".
  iv. Stray dogs in the neighborhood of the house or school.

Schedule of pre-exposure vaccination

Intramuscular—Three doses of any CCRV (1 mL or 0.5 mL depending on the brand) administered on the anterolateral thigh or deltoid region on days 0, 7 and 28.

Intradermal—The dose (0.1 mL) is same for all vaccine brands and 0.1 mL is administered intradermally over the deltoid on days 0, 7 and 28.

Further Reading

1. Association for Prevention and Control of Rabies in India. Assessing Burden of Rabies in India, WHO Sponsored National Multi-centric Rabies Survey, Bangalore, India. www.apcri.org.
2. Sudarshan MK. Rabies. In: Parthasarathy A, Kundu R, Agrawal R, et al. (Eds). Textbook of Pediatric Infcetious Diseases, 1st edition. New Delhi, Jaypee Brothers; 2013.
3. World Health Organization. WHO expert consultation on rabies, First report, Technical Report Series: 931, Geneva, Switzerland; 2005.
4. World Health Organization. WHO recommendations on rabies post-exposure treatment and the correct technique of intra-dermal immunization against rabies. Geneva, Switzerland; 1997.

22

Viral Hepatitis

Malathi Sathiyasekaran

1. What is the epidemiology, mode of transmission and important characteristic features of the different hepatitis viruses?

The major hepatotropic viruses are Hepatitis A, B, C, D and E (HAV, HBV, HCV, HDV, HEV) of which all are RNA viruses except HBV which is a DNA virus. In this "hepatitis alphabet" HAV and HEV share some similarities, whereas HBV and HCV have some common features.

In India, sporadic Acute Viral Hepatitis (AVH) is caused by the two enterally transmitted viruses namely hepatitis A (60-70%) and hepatitis E (10-20%). Improvement in socioeconomic status has made an epidemiological shift in HAV with older children being more susceptible to the infection. Hepatitis E virus is prevalent in regions around the river Ganges and has been identified with the major hepatitis epidemics in India. The viruses HAV and HEV have an incubation period of 15 to 40 days and are spread by the orofecal route. They can present as acute hepatitis and acute liver failure but do not cause chronic infection. HEV infection during pregnancy is associated with a high maternal mortality and fetal deaths.

The two parenterally transmitted viruses namely HBV (10-15%) and HCV (<1%) are less common causes of acute sporadic hepatitis and have a long incubation period of 50 to 180 days. The prevalence of hepatitis B surface antigen (HBsAg) positivity in India is approximately 2 to 7%, whereas HCV is 1 to 2.5%. HBV is more infectious than HCV and is spread by blood, blood products and body fluids (cervico-vaginal secretions, semen, breast milk, saliva, tears). Perinatal transmission is also more common in HBV. Apart from mother to infant transmission, HCV is prevalent in those requiring multiple blood/blood product transfusions, IV drug users, hemodialysis and post organ transplant. These two viruses can present with acute hepatitis, acute liver failure, chronic hepatitis (persisting for more than 6 months) or cirrhosis. The incidence of chronicity in HBV is inversely proportional to the age of acquisition of the infection. A high incidence of 90% is seen in young infants following perinatal transmission, 25 to 40% in older children (less than 5 years of age) and 5 to 10% in teens and adults. HCV is a more sinister virus than HBV, but both result in chronicity, cirrhosis and hepatocellular carcinoma (HCC). HCV related complications present several years (15 to 20 years) following infection and are rarely seen in children compared to HBV infection. The several genotypes identified in HBV and HCV may modify the course of illness and response to therapy.

Hepatitis D

Hepatitis D virus cannot produce infection without a concurrent HBV infection because the virus cannot replicate without the help of Hepatits B Virus. Hepatits B virus, causing infection simultanously in a person is called as co-infection. If Hepatits D infects a person who is already infected with HBV, it is called super infection. Transmission occurs via parenteral route (in low endemic area) or through intimate contact (in high endemic area). Hepatits D virus infection must be considered in all causes of severe liver disease or acute liver failure. In coinfection, acute hepatitis is more severe than Hepatits B alone, but chronicity is rare, whereas in super infection chronic hepatitis is common.

2. **How do we interpret serological markers of various hepatitis viruses?**

I. Interpretation of serological markers in HAV and HEV infection

Virus	Test	Interpretation
Hepatitis A	Anti HAV IgM	Recent HAV infection/acute hepatitis A
Hepatitis A	Anti HAV IgG	Past HAV infection
Hepatitis E	Anti HEV IgM	Recent HEV infection/acute hepatitis E
Hepatitis E	Anti HEV IgG	Past HEV infection

II. Interpretation of HCV serology

Anti HCV	HCV RNA Quantitative/ SGPT	Interpretation
+ Appears later	Detectable + high SGPT	Acute hepatitis C (AHC)
+>6 m Positive for > 6 mth	+ > 6m + SGPT normal or > 2ULN Positive for >6 mth	Chronic hepatitis C
+	–	Resolution of infection/ Acute hepatitis period of low viremia
–	+	Early AHC/ Chronic infection in immunocompromised/ false positive

III. Interpretation of HBV serology along with SGPT

HBsAg	HBeAg	antiHBe	antiHBc	antiHBS	HBV DNA/ SGPT	Interpretation
+ +>6 m	+	–	IgM	–	High HBV DNA/SGPT ↑	Acute hepatitis
Positive for > 6 month	+	–	IgG	–	>20,000 IU/L, SGPT normal	Chronic hepatitis. Immune tolerance
+>6 m	+	–	IgG	–	>20,000 IU/L, SGPT >1.5 times UL/N > 3 m, Upper limit more than of normal for > 3 month	Chronic hepatitis- HBeAg +ve. immune active
+>6 m.	–	–	IgG	–	>2000 IU/L, SGPT >1.5 ULN	Chronic hepatitis HBeAg negative/ pre core mutant infection

Contd...

Contd...

HBsAg	HBeAg	antiHBe	antiHBc	antiHBS	HBV DNA/ SGPT	Interpretation
+>6 m	-	+	IgG	-	Low/SGPT normal >1.5 ULN	Chronic inactive HBsAg carrier
-	-	-	IgG	+	Undetected	Viral clearance following infection
-	-	-	-	+	-	Vaccination immunity

IV. Interpretation of HDV serology.
HDV infection can occur only in a HBsAg positive individual.

HBsAg	Anti HBcIgM	Anti HDV IgM	Interpretation
+	+	Low titers	Coinfection
+	-	High titers	Superinfection

3. What are the extrahepatic manifestations associated with HBV infection?

A spectrum of immune mediated extra-hepatic manifestations such as aplastic anemia, rash, leucoclastocytic vasculitis, glomerulonephritis, Guillain-Barré's syndrome, myocarditis, pancreatitis, urticaria, polyarteritis nodosa, migratory polyarthritis, cryoglobulinemia and papular acrodermatitis of childhood or Gianotti Crosti syndrome may be seen in HBV infection.

4. How can we prevent mother to child transmission (MTCT) of HBV infection?

There are some important facts to be considered in MTCT of HBV infection. If a mother is HBsAg and HBeAg positive with a high viral load, the transmission to the baby occurs not only during delivery, at the time of placental separation but may occur in 10 to 15% cases much earlier in utero. The likelihood of the newborn acquiring infection is as high as 90% when these biomarkers are present in the mother. The protective efficacy of the combined Hepatitis B immunoglobulin (HBIG) and vaccine also decreases in this group and 10 to 15% acquire infection inspite of the approved schedule. Hence in addition to administering HBIG and vaccine to the new born, antivirals are now recommended for a select group of pregnant mothers to prevent MTCT.

Combined Active and Passive immunization: If the mother is HBsAg positive, the neonate is given both passive immunization with Hepatitis B Immunoglobulin 0.5 mL and active immunization with Hepatitis B vaccine soon after birth or at least within 6 hours. The active immunization is then completed as per schedule.

In the majority of pregnant women with HBV infection, HBsAg is incidentally detected to be positive. Biochemical tests of the liver, HBeAg, anti HBe and HBV DNA viral load are included in the evaluation of these mothers. Based on the results, the algorithm (Flow chart 1) may be followed to prevent MTCT.

If SGPT is elevated more than 2 ULN, the mother is treated with antivirals.

5. What are the other indications for hepatitis B immunoglobulin?

Hepatitis B immunoglobulin is indicated in two situations apart from its use in preventing perinatal transmission.

I. Post Exposure prophylaxis: Occupational exposure and non occupational exposure.

Occupational exposure: Those who are occupied in high risk areas such as hemodialysis unit, transplant centers, blood banks are usually immunized, and therefore, may need only a booster with active immunization. In case they have not been immunized, HBI g 0.06 mL/kg along with active immunization is given at different sites within 24 hours of exposure. The immunization is completed in accordance with the age appropriate vaccine dose schedule.

Flow chart 1: Preventing MTCT in an infant of a HBsAg positive mother

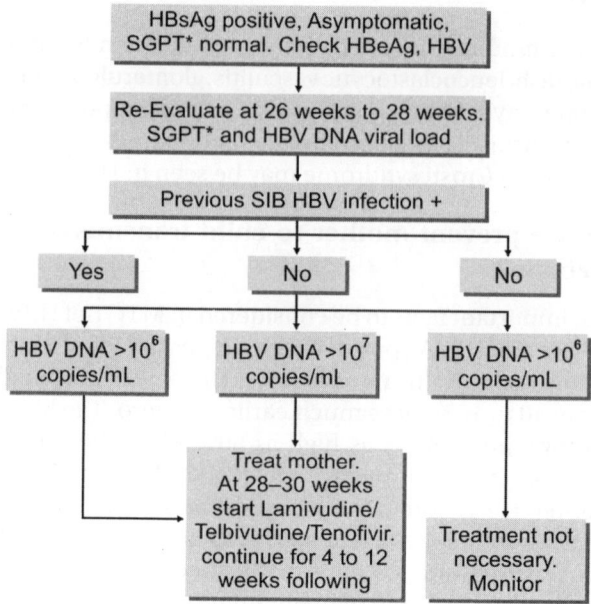

Nonoccupational exposure: If the exposure occurs to a known HBsAg positive source and the individual has a written documentation of immunization a booster dose of vaccine is sufficient. If the individual has neither completed the schedule nor has been immunized, both HBIg and vaccine are given at different sites within 24 hours of exposure. HB vaccine is then completed in accordance with the age appropriate vaccine dose and schedule.

II. Prophylaxis in Post liver transplant HBV infection: The prevention of HBV reinfection following liver transplant(LT) for HBV related liver disease is done by administering low- to high-dose HBIg with or without antivirals.

6. What are the long term complications of HBV infection?

The long term complications of HBV are chronic infection (HBeAg positive chronic hepatitis, HBeAg negative chronic hepatitis) cirrhosis, endstage liver disease, hepatocellular carcinoma and death. The outcome of HBV infection may be seen within 5 to 50 years and is shown in Flow chart 2.

7. What are the treatment options for the spectrum of hepatitis B infection?

Pediatric HBV infection is usually diagnosed incidentally or during antenatal screening or while evaluating acute and chronic liver disease. The common HBV related case scenarios which require management guidelines are perinatal infection, acute hepatitis, acute liver failure, chronic immune tolerant,

Flow chart 2: Outcome of HBV infection

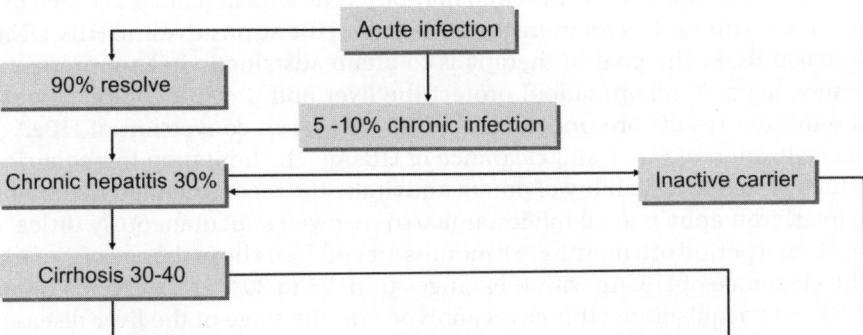

chronic inactive carrier, chronic HBeAg positive hepatitis, chronic HBeAg negative hepatitis, compensated cirrhosis, decompensated cirrhosis and special situations. The management of perinatal infection has been discussed in the previous paragraph.

Acute hepatitis: The child with acute hepatitis may be icteric or anicteric, with high transaminases > 20 ULN and is HBsAg positive, anti-HBcIgM positive with high viral load. During the illness, only supportive treatment is recommended and there is no role for antivirals. HBsAg and anti HBs are checked after 6 months, if HBsAg is negative and antibodies are present the child is considered to have cleared the virus and seroconverted naturally. If HBsAg continues to be positive even after 6 months, the child is considered to have chronic infection and is managed accordingly.

Acute liver failure: Liver transplant is the definitive management of children presenting with acute liver failure who do not respond to supportive treatment. Nucleoside analogs have been suggested for this group with progressive deterioration of liver function but this is controversial.

Chronic immune tolerant phase: This phase (high DNA with normal SGPT) may last upto 20 to 30 years in individuals infected perinatally. There is no role for antivirals or interferon in this phase even though the HBV DNA is very high. However, if the transaminases are fluctuating, a liver biopsy is done to document activity before considering therapy. If by the age of 40 years, the SGPT is still normal but there is a persistent high viral load, antivirals are recommended after liver biopsy.

Chronic inactive HBsAg carrier: This phase (normal SGPT, HBeAg negative and low viral load) does not warrant any therapy but needs regular monitoring of SGPT and HBV DNA. Since HBV infection is a dynamic disease reactivation may occur in 20 to 30% of inactive carriers and present as precore mutant infection/HBeAg negative chronic hepatitis.

Chronic HBeAg positive hepatitis: This is the phase where definitive therapy is recommended. The child may be icteric with hepatosplenomegaly, SGPT is 1.5 times ULN for more than 6 months, HBeAg positive and HBV DNA > 20,000 IU/L. The goal of therapy is to attain sustained viral suppression, reduce hepatic inflammation, protect the liver and prevent complications. The desired results are undetectable HBV DNA, seroconversion of HBeAg, normalization of SGPT and clearance of HBsAg. The limitation in pediatrics is the restricted availability of potent antivirals. The recommended treatment is interferon apha 6 to 10 million units/sq m, given subcutaneously thrice a week for a period of 6 months to 8 months for children above the age of 2 years. The clearance of HBsAg with IFN ranges from 25 to 30% and depends upon the age of acquisition, ethnicity, genotype and the stage of the liver disease. The introduction of lamivudine either in combination with interferon or post interferon has not shown consistent results. Lamivudine at a dose of 3 mg/kg is well tolerated but the high incidence of drug resistance makes it a poor candidate for therapeutic use. The other nucleos(t)ide analogs (NA) such as entecavir, tenofivir, telbivudine have better antiviral properties and less drug resistance but are recommended only in patients more than 16 years of age. The duration of therapy with NAs is not well defined. The recommended end point is twice undetectable HBV DNA levels 6 months apart in HBeAg positive and thrice undetectable levels at 6 months intervals in HBeAg negative hepatitis. The ideal end point would be to clear HBsAg if possible or to attain very low levels of HBsAg as assessed by quantitative HBsAg (qHBsAg).

Chronic HBeAg negative hepatitis: In this phase, therapy is recommended even when the viral load is > 2000 IU/L, HBeAg is negative, SGPT is >1.5 ULN. The response to therapy is less than in HBeAg positive hepatitis. The recommended dose of interferon is the same as for HBeAg positive chronic hepatitis but the duration of therapy is longer varying from 12 months to 24 months.

Compensated cirrhosis: In children with HBV related compensated cirrhosis if the HBV DNA is less than 2000 IU/L, no treatment is recommended. They should be monitored regularly with HBV DNA and SGPT and therapy initiated when necessary. If the HBV DNA is more than 2000 IU/L with SGPT more than 5 ULN then antivirals are indicated whereas if SGPT is less than 5 times ULN interferon, antivirals are recommended.

Decompensated cirrhosis: In HBV related decompensated cirrhosis, there is no role for interferon therapy. Irrespective of HBV DNA levels, NAs are prescribed and the patient is registered for liver transplantation.

Special Situations: Children who are HBsAg positive and are on chemotherapy or immunosuppression irrespective of HBV DNA levels should be started on antivirals and continued for 12 months after the cessation of therapy. The other conditions where either short or long term antivirals should be considered are glomerulonephritis due to HBV infection, prevention or treatment of recurrent HBV infection after liver transplantation, recipient of a liver graft from an anti-hepatitis B core antigen (anti-HBc)-positive donor, presence of coinfections (HBV/HIV, HBV/HCV, HBV/HDV) and those who are in the immune active phase with a strong family history of HCC (hepatocellular carcinoma).

8. How should we manage a child who is incidentally detected to be HBsAg positive?

When an asymptomatic child is incidentally detected to be HBsAg positive, he should be considered as an individual who is at risk not only for presenting with the disease at any point in his life time but also the one who can transmit the infection to susceptible individuals. Knowing the dynamic nature of the disease, he should be evaluated methodically using seven simple steps:

1. The first step is the basic evaluation which includes a detailed history (surgery, blood transfusion, tattoo, family history of jaundice) and physical examination (hepatosplenomegaly, clubbing, abdominal veins). If there are features of liver disease then further investigation such as prothrombin time, US abdomen, alpha fetoprotein and upper GI endoscopy are done.
2. Check the status of the liver using SGPT as a surrogate marker and also the viral status whether infection is recent or a past exposure. If the infection is recent, i.e. anti HBcIgM positive with normal or elevated SGPT he should be observed and reviewed after 6 months. If he continues to be HBsAg positive after 6 months then he should be evaluated in detail and treated accordingly. If he is anti HBcIgM negative then the other viral markers are done.
3. The third step is the classification into the various groups mentioned above according to the SGPT, HBeAg and HBV DNA viral load. Hence, HBV DNA becomes a very essential test in the evaluation of all children who are HBsAg positive.
4. The fourth step is the therapy of the specific groups and in special situations.
5. Education of the child and the family regarding the modes of transmission and prevention including screening of contacts and immunization of those who are HBsAg negative.
6. Prevention of further liver damage by viruses (Hepatitis A vaccine to be advised) medication, alcohol and obesity.
7. Regular follow up and monitoring of all children who are incidentally detected to be HBsAg positive.

9. How do we identify and manage pediatric hepatitis C infection?

Children with HCV infection differ from adults in several ways including some modes of transmission, rates of clearance, progression of fibrosis, and the duration of potential chronic infection when infection is acquired at birth.

Neonatal hepatitis C infection is defined as detectable HCV RNA in an infant's blood in the first 1 to 6 months of life following maternal-to-infant transmission of HCV infection.

Perinatal transient viremia is the detection of HCV RNA in peripheral blood within 0 to 5 days of birth.

Acute hepatitis (AHC) is usually asymptomatic and not perceived clinically. High transaminases >20 ULN and presence of HCV RNA with anti HCV appearing later are characteristic of AHC.

Chronic HCV infection (CHC) is evident by active viral infection with detectable HCV RNA for at least 6 months.

A striking feature of pediatric HCV infection is the spontaneous resolution of neonatal AHC which occurs in 25 to 40% by 24 months. These children are therefore rechecked for HCV RNA at 18 months of age. Chronic HCV infection acquired either through mother to child transmission or blood transfusion also has a tendency to resolve by 7 years of age. The infection is mild in those where resolution does not occur with mild elevation of transaminases and minimal changes on histopathology.

Management: Since HCV infection in children seems to be mild with a slow progression, postponing therapy and following up these children until adulthood seems to be a valid therapeutic option. Conversely, treatment may be justified because it allows definitive resolution in a subgroup of patients. North American society for pediatric gastroenterology, hepatology and nutrition (NASPGHAN) recommends that children with hepatitis C who demonstrate persistently elevated serum aminotransferases or those with progressive disease (ie fibrosis on liver histology) should be considered for treatment. The American association for the study of liver diseases (AASLD) recommends the combination of PEG-IFN-α with ribavirin as first-line treatment for CHC in children of ages 3 to 17 years. The duration of therapy is 48 weeks for genotypes 1 or 4 and 24 weeks for genotypes 2 or 3. Children are susceptible to deficits in growth in both weight and height while receiving PEG-IFN-and ribavirin and therefore need to be monitored. The sustained viral response (SVR) as seen in adults is 90% in genotype 2 and 3 and 53% for children with genotype I. Preventing perinatal transmission and screening of blood products for HCV prior to transfusion and education of IV drug users, will help in reducing the global burden of HCV.

Further Reading

1. Bortolotti F, Verucchi G, Camma C, et al. Long-term course of chronic hepatitis C in children: from viral clearance to end-stage liver disease. Gastroenterology 2008;134:1900-7.
2. Centers for Disease Control and Prevention (CDC). Updated CDC recommendations for the management of hepatitis B virus-infected health-care providers and students. MMWR Recomm Rep. 2012;61:1.
3. European Association for the Study of the Liver. EASL clinical practice guidelines: Management of chronic hepatitis B virus infection. J Hepatol. 2012; 57:167.
4. Ghany MG, Nelson DR, Strader DB, et al. An update on treatment of genotype 1 chronic hepatitis C virus infection: 2011 practice guideline by the AASLD. Hepatology 2011;54:1433-44.

5. Ghendon Y. Perinatal transmission of hepatitis B virus in high-incidence countries. J Virol Methods. 1987;17(1-2):69-79.
6. Jonas MM, Block JM, Haber BA, Karpen SJ, London WT, Murray KF, et al.Treatment of children with chronic hepatitis B virus infection in the United States: patient selection and therapeutic options. Hepatology 2010;52:2192-2205.
7. Jonas MM, Little NR, Gardner SD. Long-term lamivudine treatment of children with chronic hepatitis B: Durability of therapeutic responses and safety. J Viral Hepat 2008;15:20-7.
8. Kamath SR, Sathiyasekaran M, Raja TE. Profile of viral hepatitis A in Chennai. Indian Pediatr. 2009;46:642-3.
9. MackCara L, Gonzalez-PeraltaRegino P, Nitika G, Daniel L, Narkewicz Michael R, Roberts Eve A, Philip R, Kathleen BS. NASPGHAN Practice Guidelines: Diagnosis and Management of Hepatitis C Infection in Infants, Children, and Adolescents. J Pediatr Gastroenterol Nutr. 2012;54:838-55.
10. Mast EE, Weinbaum CM, Fiore AE, et al. A comprehensive immunization strategy to eliminate transmission of hepatitis B virus infection in the United States: Recommendations of the Advisory Committee on Immunization Practices (ACIP) Part II: Immunization of adults. MMWR Recomm Rep. 2006;55:1.
11. Payam D, Mohamad JS, Moayed AS. Hepatitis B Immune Globulin in Liver Transplantation Prophylaxis: An Update. Hepat Mon. 2012;12(3):168-76.
12. Rong HG, Lu XC, Wei Z, Feng YY. Management of chronic hepatitis B in pregnancy. World J Gastroenterol. 2012 ; 18(33): 4517-21.
13. Shah U, Kelly D, Chang MH, Fujisawa T, Heller S, González-Peralta RP, Jara P, Mieli-Vergani G, Mohan N, Murray KF. Management of chronic hepatitis B in children. J Pediatr Gastroenterol Nutr. 2009 Apr;48(4):399-404.
14. Shi Z, Yang Y, Ma L, Li X, Schreiber A. Lamivudine in late pregnancy to interrupt inutero transmission of hepatitis B virus: A systematic review and meta-analysis. Obstet Gynecol. 2010 Jul;116(1):147-59. doi: 10.1097/AOG.0b013e3181e45951.
15. Tagle M, Marioa MD, Schiff ER. Hepatitis A and E. In: Bacon BR, O'Grady JG, Di Bisceglie AM, Lake JR (Eds). Comprehensive Clinical Hepatology, 2nd edition. Mosby Elseiver; 2010. p. 205-12.
16. Wirth S, Lang T, Gehring S, et al. Recombinant alfa-interferon plus ribavirin therapy in children and adolescents with chronic hepatitis C. Hepatology 2002;36:1280-4.

23

Chikungunya

Rajniti Prasad

1. What is the epidemiology of chikungunya?

Chikungunya is a viral fever caused by an Alphavirus (RNA) of Togaviridae family and spread by infected *Aedes aegypti* mosquito. Other reported vectors are *Aedes albopictus, Aedes polynesiensis* and *culex*. Chikungunya virus (CHIKV) was probably an infection of primates in forests of savannahs of Africa. However chikungunya fever is endemic in large parts of Africa and Asia. In India, recent outbreak has started from coastal areas of Andhra Pradesh and Karnataka and involved all states.

Chikungunya is transmitted through the bite of infected aedes mosquito to humans during daytime. Mother-to-child transmission, occupational exposure and occurrence among heath workers due to careless handling of patient's blood has also been reported. Monkeys and other wild animals may be the reservoir of infection. Mosquito breeds mainly in manmade containers.

The incubation period is usually 2-4 days (range—1-12 days).

2. What is the typical clinical presentation of chikungunya?

Chikungunya is characterized by triad of fever, arthralgia and rash. Fever is usually abrupt onset with chills, myalgia, headache and photophobia that lasts for 2-3 days. Fever may remit for 1-2 days after a gap of 4-10 days, typically described as saddle back fever.

The arthralgias are polyarticular, migratory and mainly affect the small joints of hands, wrists, ankles and feet. Pain is worse in the morning improved by mild exercise and worsens by heavy exercise. Fluid accumulation is uncommon.

The cutaneous manifestations include flushing of face and trunk followed by maculopapular rashes. Trunks and limbs are primarily involved but may involve face, palms and soles. Rashes may fade or desquamate.

Other manifestations are iridocyclitis, retinitis, diarrhea, vomiting, abdomninal pain, encephalopathy, encephalitis, febrile seizures, and Guilain Barre syndrone.

3. What are the laboratory tests to confirm diagnosis?

Three main laboratory tests are used for diagnosing chikungunya fever:
  i. Isolation of the virus in cell culture is the gold standard. Recently reverse transcriptase PCR (RTPCR) is developed and results can be obtained within 1–2 days.
  ii. Serological diagnosis: The demonstration of fourfold rise in antibody in acute or convalescent sera or demonstrating IgM antibody specific for the virus. A commonly used test is the IgM antibody capture enzyme linked immunosorbent assay (MAC-ELISA). Its result can be available within 2-3 days.
  iii. Polymerase chain reaction(PCR) for E1 and C genome either singly or together constitute a positive result.

4. What are differential diagnosis of chikungunya?

The differential diagnosis include dengue fever, rubella, parvovirus B19 infection, herpes virus infection, leptospirosis, falciparum malaria and mumps.

5. What are the diagnostic criteria of chikungunya?

The diagnostic criteria of chikungunya fever are mentioned below:

Suspected case

A patient presenting with acute onset of fever usually with chills/rigors, which lasts for 3–5 days with multiple joint pains/swelling of extremities that may continue for weeks to months.

Probable case

A suspected case (see above) with any one of the following:
- History of travel or residence in areas reporting outbreaks
- Ability to exclude malaria, dengue and any other known cause for fever with joint pains.

Confirmed case

- Any patient who meets one or more of the following findings irrespective of the clinical presentation
- Virus isolation in cell culture or animal inoculations from acute phase sera
- Presence of viral RNA in acute phase sera by RT-PCR
- Presence of virus-specific IgM antibodies in single serum sample in acute or convalescent stage
- Four fold increase in virus-specific IgG antibody titer in samples collected at least three weeks apart.

RNA: Ribonucleic acid; RT-PCR: Reverse transcription polymerase chain reaction; IgM: Immunoglobulin M; IgG: Immunoglobulin G.

6. What are the long-term effect of chikungunya fever?

Most of the symptomatic patients have a chronic stage of disease characterized by pain in joints (persistent arthralgias) and arthritis or both. The pain was continuous or intermittent with frequent clinical remission and relapses.

Further Reading

1. Burt FJ, Rolph MS, Rulli NE, Mahalingam NE, Heise MT. Chikungunya: a re-emerging virus. Lancet 2012;379:662-71.
2. Chhabra M, Mittal V, Bhattacharya D, Rana U, Lal S. Chikungunya fever: A re-emerging viral infection. Indian J Med Microbiol. 2008;26:5-12.
3. Inamadar AC, Palit A, Sampagavi VV, Raghunath S,Deshmukh NS. Cutaneous manifestations of chikungunya fever: observations made during a recent outbreak in south India. Intern J Dermatol. 2008;47:154-9.
4. Khan AH, Morita K, Parquet MC, Hasebe F, Mathenge EG, Igarashi A. Complete nucleotide sequence of chikungunya virus and evidence for an internal polyadenylation site. J Gen Virol. 2002;83:3075-84.
5. Lahariya C, Pradhan SK. Emergence of chikungunya virus in Indian subcontinent after 32 years: a review. J Vect Borne Dis. 2006;43:151-60.
6. Mahendradas P, Ranganna SK, Shetty R, Balu R, Narayana KM, Babu RB, et al. Ocular manifestations associated with chikungunya. Ophthalmology. 2008; 115(2):287-91.
7. Mohan A. Chikungunya fever: clinical manifestations and management. Indian J Med Res. 2006; 124:471-4.
8. Parola P, Lamballerie X, Jourdan J, et al. Novel chikungunya virus variant in travelers returning from Indian Ocean Islands. Emerg Infect Dis. 2006; 12:1493-99.
9. Pialoux G, Gauzere BA, Strobel M. Chikungunya virus infection: review through an epidemic. Med Mal Infect. 2006; 36: 253-63.
10. Powers AM, Brault AC, Tesh RB, et al. Re- emergence of Chikungunya and O' nyong-nyong viruses: evidence for distinct geographical lineages and distant evolutionary relationships. J Gen Virol. 2000;81:471-9.
11. Queyriaux B, Simon F, Grandadam M, Michel R, Hugues Tolou, Jean-Paul Boutin. Clinical burden of chikungunya virus infection. Lancet Infect Dis. 2008;1:2-3.
12. WHO. Disease outbreak news. Chikungunya and dengue in the southwest Indian Ocean, Geneva. 17 March 2006.

PART C: FUNGAL AND PROTOZOAL INFECTIONS

24
Common Fungi

Kheya Ghosh Uttam

1. What are the common fungal species which affect children?

Fungal infections can be superficial or systemic. Superficial fungal infection is commonly caused by dermatophytes, *Malassezia* and *Candida*. Systemic fungal infection in immunocompetent host is mostly due to histoplasma, coccidioides and blastomyces. Systemic fungal infection in immunocompromised host may be due to *Candida*, *Aspergillus*, pneumocystis, *Cryptococcus*, *Mucorales*, *Malassezia*. Subcutaneous fungal infections by *Sporothrix* are relatively uncommon.

2. When to suspect fungal infection in neonatal intensive care unit and pediatric intensive care unit?

Nosocomial fungal infection in intensive care unit is rising. It should be suspected in any neonate who is not recovering adequately inspite of sensitive antibiotic in proper doses with any of the risk factors. The risk factors for invasive fungal disease in a neonates are low birth weight (especially birth weight < 1,000 grams), delay in enteral feeding and exposure to 3rd generation cephalosporins, prolonged intubation, presence of central venous catheters, parenteral nutrition, intralipid infusion, shock and DIC.

Fungal infection should be suspected in a PICU if fever remains unresponsive to antibiotics in adequate dose and the child has any one or more of the following:
  i. Poor or worsening clinical stability.
  ii. Prolonged prior exposure to antibacterial agents.
  iii. Prolonged central venous or foley catheterization.
  iv. Recent history of abdominal perforation.
  v. T-lymphocyte dysfunction.

3. What are the different clinical types of candidiasis?

Candidiasis can affect different organ systems varying from benign superficial infections to deep invasive or systemic infections. Candida species causing systemic infection are *C. albicans*, *C. tropicalis*, *C. parapsilosis* and *C. glabrata*, *C. kruzei*. Normally *C. albicans* can be present in small numbers on skin, mucous membranes, or in the intestinal tract Intact epithelial barriers, normal neutrophils lymphocyte and macrophage function, adequate antibody and complement level, and normal bacterial flora are the host factors, which prevent invasion.

Superficial candidiasis

Oral thrush

Typically the lesions are few or extensive adherent creamy white painful plaques on the buccal, gingival, or lingual mucosa. Oral thrush may be asymptomatic or it may cause pain and decreased feeding. Thrush is very common in otherwise normal infants in the first weeks of life; it may last weeks despite topical therapy. Spontaneous thrush in older children is unusual unless they have recently received antimicrobials or are immunosuppressed. Corticosteroid inhalation is the most common predisposing factor. Angular cheilitis is caused by *Candida* at the corners of the mouth, often in association with a vitamin or iron deficiency.

Diaper dermatitis

It occurs most commonly due to Candida. The lesions are confluent erythematous and satellite lesions are common . Pustules, vesicles, papules, or scales may be seen. Weeping, eroded lesions with a scalloped border are common. Moist areas, such as axillae or neck folds are frequently involved.

Vaginal infection

Vulvovaginitis occurs in sexually active girls, pregnant women, diabetic patients, and in those on prolonged antibiotic or oral contraceptive therapy. Patients present with thick, odorless, cheesy discharge with intense pruritus. The vagina and labia are erythematous and swollen.

Congenital cutaneous candidiasis

These lesions may be seen in infants born to women with Candida amnionitis or after prolonged rupture of membranes in an affected mother. A red maculopapular or pustular rash or erythema is characteristically present at birth.

Paronychia and onychomycosis

These conditions may occur in immunocompetent children but are more commonly associated with immunosuppression, diabetes mellitus, hypoparathyroidism, or adrenal insufficiency (Candida endocrinopathy syndrome). Paronychia and onychomycosis is usually caused by trichophyton and epidermophyton but can also be due to candida, which usually involves the fingernails and not the toe nails.

Systemic candidiasis

Enteric infection

Esophageal involvement is most common in immunosuppressed. It is manifests as substernal pain, dysphagia, painful swallowing, and anorexia.

Nausea and vomiting are common in young children. Most patients do not have thrush. Stomach or intestinal ulcers also occur. Atrophic glossitis, chronic hyperplastic candidiasis may occur in critically ill children. A syndrome of mild diarrhea in normal individuals who have predominant *Candida* on stool culture has also been described, although *Candida* is not considered a true enteric pathogen. Its presence more often reflects recent antimicrobial therapy.

Pulmonary infection

Because the organism frequently colonizes the respiratory tract, it is commonly isolated from respiratory secretions. Thus, demonstration of tissue invasion is needed to diagnose Candida pneumonia or tracheitis. It is rare, being seen in immunosuppressed patients and patients intubated for long periods, usually while taking antibiotics. The infection may cause fever, cough, abscesses, nodular infiltrates, and effusion.

Urinary tract infection

Candiduria may be the only manifestation of disseminated disease. More often, candiduria is associated with instrumentation, an indwelling catheter, anatomic abnormality of the urinary tract or immunosupressed host especially in diabetics. It is usually asymptomatic but symptoms of cystitis may be present. Masses of Candida (fungal balls) may obstruct ureters and cause obstructive nephropathy. Candida casts in the urine suggest renal tissue infection.

Other infections

Endocarditis, myocarditis, meningitis, and osteomyelitis may occur in immunocompromised patients or neonates.

Disseminated candidiasis

This occurs in neonates, especially in premature infants, in an intensive care setting, and is recognized when the infant fails to respond to antibiotics or when candidemia is documented. These infants have unexplained feeding intolerance, cardiovascular instability, apnea, new or worsening respiratory failure, glucose intolerance, thrombocytopenia, or hyperbilirubinemia. Treatment for presumptive infection is often undertaken because candidemia is not identified in many such patients.

Hepatosplenic candidiasis occurs in immunosuppressed, severely neutropenic patients with chronic fever, variable abdominal pain, and abnormal liver function tests. Symptoms persist even when neutrophils return. It may occur with or without fungemia. Ultrasound or CT scan of the liver and spleen demonstrates multiple round lesions. Biopsy is confirmative.

4. What is the epidemiology of histoplasmosis?

The dimorphic fungus *Histoplasma capsulatum* is found in soil rich in nitrates such as soil contaminated with feces of bat or bird, or decayed wood. The small yeast form (2-4 m) is seen in tissue, especially within macrophages. Infection is acquired by inhaling spores that transform into the pathogenic yeast phase in the alveoli. Reactivation is very rare in children. Re-infection also occurs. The extent of symptoms with primary or reinfection is influenced by the size of the infecting inoculum. Human-to-human transmission and congenital infection does not occur.

5. What are the clinical manifestation of histoplasmosis?

Asymptomatic infection

About 90% cases presents as asymptomatic infections. Asymptomatic histoplasmosis is usually diagnosed by the presence of scattered calcifications in lungs or spleen and a positive skin test, with its nearest differential being Gohn's focus.

Pneumonia

Approximately 5% of patients have mild to moderate disease. Acute pulmonary disease may resemble influenza, with fever, myalgia, arthralgia, and cough occurring 1-3 weeks after exposure; the subacute form resembles infections such as tuberculosis, with cough, weight loss, night sweats, and pleurisy. Most children have a normal chest X-ray but may have patchy bronchopneumonia and hilar lymphadenopathy. Chronic disease is unusual in children. The usual duration of the disease is less than 2 weeks, followed by complete resolution. Symptoms may last several months and still resolve without antifungal therapy.

Disseminated infection

About 5% are disseminated infections. Fungemia during primary infection probably occurs in the first 2 weeks of all infections, including those with minimal symptoms. Resolution is the rule in immunocompetent individuals. Dissemination may occur in otherwise immunocompetent children; especially in younger children of less than 2 years. The majority presents with hepatosplenomegaly, enlarged lymph node, anemia and thrombocytopenia. pneumonia and pancytopenia are variably present.

Other forms

Ocular involvement consists of multifocal choroiditis and is common in adults. Brain, pericardium, intestine, and skin (oral ulcers and nodules) are other involved sites. Adrenal gland involvement is common with systemic disease.

6. What are the common opportunistic fungal infections and how they present? How they are treated?

Opportunistic fungal infections are always included in the differential diagnosis for immunocompromised patients with unexplained fever or pulmonary infiltrates. These pathogens should be aggressively pursued with imaging studies and with tissue sampling when clues are available. These infections occur most commonly when patients are treated with corticosteroids, antineoplastic drugs, or radiation, thereby reducing the number or function of neutrophils and competent lymphocytes. Inborn errors in immune function (combined immune deficiency or chronic granulomatous disease) may also be complicated by these fungal infections.

Aspergillus species (usually fumigatus) and Zygomycetes (usually Mucorales) cause subacute pneumonia and nasopharyngeal infection and should be considered when these conditions do not respond to antibiotics in immunocompromised patients.

Systemic aspergilosis is the second most common invasive fungal infection in critically ill child. Aspergilosis may manifest as relatively noninvasive disease (an aspergilloma in a pre-existing pulmonary cavity, or allergic bronchopulmonary aspergillosis in patients with bronchiectasis) or invasive disease as necrotizing bronchopneumonia with invasion of the pulmonary vessels. This may results in widespread fungal embolization to heart, GI tract, skin, kidney, liver and CNS. Aspergillus rhinosinusitis should be suspected when a neutropenic patient develops fever with signs and symptoms of rhinitis or sinusitis. Cavernous sinus thrombosis and CNS involvement may occur as a complication.

Mucormycosis is especially likely to produce severe sinusitis in patients with chronic acidosis, usually because of poorly controlled diabetes. This fungus may invade the orbit and cause brain infection. Mucormycosis also occurs in patients receiving iron chelation therapy. These fungal infections may disseminate widely. Imaging procedures may suggest the etiology, but they are best diagnosed by aspiration or biopsy of infected tissues.

Cryptococcus, which can cause disease in the immunocompetent host, is more likely to be clinically apparent and severe in immunocompromised patients with T cell immune defect, such as those seen in HIV infection or acute lymphoblastic leukemia. This yeast causes pneumonia or it may disseminate hematogenously to any organ system. The CNS is the most common site of infection and it presents with features of chronic meningitis.

Malassezia furfur is a yeast that normally causes the superficial skin infection known as tinea versicolor. This organism is considered an opportunist when it is associated with prolonged intravenous therapy, especially central lines used for hyperalimentation. The yeast, which requires skin lipids for its growth, can infect lines when lipids are present in the infusate. Some species will grow in the absence of lipids. Unexplained fever and thrombocytopenia are common. Pulmonary infiltrates may be present. The diagnosis is facilitated by alerting the bacteriology laboratory to add olive oil to culture media. The infection will respond to removal of the line or the lipid supplement. Amphotericin B may hasten resolution.

Pneumocystis jiroveci, though classified as a fungus on the basis of structural and nucleic acid characteristics, it responds readily to antiprotozoal drugs. It is a ubiquitous pathogen. Initial infection is presumed to occur asymptomatically via inhalation and tends to become a clinical problem upon reactivation during immune suppression. Severe signs and symptoms occur chiefly in patients with abnormal T-cell function, such as occurs with HIV infection, hematologic malignancies, and organ transplantation. It is one of the AIDS defining illnesses. Prophylaxis with trimethoprim and sulfamethoxazole (TMP-SMZ) usually prevents this infection. Infection is generally limited to the lower respiratory tract. In advanced disease, spread to other organs occurs.

Opportunistic fungal infections are difficult to treat. Amphotericin B and appropriate triazole drugs are usually indicated. The echinocandins and voriconazole are now used to treat Candida and Aspergillus infections. Combinations of current antifungal drugs are being tested to improve the outcome. *Pneumocystis jiroveci* infection is treated with TMP-SMZ (initially IV) and corticosteroids. The alternative therapy is with IV pentamidine.

7. How to treat invasive fungal infections?

Empiric therapy for invasive fungal infections should be intravenous amphotericin B or its lipid preparations which are less nephrotoxic. Central venous catheters should be promptly removed, if feasible, for faster resolution of infections and to prevent further blood borne dissemination and endocarditis. Definitive treatment should be based on site of infection, type and sensitivity pattern of the identified fungus. The drugs for invasive fungal infection with their doses have been summarized in Table 1.

Table 1: Dosing of the drugs in invasive fungal infections

Drug	Suggested dose
Amphotericin B deoxycholate	1 mg/kg/day
Liposomal amphotericin B	5 mg/kg/day
Fluconazole	12 mg/kg/day
Voriconazole*	7 mg/kg every 12 hour
Micafungin	4-10 mg/kg/day
Caspofungin**	50 mg/m^2/day
Anidulafungin**	1.5 mg/kg/day

* Voriconazole dose for neonates has not been investigated.
** Caspofungin and anidulafungin should be avoided in neonates and infants.

Treatment options according to fungal isolates

Candida

Fluconazole should be used for susceptible organism and less critically ill children. Fluconazole should not be used for *Candida krusei* and few isolates of *Candida glabrata*. Newer azoles like itraconazole and voricanazole are acceptable second line drugs for systemic fungal infections. Amphotericin B is traditionally used for systemic fungal infection. It is inactive against few strains of *C. Lusitaniae*. Lipid formulations are used for patients with renal problems. Echinocandins are favored for severely ill children.

Cryptococcus

Immunocompetent patients with pulmonary diseases are treated with oral fluconazole or itraconazole for 3-12 months. Immunocompetent children with serious diseases (bone or CNS infections) should be treated with amphotericin B plus flucytosine for 6-8 weeks.

Immunocompromised children treated with induction therapy with Amphotericin B plus flucytosine for minimum 2 weeks and as long as 6-10 weeks depending on the clinical response. A lumbar puncture is performed after 2 weeks of therapy and if CSF study is positive a longer treatment is required. Induction is followed by a consolidation phase with oral fluconazole for a minimum of 6-12 months. Lifelong therapy is required if the child remains immunocomprmised or in HIV infected patients. Itraconazole may also be used provided there is no CNS infection and the child is not HIV infected.

Invasive aspergillosis

According to 2008 guidelines of Infectious Disease Society of America, primary therapy for Invasive Aspergillosis is now voriconazole. Posaconazole may be an alternative agent but pharmacokinetic studies in pediatric patients is lacking. Amphotericin B and its lipid preparation, used earlier, may still have a role as first line therapy for Invasive Aspergillosis in certain patients.

Echinocandins in Invasive Aspergillosis is considered as second line medication.

Histoplasmosis

Asymptomatic or mildly symptomatic requires no treatment. Symptomatic for more than one month—oral itraconazole or fluconazole for 6-12 months.

Moderate to severe form or hypoxemic patients requiring respiratory support. Amphotericin B should be used until improvement (2 weeks-6 weeks) followed by oral itraconazole for 12 weeks. Sometimes prolonged therapy may be needed depending upon the severity. In HIV patients, lifelong suppressive therapy with daily itraconazole is required.

Coccidioidomycosis

Treatment will depend upon the severity of the disease. Mild acute pneumonia may not require treatment. First line drugs for uncomplicated pneumonia include oral and intravenous preparation of fluconazole and itraconazole. Serum level of itraconazole should be monitored.

In severe and progressive infections (disseminated disease, meningitis, diffuse pneumonia and in immunocompromised patients), amphotericin B is preferred for initial treatment and maintained by prolonged azole therapy. Duration of therapy varies from 3 to 6 months to one year or more, with follow up at 1-3 months.

Blastomycosis

In newborn infection should be treated with amphotericin B. Mild-to-moderate infection is treated with Itraconazole for 6–12 months. In case of severe and CNS blastomycosis initial treatment should be with amphotericin B followed by itraconazole. Serum level of itraconazole should be monitored.

Further Reading

1. Balasubramanian S. Protozoal, parasitic and Fungal infections. In: Parthasarathy A (ed). Textbook of Pediatric Infectious Diseases, 1st edition. New Delhi: Jaypee Brothers. 2013.
2. Burgos A, et al. Pediatric invasive aspergillosis: a multicenter retrospective analysis. Pediatrics. 2008;121:e1286-94.
3. Maschmeyer G, et al. Invasive aspergillosis: Epidemiology, diagnosis and management in immunocompromised patients. Drug. 2007;67:1567 [PMID: 17661528].
4. Mennink-Kersten M, Verweij PE. Non-culture-based diagnostics. Infect Dis Clin N Am. 2006;20:711-27.
5. Sharma A. Fungal infection in critically ill Children. In: Nadel S (ed). Infectious Diseases in the Pediatric Intensive Care Unit, 1st edition. Springer-Verlag London limited. 2008.
6. Silveira FP, Hussain S. Fungal infections in solid organ transplantation. Med Mycol 2007;45:305. [PMID: 17510855] Kyle C (ed). A handbook for the interpretation of laboratory tests. 4th Ed. Auckland: Diagnostic Medlab; 2008.

25
Kala-azar

Nigam P Narain

1. What are the common clinical presentations of Kala-azar?

Clinical Features of Kala-azar

Fever: It is intermittent with double rise in a day.

Splenomegaly: Massive but usually of gradual onset and may take more than 6 months to enlarge that big.

Hepatomegaly: Not very prominent.

Weight loss

Darkening of Skin: Over face, hands, feet, and abdomen (common in India) which characteristically gives its name Kala-azar ('Black fever').

Features of secondary infections: Due to immunosuppression, infection is common particularly tuberculosis.

In India, the course can be quite rapid and sometimes fatal with lymphadenopathy, anasarca, and fever with rigor and vomiting.

Atypical features
   i. Lymphadenopathy
   ii. Post kala-azar dermal leishmaniasis (PKDL)—Occurs several years after apparent cure of kala-azar, multiple nodular infiltration of the skin usually without ulceration. Parasites are numerous in the lesion.

2. What are the suggestive and confirmatory laboratory tests available for kala-azar?

Direct evidence

Peripheral blood films do not show the parasites and hence following tissues are examined for parasites:
- Bone marrow examination—By sternal/iliac puncture (amastigotes), 60–85% sensitivity
- Splenic puncture—98% sensitivity, an extremely important procedure if done with proper precaution.

Indirect evidences

- Changes in blood picture as suggested by blood count (leukopenia) with relative increase of lymphocytes and monocytes. Eosinophils may be absent
- Erythrocytes are decreased in number
- Proportion of leukocytes: erythrocytes = 1:2000 to 1000 (normal = 1:750)
- Increased ESR
- Rise in serum gamma-globulin.

Among all the tests mentioned above, finding of parasite remains the gold standard for diagnosis of the individual patient.

Newer diagnostic tools

rK 39 Strip test: A dipstick test, is based on the cloned antigen of a 39 amino acid repeat that is part of a 230 kDa protein encoded by a kinesin-like gene of *L chagasi*. A recombinant antigen, rK39, has been shown to be specific for antibodies in patients with visceral leishmaniasis caused by members of the *L. donovani* complex. This antigen is highly sensitive and predictive of the onset of acute disease. Recently, this test has been evaluated in diagnosis of Kala-azar. ELISA using K39 antigen has been found to be about 82–100% specific and 85-100% sensitive in the diagnosis of Kala-azar. A ready to use strip test has been developed for rapid testing in field conditions. The reading of the test is done after exactly 10 minutes. A dipstick test is considered positive when both the internal control and the test band are stained (irrespective of the intensity of the staining).

2. **When to avoid Splenic puncture in Kala-azar?**

Splenic puncture is one of the most valuable methods for diagnosis with sensitivity exceeding 95% but it carries a risk of fatal hemorrhage in inexperienced hands. Splenic aspiration should not be done if the prothombin time is more than 5 seconds longer than that of the control or if the platelet count is below 40×10^9/L (40,000/cu mm).

The two important factors for safety are that the needle remains within the spleen for less than 1 second and the entry and exit axis of the aspirating needle are identical to avoid tearing of splenic capsule.

3. **What is the clinical manifestation of Kala-azar in HIV-infected child? How to treat these children?**

Atypical clinical presentation of visceral leishmaniasis in HIV-infected patients pose a considerable diagnostic challenge.
- Diagnostic principles remain essentially same
- Amastigotes may be demonstrated in buffy coat preparation
- Amastigotes can be demonstrated in bone marrow
- Sensitivity of antibody based immunologic tests is low

- Leshmania amastigotes can be found at unexpected locations like the stomach, colon or lungs
- PCR analysis of the whole blood or its buffy coat preparation may prove a useful screening test for these patients
- Treatment options which have been tried largely in adult population consist of liposomal amphotericin B along with combined anti-retroviral therapy. Oral miltefosine also has been tried with varying success.

4. How to treat Kala-azar?

For more than half a century, the pentavalent antimony compounds meglumineantimonite and sodium stibogluconate remained the standard anti-leishmanial treatment world-wide except in India, where widespread resistance is now being observed. The current alternative treatment of choice is amphotericin B, an antifungal agent that is highly effective in cases resistant to antimony compounds. Miltefosine, a new oral agent, is a highly effective drug, is safe, and affordable.

Pentavalent antimony drugs (sodium stibogluconate, SSG)

The drug is given as 20 mg/kg/day IM/IV, once daily for 20–30 days. Total dose may be divided equally and given at an interval of 8–12 hours. The drug is given in the same dose for double duration in case of relapse. Most children improve and become afebrile in less than a week, whereas hematological restoration and significant subsidence of splenomegaly usually occur within 2 weeks. While active elsewhere in India, SSG is no longer useful in north eastern state of Bihar, where as many as 65% of the previously untreated patients fail to respond to or promptly relapse after therapy with SSG. Disadvantages of SSG include parenteral mode of administration, the long duration of therapy and the adverse reactions. Systemic toxicity normally relates to total dose administered. Secondary effects (such as fatigue, body ache, abdominal discomfort ECG abnormalities, raised aminotransferase levels and chemical pancreatitis) are frequent, albeit usually reversible. It is not recommended at present day situation.

Amphotericin B

The current alternative treatment of choice is amphotericin B which has become the first-line treatment for Kala-azar and 90–95% long-term cure rate has been obtained in both antimonial-unresponsive and previously untreated patients. The dose is 1 mg/kg IV on an alternate-day schedule over a 30-day period (cumulative dose 7–20 mg/kg). The drug is administered as IV infusion in 5% dextrose solution at a concentration of 0.1 mg/mL over 6–8 hours, with a close vigil on feBrile and allergic reactions. Adverse effects of this drug are mainly infusion-related fever, chill and bone pain. It is also associated with renal toxicity necessitating monitoring of renal function. The drawbacks of amphotericin B are its high cost and toxicity. Three new lipid-associated formulations of amphotericin B with improved therapeutic indices have been developed in the last decade and have been proven to increase the efficacy and to limit the toxicity of conventional amphotericin B. These formulations allow administration of considerably higher daily doses and simultaneously appear to target infected tissue macrophages via enhanced phagocytic uptake. Three lipid formulations are available:

i. *AmBisome*®, (liposomal Amphotericin B) which is a formulation using spherical, unilamellar liposomes that are less than 100 nm in size.
ii. *Amphocil*®, (Amphotericin B cholesterol dispersion) which is dispersion with cholesterol sulfate in 1:1 molar ratio.
iii. *Abelcet*®, (Amphotericin B lipid complex) which is a ribbon-like lipid structure using a phospholipid matrix.

In 1997, the US FDA approved AmBisome (in the dose of 3 mg/kg/day on days 1-5, 14, and 21) for the treatment of visceral leishmaniasis in immunocompetent children. Amphocil is given at dose of 2-4 mg/kg/day for 7-10 days in children with Kala-azar. Abelcet is given at 5 mg/kg/day for 2 days.

By using the lipid formulations of Amphotericin B, drug toxicity is minimized, and hospital stay can be reduced to 2-5 days from 30-40 days, which can offset the high cost of these drugs, however these drugs still remain beyond reach of most of the Indian patients or those from other developing countries.

Aminosidine

Aminosidine is an aminoglycoside antibiotic identical to Paromomycin. An injectable formulation of 500 mg aminosidine sulfate has been on the market in several countries for over 30 years for treating bacterial and parasitic infections. Aminosidine given IM at 16 to 20 mg/kg/day for 21 days was significantly more effective in producing final cure than sodium stibogluconate 20 mg/kg/day for 30 days. Aminosidine has low incidence of adverse reactions, including ototoxicity and renal toxicity, and is well-tolerated.

Miltefosine

Treatment with this agent has been almost 100% effective and well-tolerated in various studies conducted in India among newly diagnosed patients or patients unresponsive to pentavalent antimonial agents.

The recommended dose of miltefosine for the treatment of visceral leishmaniasis is 2.5 mg/kg per day for 28 days. The dose should be adjusted based on patient's weight so that a dose of 4 mg/kg per day is not exceeded. Miltefosine is well-tolerated with considerably fewer adverse effects as compared to antimonials and amphotericin. The most commonly seen adverse effects are nausea and vomiting. There is an increase in AST and creatinine and/or BUN level, which is mild. Grade III hepatotoxicity and renal damage, has also been reported in some cases. However, these changes are reversible in the face of continued treatment or after discontinuation of treatment. Miltefosine is now available in under the name impavido,

(10, 50 and 100 mg capsules). Based on the results available with this drug, it is hoped that this drug will eventually become the firstline treatment for Kala-azar in India.

Thus, the current status of diagnosis and treatment of Kala-azar in endemic regions, including India, remains far from satisfactory. The development of rapid rK 39 strip test is a good sign and its widespread use is expected to improve the diagnostic capabilities to a large extent. Therapy of Kala-azar remains far from ideal. SSG is no more useful in India due to development of widespread resistance to this drug.

Response to therapy

Evaluation of effectiveness of therapy of Kala-azar is very important. Response to therapy can be assessed clinically and a repeat bone marrow/splenic examination. Acute phase reactants like C-reactive protein, serum amyloid A protein, and alpha-1 acid glycoprotein are less invasive tests for monitoring of therapy. The role of rK 39 test in predicting response to therapy is also being evaluated.

Splenectomy

It should be reserved for cases that are unresponsive to both first and second line drugs to kill the residual parasites. Splenectomy should be followed by SSG in recommended dose schedule.

Further Reading

1. Behrman RE, Kleigman RM, Arvin AM, Wyler GJ, Hammer DH. Leishmaniasis. Nelson's textbook of pediatrics, 15th Ed.
2. Berman JD. Human Leishmaniasis: clinical diagnostic and chemotherapeutic in the last 10 years. Clin Infect Dis. 1997;24:684-703.
3. Chatterjee KD. Parasitology. 12th Ed. 1981.p.54-65.
4. Jha TK, Olliaro P, Thakur CPN, Kanyok TP, Singhania BL, Singh IJ, et al. Randomised controlled trial of aminosidine (paromomycin) vs sodium stibogluconate for treating visceral leishmaniasis in North Bihar, India. BMJ. 1998;316:1200-5.
5. Jha TK. Refractory Kalazar- diagnosis and management. Medicine update, 1998.p.137-44.
6. Kuhlencord A, Maniera T, Eibl H, Unger C. Oral treatment of visceral leishmaniasis in mice. Antimicrob Agents Chemother. 1992;36:1630-4.
7. Manson Bahr PEC. Leishmaniasis. Manson's Tropical diseases, 19th Ed. London: BailiereTindall. 1987: p.90-113.
8. Park's textbook of preventive and social medicine. 14th Ed. 1994.p.215-8.
9. Prasad LSN. Kalazar in Indian children. Asian J Peditr Practice 1977.p.31-8.
10. Schallig H, Canto-Cavalheiro, da Silva ES. Evaluation of the Direct Agglutination Test and the rK39 Dipstick Test for the Sero-diagnosis of Visceral Leishmaniasis. MemInstOswaldo Cruz, Rio de Janeiro. 2002;97(7):1015-8.
11. Sinha PK, Bhattacharya SK, Thakur CP, Jha TK, Sundar S. Rajendra Memorial Research Institute of Medical Sciences and Kalazar Research Centre, Patna, India;

Kalazar Research Centre and Kala-azar Medical Research Centre, Muzzafarpur, India. Presented at the 3rd International Congress on Leishmaniasis. Palermo, Sicily; 2005.
12. Sundar S, Makharia A, More DK. Short course of oral Miltefosine for treatment of visceral leishmaniasis. Clin infect Dis. 2000;31:1110-3.
13. Sundar S, Reed SG, Singh VP, Kumar PC, Murray HW. Rapid accurate field diagnosis of Indian visceralleishmaniasis. Lancet. 1998;351:563-5.
14. Valenzuela JG, Belkaid Y, Garfield MK, Mendez S, Kamhawi S, Rowton ED, et al. Ex Med. 2001;194(3):331-42.
15. WHO. Tech Rep Ser No 637;1979.p.41.
16. WHO. Tech Rep Ser No 701;1984.
17. WHO. The world health situation of the global strategy for health for all by the year 2000. 8th report, 2nd evaluation. Vol 1, global reviews, Geneva.

26

Malaria

Jaydeep Choudhury

1. What is the current epidemiology of malaria in India?

In India, there were about 3 million cases of malaria in 1996. Since then, the incidence of malaria is declining. In 2006, there were about 2 million cases of malaria and in 2010 there were 1.7 million cases. The incidences of *Plasmodium vivax* were about 2 million in 2006 and it has come down to 1.5 million in 2010. There have been hardly any change in the incidence of *Plasmodium falciparum* cases over the years, it is around 1 million cases per year in India. What is more alarming is the increase in the *P. falciparum* to *P. vivax* ratio. The ratio was 0.6 in 1990s. During 2000 to 2008 it was around 1, and then in 2008–2009, it has reached 1.2.

According to the National Vector Borne Disease Control Program, chloroquine resistance to falciparum malaria is observed in 117 districts in India. In large parts of North-Eastern states, there is not only resistance to chloroquine but also to sulfadoxin-pyrimethamine (SP). Out of the 117 districts that have reported chloroquine resistance, many districts are endemic to *P. falciparum* cases.

2. What are RDT? What are the advantages and disadvantages?

Rapid Diagnostic Tests or RDT are immunochromatographic test (ICT) to detect *Plasmodium* specific antigens in blood sample. These tests employ monoclonal antibodies directed against the targeted parasite antigens. The following are the targeted antigens which are currently available RDTs.
  i. *Histidine rich protein II (HRP-II)*—It is actively secreted by asexual stages and young gametocytes of *P. falciparum* but not by mature gametocytes.
  ii. A metabolic enzyme *parasite lactate dehydrogenase (pLDH)*—It is produced by all four species of *Plasmodia* in both asexual and sexual (gametocytes) stages when they are viable. Monoclonal antibodies produced against this antigen are of three groups. One specific for *P. falciparum* and the second specific for *P. vivax*. The other is pan specific antibody which reacts with all the four species of *Plasmodia* but it cannot separate them individually. Commercially available kit can detect *P. falciparum, P. vivax* and other malaria but cannot differentiate *P. ovale* and *P. malariae*.

iii. Certain new antigens like plasmodium aldolase, an enzyme of the glycolytic pathway produced by all four species have been recently developed.

Laboratory confirmation of malaria is an essential component of disease management. In our country, *P. falciparum* and *P. vivax* malaria parasite often co-circulate, typically occurring as a single species infection. An RDT which can detect both *P. falciparum* and *P. vivax* malaria and distinguish between them is essential. There are some commercially available kits which detects *P. falciparum* specific LDH and panspecific LDH. So they can distinguish between *P. falciparum* from non *P. falciparum* malaria. But these kits can not distinguish *P. falciparum* malaria from mixed infection, and secondly as P vivax malaria is almost the only non *P. falciparum* malaria in our country so often they equate non *P falciparum* malaria with *P. vivax* malaria.

Role of RDTs in the diagnosis of malaria—In comparison to high transmission areas, malaria in our country occurs less frequently, it occurs in all age groups and it is almost always symptomatic. Drug resistances including multidrug resistance are being reported in India, so laboratory confirmation of malaria is an essential component of disease management. Expert microscopic diagnosis is available in some central health care facilities like major cities, but it is often unreliable or unavailable in peripheral areas with poor health facilities. So RDTs may be useful in the following situations in our country:

i. In communities with poor health care facilities where microscopic diagnosis is not available. In areas, where laboratory service is inadequate, it is of unacceptable standard or not available round the clock.
ii. In places where quality microscopy is available, RDTs and microscopy can run in tandem. RDTs will provide rapid or screening diagnosis whereas microscopy is reserved for resolution of confusing cases, confirmation of negative result in RDTs with high clinical suspicion of malaria.
iii. In some cases of severe and complicated malaria, peripheral parasitemia may be negative due to sequestration but RDTs are expected to provide evidence of antigenemia.
iv. According to the new National drug policy of malaria, any fever cases clinically suspected to be malaria should preferably be investigated for confirmation of malaria by microscopy or RDT so as to insure full therapeutic dose with appropriate drug to all confirmed cases.

RDTs permit on the spot confirmation of malaria even at the peripheral health care system by unskilled health worker with minimal training. Rational use of RDTs as a complement to microscopy might offer following benefits:

i. Early treatment will reduce mortality and morbidity.
ii. In multidrug resistance areas, expensive drugs and drug combination will be given only to those who need them.
iii. Avoidance of unnecessary treatment will reduce drug pressure and delay progress of drug resistance.

The main disadvantage of RDT is the cost involved.

3. How microscopy can be used in malaria?

Light microscopy of well stained thick and thin films by a skilled person is the "gold standard" for diagnosis of malaria. Thick films are more sensitive for diagnosis of malaria due to larger amount of blood in the given area as compared to thin films. But species identification is better done with thin films as morphology of the parasite and RBC are well preserved. Smears should be prepared soon after collection, which enables better adherence of films to the slide and cause minimal distortion of parasites and red cells.

Blood can be collected any time irrespective of fever and not necessarily only at the height of fever. Blood collection should be before administration of antimalarial medication as it causes morphologic alteration of parasites.

Smear should be examined with 100X oil immersion objective. A minimum of 100 fields should be examined before concluding the slide to be negative. Once negative, blood smear may be examined for at least three consecutive days where clinical suspicion of malaria is high.

4. What is severe and complicated malaria? What are the common manifestations of it in pediatric age group?

The clinical and laboratory criteria for diagnosis of severe malaria are shown in Table 1.

Table 1: Clinical and laboratory criteria for severe malaria

Clinical:
- Impaired consciousness or unarousable coma
- Severe prostration
- Failure to feed
- Recurrent convulsion
- Respiratory distress from metabolic acidosis
- Circulatory collapse or shock
- Clinical jaundice plus evidence of other vital organ dysfunction
- Hemoglobinuria
- Abnormal spontaneous breathing.

Laboratory:
- Hypoglycemia (blood glucose <40 mg/dL)
- Metabolic acidosis (plasma bicarbonate < 15 mmol/L)
- Severe normocytic anemia (Hb <5 g/dL)
- Hyperparasitemia (>2% or 100,000/mL)
- Renal impairment (serum creatinine >3 mg/dL)
- Pulmonary edema
- Hyperlactemia (lactate>5mmol/L).

High degree of suspicion of severe malaria is of utmost importance and any delay in initiation of treatment can be fatal. Severe life threatening malaria is almost always due to *P. falciparum* and is to be treated with injectable antimalarials, irrespective of the species. It should be treated as a medical emergency preferably in an intensive care setting. Confirmation of the diagnosis is preferable but one should not delay the treatment if it needs more than 1 hour.

In cases of strong clinical suspicion, prompt antimalarial therapy is needed even if parasite is not found in the initial blood examination. Effective therapy in children with severe malaria includes antimalarial chemotherapy, supportive management and management of complications. All these three interventions are equally important and to be taken care of simultanously.

5. How to treat uncomplicated malaria?

According to the National Vector Borne Disease Control Program, it has been suggested that all *P. falciparum* cases should be treated with Artemisinin Combination Therapy (ACT) to overcome the chance of drug resistance.

Treatment of P. vivax malaria

Confirmed *P. vivax* cases should be treated with chloroquine in full therapeutic dose of 25 mg/kg divided over three days. Chloroquine 10 mg base/kg stat orally followed by 10mg/kg at 24 and 5 mg/kg at 48 hours (total dose 25 mg/kg). Chloroquine should not be given in empty stomach and in presence of high fever. Temperature should be brought down first. If vomiting occurs within 30 minutes of a dose of chloroquine that particular dose is to be repeated after taking care of vomiting by using antiemetic medications (domperidone or ondansetron).

In order to prevent relapse, primaquine should be given at a dose of 0.25 mg/kg body weight daily for 14 days. Primaquine is contraindicated in known G6PD-deficient patients, infants and pregnant women. As primaquine can lead to hemolysis in G6PD deficiency, caution should be exercised before administering primaquine in areas known to have high prevalence of G6PD deficiency. G6PD should be tested if facilities are available. Patient should be advised to stop primaquine immediately if he/she develop symptoms like dark colored urine, yellow conjunctiva, bluish discoloration of lips, abdominal pain, nausea, vomiting, etc and should report to the doctor immediately. As infants are relatively G6PD-deficient, it is not recommended in children below 1 year. In cases of borderline G6PD deficiency, once weekly dose of primaquine 0.6–0.8 mg/kg is given for 6 weeks.

Treatment of uncomplicated P. falciparum malaria

Artemisinin Combination Therapy (ACT) should be given to all confirmed *P. falciparum* cases found positive by microscopy or RDT. A single dose primaquine (0.75 mg/kg body weight) should be given on Day 2 for gametocytocidal action.

ACT consists of an artemisinin derivative combined with a long acting antimalarial (lumefantrine, or sulfadoxine-pyrimethamine). The ACT recommended in the National Program of India is artesunate (4 mg/kg body weight) daily for 3 days and sulfadoxine (25 mg/kg body weight) -pyrimethamine (1.25 mg/kg body weight) on day 0. Oral artesunate monotherapy is not recommended. Also mefloquine is not advocated for use in India due to risk of neuropsychiatric complications.

Co-formulated tablets containing 20 mg of artemether and 120 mg of lumefantrine can be used as a six-dose regimen orally twice a day for 3 days. Lumefantrine absorption is enhanced by co-administration with fatty food like milk.
- 5–14 kg body weight—1 tablet twice daily for 3 days
- 15 to 24 kg body weight—same schedule with 2 tablets.
- 25-35 kg body weight and above—same schedule with 3 and 4 tablets respectively.

In North-Eastern states of India where resistance to SP is present, the ACT of choice is artemether plus lumefantrine instead of artesunate-SP.

6. How to treat mixed infections?

Mixed infections with *P. falciparum* should be treated as falciparum malaria. However, treatment with primaquine should be given for 14 days, if indicated.

7. How to treat complicated malaria?

According to the National Anti-Malaria Program (NAMP), all cases of severe malaria is an emergency and treatment should be given promptly. Parenteral artemisinin derivatives or quinine should be used, irrespective of chloroquine sensitivity. Severe malaria caused by *P. vivax* should be treated like severe *P. falciparum* malaria.

Artesunate

Artesunate 2.4 mg/kg body weight IV or IM given on admission, then at 12 hours and 24 hours, then once a day. Artesunate powder should be diluted in 5% sodium bi-carbonate provided in the pack.

Quinine

Quinine 20 mg salt/kg body weight on admission as IV infusion in 5% dextrose or dextrose saline over a period of 4 hours followed by maintenance dose of 10 mg/kg body weight 8 hourly, infusion rate should not exceed 5 mg/kg body weight per hour. Loading dose of 20 mg/kg body weight should not be given, if the patient has already received quinine. If parenteral quinine therapy needs to be continued beyond 48 hours, dose should be reduced to 7 mg/kg body weight, 8 hourly.

Parenteral treatment should be given for minimum of 24 hours once started. Once the patient can take oral therapy, further follow-up treatments should be as given below:
- Patients receiving parenteral quinine should be treated with oral quinine 10 mg/kg body weight three times a day to complete a course of 7 days, along with doxycycline 3 mg/kg body weight per day for 7 days (Doxycycline is contraindicated in pregnant women and children under 8 years of age; instead, clindamycin 10 mg/kg body weight 12 hourly for 7 days should be used)

- Patients receiving artemisinin derivatives should get full course of oral ACT as in the treatment of uncomplicated falciparum malaria.

Supportive management

- Regular clinical assessment—Level of consciousness, blood pressure, rate and depth of respiration, anemia, hydration and temperature. Oxygen therapy and respiratory support, if necessary
- Proper positioning, meticulous attention to airways, eyes, mucosa and skin should be done. Monitoring of the vital signs preferably every 4 hours, till the patient is out of danger. Also maintain intake output chart and watch for hemoglobinuria
- For unconscious child—Nasogastric tube in situ to reduce the risk of aspiration
- Management of shock—Normal saline or Ringer's lactate by bolus infusion. Overhydration should be avoided
- Hyperpyrexia should be treated with tepid sponging, fanning and paracetamol
- Monitoring of the response to treatment is essential. Blood smear examination every 6 to 12 hours for parasitemia, and parasite density for the first 48 hours
- In case of treatment with artemisinin derivatives, parasite count usually comes down within 5 to 6 hours of starting therapy. Asexual parasitemia generally disappears after 72 hours of therapy
- In case of quinine, parasite count may remain unchanged or even rise in first 18-24 hours which should not be taken as an indicator of quinine resistance. However, parasite count should fall after 24 hours of quinine therapy and should disappear within 5 days.

Management of complications of malaria

Of the various complications of *P. falciparum* malaria, the common and important ones in children are the following:

Cerebral malaria—Presentation is usually with fever followed by inability to eat or drink. The progression to coma or convulsion is usually very rapid within one or two days. Good nursing care is essential. Convulsions should be treated with diazepam or midazolam and harmful adjuvant treatment like corticosteroids, mannitol, adrenaline and phenobarbitone should be avoided.

Severe anemia—Children with hyperparasitemia due to acute destruction of red cells may develop severe anemia. Packed red cell transfusion should be given cautiously when PCV is 12% or less, or hemoglobin is below 4 g%. Transfusion should also be considered in patients with less severe anemia in the presence of respiratory distress (acidosis), impaired consciousness or hyperparasitemia (>20% of RBCs infected).

Lactic acidosis—Deep breathing with indrawing of lower chest wall without any localizing chest signs suggest lactic acidosis. It usually accompanies cerebral malaria, anemia or dehydration. Correction of hypovolemia, treatment of anemia and prevention of seizures are the mainstay. Monitor acid base status, blood glucose and urea and electrolyte level.

Hypoglycemia—It is common in children below 3 years specially with hyperparasitemia or with convulsion. It also occurs in patients treated with quinine. Manifestations are similar to those of cerebral malaria so it can be easily overlooked. Blood sugar level should be monitored every 4 to 6 hours. Hypoglycemia is corrected with IV dextrose (25% dextrose 2 to 4 mL/kg by bolus) and it should be followed by slow infusion of 5% dextrose containing fluid to prevent recurrence.

Further Reading

1. Guidelines for Diagnosis and Treatment of Malaria in India. National Vector Borne Disease Control Program. New Delhi: Ministry of Health, Government of India, 2011.
2. Kundu R. Arthropod Borne Infection—Malaria, Dengue, Japanese Encephalitis. In: Choudhury J, Kundu R, editors. Pediatric Infectious Diseases, 1st edition. New Delhi: Jaypee Brothers, 2012.
3. National drug policy on malaria. Ministry of Health and Family Welfare/Directorate of National Vector Borne Disease Control Program, Government of India; 2010. http://www.nvbdcp.gov.in
4. WHO Guidelines for the Treatment of Malaria, second edition. Geneva, World Health Organization (2010). http://www.who.int/malaria/publications/atoz/9789241547925/enindex.html.

27. Amebiasis and Giardiasis

Ajay Kalra

1. When should we suspect amebic dysentery?

Amebiasis is a very rare cause of dysentery (bloody stools) in children. The overall incidence of disease with *Entameba histolytica* itself is less than 2% in children. It should be suspected as a cause of dysentery when (i) blood is separate and not mixed with mucus or fecal matter unlike what occurs in bacillary dysentery; and (ii) if two different antibiotics usually effective for *Shigella* in the area have been given sequentially and the child having dysentery has not shown signs of clinical improvement.

2. Will examination of stool be helpful in the diagnosis of amebiasis?

Light microscopy is not of much help. It cannot distinguish *Entameba histolytica* from other entamebas. *Entameba dispar* (which is nonpathogenic, noninvasive ameba) is ten times more common. Only when trophozoites contain ingested RBCs, they are considered as diagnostic and not merely the visualization of cysts or non-RBC-ingested trophozoites. Moreover, this examination has to be done on a fresh stool. At least 3 and preferably 6 samples on successive days need to be examined using Trichrome or Lugol's iodine for staining. Therefore, it is not a very sensitive investigation and WHO recommends that no treatment be given only on the basis of microscopic examination. Moreover, the organism cannot be detected in stool once it goes into the extraintestinal tissues. An enzyme immunoassay kit using antibody-coated strips to specifically detect *E. histolytica* antigen is more reliable, although not easily available. Polymerase chain reaction-based diagnostic tests are not widely available and not better than the antigen detection tests. Absence of fecal leukocytes and presence of heme and Charcot Leyden crystals in stools may provide collaborative evidence.

3a. How does amebic liver abscess present?

Amebic liver abscess is the most common form of extraintestinal amebiasis. It is emerging as a problem in HIV patients. In children, amebic hepatitis presenting with jaundice is more common than liver abscess. Liver involvement results from spread of the organisms from the intestinal submucosa to the liver via the portal system. Liver abscess occurs in as many as 5% of patients with symptomatic intestinal amebiasis and is ten times as frequent in males as compared to females. Approximately, 40% of the patients, who have amebic liver abscess, do not have a history of prior bowel symptoms. Nearly 80% of patients with amebic liver abscess present within 2-4 weeks of infection. Common modes of presentation are fever and constant, dull, upper right abdominal or epigastrium pain. Right-sided pleuritic pain or referred shoulder pain may occur in involvement of the diaphragmatic surface of the liver. Associated gastrointestinal symptoms occur in 10-35% of patients and include nausea, vomiting, abdominal distention, diarrhea and constipation. A small number of patients with amebic liver abscess have a subacute presentation with vague abdominal discomfort, weight loss and anemia. Roughly 2-7% of liver abscess ruptures into the peritoneum. When it occurs, it may lead to amebic peritonitis, which presents with fever and rigid distended abdomen. When an abscess from the left liver lobe ruptures into the pericardium, it leads to amebic pericarditis. This occurs in 3% of patients with hepatic amebiasis and may present with chest pain and features of congestive heart failure.

3b. How to manage amebic liver abscess?

Diagnosis

Diagnosis of liver abscess is mostly by radiological means. Chest radiography may reveal an elevated right hemidiaphragm and a right-sided pleural effusion. Ultrasonography is preferred for evaluation of amebic liver abscess because of its low cost, rapid reports and lack of adverse effects. Computed tomography (CT) and magnetic resonance imaging (MRI) may be slightly more sensitive than ultrasonography. Repeat imaging is not indicated if the patient is doing well because complete resolution of liver abscess may take as long as 2 years. Liver function tests reveal elevated alkaline phosphatase levels, transaminase levels, mild elevation of serum bilirubin level, and reduced albumin levels. The erythrocyte sedimentation rate is elevated. The indirect hemagglutination test is positive when the titer is 1:128 or above. Detection of antiamebic antibodies (IgM) in serum (but only after two weeks of infection) has a sensitivity of 90% for liver abscess. However, antibodies may persist for two years and, therefore, the test will remain positive for this much time. Aspiration of liver abscess is occasionally required to rule out pyogenic abscess. Amebic liver abscess is anchovy paste-like (thick chocolate color or yellow grey odorless) material that lacks WBCs due to lyses by the parasite. Amebae may not be or rarely visualized in the abscess fluid because they are localized in the wall of the cavity. A bacteriologically sterile aspirate is also a collaborative evidence.

Treatment

Treatment is with tissue amebicides which are as follows (in order of preference):

i. Metronidazole (nitroimadazole compound)—20 mg/kg/day in 3 divided doses as infusion for 24–48 hours, followed by oral medication, 25–50 mg/kg/day 8 hourly for 10 days.

The IV metronidazole has an extra advantage that it takes care of the anerobic bacteroides which are likely to be present in 26% of amebic liver abscess with so called "sterile pus".

ii. Tinidazole (nitroimadazole compound)—60 mg/kg/day as single oral dose for 3 days.

iii. Chloroquine hydrochloride 10 mg/kg orally in 3 divided doses for 14 to 21 days.

iv. Dihydroemetine 1mg/kg/day IM or deep SC for 10 days (only in hospitalized patients due to the possibility of cardiac/renal toxicity).

The tissue amebicides are good for invasive amebiasis, but are not very effective in eradicating the organisms from the intestinal lumen and, thus, carry the risk of relapse. Therefore, they need to be followed with a luminal amebicide, for example, diloxanide furoate 125 mg or 250 mg 3 times daily for 10 days for children <5 years or >5 years respectively or diiodohydroxyquinolone 30–40 mg/kg/day orally in 3 divided doses for 3 weeks or tetracycline 25–50 mg/kg in 3 divided doses for 10 days.

Oral chloroquine and dehydroemetine, when given together, also bring down the relapse rate to <1%.

Therapeutically, aspiration of liver is indicated only for large abscesses (>12 own diameter), imminent abscess rupture, failure of medical therapy or presence on left lobe.

4. What are the clinical manifestations of giardiasis and how to manage it?

Diarrhea is the most common symptom of giardia infection, occurring in 90% of symptomatic subject. A small number of patients develop abrupt onset of explosive watery diarrhea. These symptoms last for 3–4 days before transition into the more common subacute syndrome. Most patients develop more insidious onset of symptoms, which are recurrent or resistant.

Stools become malodorous, mushy and greasy. Stools do not contain blood or pus. Abdominal cramping, bloating and flatulence occur in 70–75% of symptomatic patients.

Symptoms of chronic infection include chronic diarrhea, malaise, nausea and anorexia. Marked weight loss is associated with chronic diarrhea, which may continue for months. Postinfection lactose intolerance is a common finding. Extraintestinal manifestations are rare and include allergic manifestations such as urticaria, erythema multiforme, bronchospasm, reactive arthritis and biliary tract disease, probably because of host immune system activation and cross reactivity. Such children have failure to thrive or weight loss, malabsorption syndrome, zinc deficiency and growth retardation.

Diagnosis is made by microscopic examination of fresh stools. At least three fresh specimens of stools collected on alternate days should be examined to achieve a sensitivity of 90%. Only presence of trophozoites is diagnostic, not presence of cysts. Where diagnosis is strongly suspected but stool examination is negative, duodenal aspiration or biopsy may yield high concentration of giardiasis.

Treatment is given only to symptomatic cases. Asymptomatic cyst carriers are not treated except in cases from immunocompromised family members or outbreak control or prevention. Metronidazole is given in a dose of 15 mg/kg/day/q 8 hourly for 5–7 days. Its efficacy is 80–90% but it has frequent adverse effects like nausea and vomiting. Tinidazole is used as a single dose of 50 mg/kg. It has less adverse effects. Another drug is ornidazole 40 mg/kg to be given as single dose once daily for 2 days. Secnidazole can also be given in the doze of 30 mg/kg as a single dose. Nitazoxanide is a newly introduced drug used in a dose of 100 mg/kg/q bid in children aged 1–4 years and 200 mg big in children aged 4–12 years for a period of 3 days (7–10 mg/kg/dose 2 times daily). Second line alternatives include albendazole, furazolidine, paramomycin and quinacrine.

5. **What should be the management of chance detection of amebic or giardia cysts?**

No treatment is needed in such cases. Only symptomatic cases and presence of RBC-laden trophozoites in amebiasis indicate need for therapy.

Further Reading

1. Bhatnagar S. Antibicrobials in Acute Gastroenteritis. In: Handbook of Rational Antibiotic Therapy IAP Infectious Diseases Chapter Publications, Mumbai, Eds. Shivananda, Yewale, Prajapati, Kundu; 2009;15-8.
2. Dubey AP, Mukherjee SB, et al. Infectious Diseases. In: Pediatrics, New Delhi: Atlantic Publishers, Eds. Satya Gupta, AP Dubey, Praveen Kumar; 2009;352-5.
3. Ganguly S. Amebiasis and Giardiasis. In: IAP Infectious Diseases Chapter Textbook of Pediatric Infectious Diseases, Gwalior: IAP National Publication House, Jaypee Brothers Medical Publishers. Parthasarathy, Kundu, Choudhury (Eds); 2013;370-5.

SECTION 2:

SYSTEMIC INFECTIONS

28. Bacterial Meningitis
29. Encephalitis
30. Upper Respiratory Infection
31. Community Acquired Pneumonia
32. Infective Endocarditis
33. Acute Gastroenteritis
34. Urinary Tract Infection
35. Enteric Fever
36. Intra-abdominal Infections
37. Bone and Joint Infections
38. Skin and Soft Tissue Infections
39. Tuberculosis
40. Congenital Infections
41. Primary Immunodeficiency
42. Sepsis Syndrome
43. Febrile Neutropenia
44. Lymphadenitis
45. HIV Infection

28
Bacterial Meningitis

Digant D Shastri

1. **What are the causative organisms of bacterial meningitis in different age groups?**

The bacterial meningitis can be caused by different variety of organisms. The etiology differs as per the age group.

Neonates

The principal pathogens in neonates are *E. coli* and other gram negative organisms like *Klebsiella, Haemophilus influenzae, Enterobacter* species. *Staphylococcus, Listeria* and group B *Sterptococcus* are the other common pathogens in neonates. *Pseudomonas aeruginosa, Proteus* species, *Serratia marcescens* are the common etiological agents in those neonates who needs respiratory support.

Infants and children

In children beyond neonatal age *S. pneumoniae, N. meningitidis* and *H. influenzae* b are the most common etiologic agents. In countries where the conjugate *H. influenzae* b vaccine coverage is high, the incidence of Hib infection has gone down practically to level of disappearance. Of the various serotypes of *S. pneumoniae* serotypes, numbers 1, 3, 6, 7, 14, 19 and 23 are the most common serotypes causing bacterial meningitis. Of all the pathogenic serotypes of *N. meningitidis* serotypes B, C, Y and W-135 account for most of the childhood cases in developed countries, while Group A strains are most prevalent in developing countries.

2. **How to diagnose bacterial meningitis?**

Cerebrospinal fluid (CSF) study

Definitive diagnosis of bacterial meningitis is based on examination of CSF obtained by lumbar puncture (LP). It is recommended to collect the CSF before initiation of antibiotic therapy, however, antibiotic treatment must not be delayed for pending lumbar puncture The CSF is to be tested for total and differential cell counts, glucose and protein estimation, Gram stains, and culture. In suspected cases pretreated with antibiotics rapid bacterial antigen testing may be considered. In bacterial meningitis, the CSF white blood cell counts are usually higher than 1000/μL, CSF protein concentration is usually greater than 50 mg/dL, and the CSF glucose concentration is usually reduced. The CSF glucose level lower than 50% of the serum level is suggestive of bacterial meningitis. Though predominance of polymorphonuclear leukocytes (PMNs) point to diagnosis of bacterial meningitis, but is not a reliable indicator of bacterial meningitis In patients with fulminant disease and poor immune response may not show cytologic or chemical changes in CSF.

Cerebrospinal fluid culture

The confirm diagnosis of bacterial meningitis is to be made by isolation of bacteria from the cerebrospinal fluid (CSF). The CSF is transported soon and should be plated immediately onto a chocolate and blood agar media.

Gram stain

A gram stain of cytocentrifuged CSF may reveal bacterial morphology. The gram stain is positive in 97% of cases when the CSF concentration of bacteria is more than 105 CFU/mm. Although gram stain may aid in diagnosis, the diagnosis may be missed in up to 30–40% of cases of culture-proven disease. The sensitivity of a positive gram stain is 67%. The yield of gram stain may be approximately 20% lower for patients who have received previous antibiotic therapy. Smears of petechial lesions may reveal microorganisms on gram stain.

Cerebrospinal fluid PCR

In cases where antibiotic administration leads to CSF sterilization, polymerase chain reaction (PCR) testing may have a role to play in identifying the pathogen.

Apart from the CSF study, following tests will aid in diagnosis of bacterial meningitis and should be included as part of study work up:
- Complete blood count (CBC) with differential
- Blood cultures
- Blood glucose: Blood sugar should be taken before performing LP as it corresponds to the CSF sugar level
- Serum Procalcitonin (PCT): Elevated PCT concentrations have been shown to be useful in differentiating between bacterial and viral meningitis in children (cut-off >5 μg/L; sensitivity 94%; specificity 100%).
- Radio imaging studies: Mainly indicated in nonresponders and to detect the complications associated with bacterial meningitis.

3. How to distinguish between bacterial, aseptic, partially treated bacterial and tuberculous meningitis?

Based on the CSF fluid findings, one can differentiate amongst bacterial, aseptic, partially treated bacterial and tuberculous meningitis as shown in Table 1.

Bacterial Meningitis

Table 1: Cerebrospinal fluid findings in CNS Infections				
Parameter (normal)	Bacterial meningitis	Aseptic/Viral	Partially treated bacterial meningitis	Early TBM
Cells (<5/cumm) (All lymphocytes)	100–10,000, Neutrophils	10–1000 Lymphocytes> Neutrophils	5–10,000 Lymphocytes> Neutrophils	10–500, Neutrophils early and then Lymphocytes
Sugar (>60% of BSL)	Low	Normal except mumps	Low	Low/Normal
Protein (20–40 mg%)	100–500 mg%	50–200 mg%	100–500 mg%	100–1000 mg%
Gram St & C/S	Positive	Neg	Usually Neg	Neg
ADA, Lactate, LDH	High	Normal	High	High

4. How to treat bacterial meningitis?

Acute bacterial meningitis is a medical emergency and hence, patients must be treated on inpatient based in a facility where emergencies can be managed. Apart from the general supportive care, appropriate antibiotic is the main stay of treatment. Child with suspected meningitis should receive antibiotics after performing LP. In cases where LP is contraindicated, antibiotics should be given immediately.

Empirical antibiotic therapy

Empirical therapy is determined not only by the most likely etiological agent but also the pattern of antimicrobial resistance. In children more than one month of age, 3rd generation cephalosporin, ceftriaxone or cefotaxime are recommended for initial therapy. Cefotaxime 200 mg/kg/24 hours, given every 6 hours or ceftriaxone 100 mg/kg/24 hours given either every 12 hours or as a single dose is currently recommended. As India has started showing intermediate resistant pneumococci, penicillin is no longer recommended. Vancomycin has role in therapy of penicillin or cephalosporin resistant meningitis in combination with cephalosporin. Because vancomycin penetrates the central nervous system (CNS) poorly, a higher dosage (60 mg/kg/day) is recommended.

In patients who are immunocompromised and where Gram negative bacterial meningitis is suspected, empiric therapy may start with ceftazidime and aminoglycosides. In patients with CSF shunt, empirical therapy can be done with vancomycin and meropenem. Combination of third generation cephalosporin plus beta-lactamase inhibitor has no role in the treatment of pyogenic meningitis.

Pathogens specific antimicrobial therapy

Pneumococcus or meningococcus which are susceptible to Penicillin or Ampicillin (MIC ≤ 0.6 mg/mL) should be treated with Penicillin G or Ampicillin.

If they are not susceptible to penicillin but susceptible to cephalosporin, 3rd generation cephalosporin like ceftriaxone or cefotaxime must be used. Isolates that are not susceptible to penicillin and have a MIC of ≥1 mg/mL to 3rd generation cephalosporin should be treated with vancomycin plus cefotaxime or ceftriaxone. For *S. pneumoniae* with intermediate resistance to penicillin, cefepime and meropenem may be considered as alternative therapy. However, trails with cefepime are not adequate but may be tried in patients who fail with other antibiotic courses.

Duration of therapy

Duration of therapy depends upon the causative pathogen and clinical course. For *Pneumococcus* 10–14 days therapy is required, whereas *Meningococcus* and *H. influenzae* the duration of therapy will be 7 days. For *S. agalactiae* (GBS)—14–21 days course, for aerobic gram-negative bacilli—21 days or 2 weeks beyond the first sterile culture (whichever is longer) and for *Listeria monocytogenes*—21 days or longer antibiotic course is needed.

5. Is there any role of corticosteroid in bacterial meningitis?

In pediatric patients, double blind placebo-controlled studies evaluating adjunctive dexamethasone in childhood bacterial meningitis showed beneficial effects in *H. influenzae* meningitis with regard to hearing outcome and pneumococcal meningitis demonstrated benefit. Dexamethasone therapy should be started intravenously at the same time as, or slightly before, the first dose of antibiotic, at a dose of 0.15 mg per kilogram of body weight every six hours for two to four days.

6. What are the short and long term complications of bacterial meningitis?

Short-term complications

Seizures are the most common complication of bacterial meningitis, affecting almost 35% of the patients. Other complications that can be seen during the course of bacterial meningitis include—the syndrome of inappropriate antidiuretic hormone secretion (SIADH), subdural effusions, and brain abscesses. Subdural effusions are generally asymptomatic and resolve without neurologic sequelae.

Long-term complications

long-term sequelae are seen in as many as 30% of children; they vary according to the infecting organism, the patient's age, the presenting features, and the hospital course. These include nerve deafness, cortical blindness, hemiparesis/quadriparesis, muscular hypertonia, ataxia, complex seizure disorders, mental motor retardation, learning disabilities, obstructive hydrocephalus, and cerebral atrophy. Mild-to-severe impairment of hearing is noted in as many as 20–30% of affected children with *H. influenzae* disease but is less common with other pathogens.

Further Reading

1. Chavez-Bueno S, McCracken GH. Bacterial meningitis in children. Pediatr Clin North Am. 2005;52:795-810.
2. Prober CG. Central nervous system infections. In: Behrman RE, Kliegman RM, Jenson HB(Eds). Nelsons Textbook of Pediatrics, 6th edition. Saunders, Philadelphia: Saunders; 2004: p. 2038-47.
3. Prospective multicentre hospital surveillance of *Streptococcus pneumoniae* disease in India. Invasive Bacterial Infection Surveillance (IBIS) Group, International Clinical Epidemiology Network (INCLEN). Lancet. 1999;353:1216-21.
4. Pyogenic Meningitis. IAP Infectious Diseases Chapter Protocol for Diagnosis and Management of Pyogenic Meningitis in Children. IAP Infectious Diseases Chapter Publication, 2008.
5. Saez-LlorensX, McCracken JrGH. Antimicrobial andanti-inflamatory treatment of bacterial meningitis. Infect Dis Clin North Am. 1999;13:619-36.
6. Tunkel AR, Hartman BJ, Kaplan SL. Practice guideline for the management of bacterial meningitis. Clin Infect Dis. 2004;39:1267-84.
7. Tunkel AR, Hartman BJ, Sheldon LK, Koufman BA, Ross KL, Scheld WM, et al. Practice Guidelines for the Management of Bacterial Meningitis. Clin Infect Dis. 2004;39:1267-124.
8. Tunkel AR, Sinner SW, Antimicrobial agents in the treatment of bacterial meningitis. Infect Dis Clini North Am. 2004;18.

29

Encephalitis

Abhay K Shah

1. What is acute encephalitis syndrome (AES)? How is it classified?

Acute Encephalitis Syndrome (AES) is defined as a person of any age, at any time of year with the acute onset of fever and a change in mental status (including symptoms such as confusion, disorientation, come, or inability to talk) AND/OR new onset of seizures (excluding simple febrile seizures). Other early clinical findings may include an increase in irritability, somnolence or abnormal behavior greater than that seen with usual febrile illness. It is a group of clinical neurologic manifestation caused by wide range of viruses, bacteria, fungi, parasites, spirochetes, chemicals and toxins.

It may be sporadic like herpes simplex encephalitis (HSE) or epidemic such as Japanese B encephalitis (JE).

Case classification

A case that meets the clinical case definition for AES (i.e. suspected case) should be classified in one of the following four ways:

a. Laboratory-confirmed JE: A suspected case that has been laboratory-confirmed as JE.
b. Probable JE: A suspected case that occurs in close geographic and temporal relationship to laboratory-confirmed case of JE, in the context of an outbreak.
c. Acute encephalitis syndrome (due to an agent other than JE): A suspected case in which diagnostic testing is performed and an etiological agent other than JE virus is identified.
d. Acute encephalitis syndrome (due to an unknown agent): A suspected case in which no diagnostic testing is performed or in which testing was performed but no etiological agent was identified or in which the test results were indeterminate.

2. What is the epidemiology of JE?

Japanese encephalitis (JE) is a major cause of childhood mortality and morbidity in the countries of South-East Asia and Western Pacific regions. JE virus is neurotropic and primarily affects the central nervous system. It is the most important cause of arboviral encephalitis. An estimated 3 billion persons live in the countries where JE is endemic. Annual incidence of the disease ranges from 30,000 to 50,000. Case-fatality rates range from 0.3% to 60%.

Broadly speaking, two epidemiological patterns of Japanese encephalitis are recognized. In the northern areas (northern Vietnam, northern Thailand, Taiwan, China, Republic of Korea, Japan, China, Nepal and northern India), large epidemics occur during the summer months, whereas in southern areas (southern Vietnam, southern Thailand, Indonesia, Malaysia, Philippines, Sri Lanka and southern India), Japanese encephalitis tends to be endemic, and the cases occur sporadically throughout the year with a peak after the start of the rainy season.

The countries, which have had major epidemics in the past, but which have controlled the disease primarily by vaccination, include China, Korea, Japan, Taiwan and Thailand. Other countries that still have periodic epidemics include Vietnam, Cambodia, Myanmar, India, Nepal and Malaysia.

JE is one of the most important causes of viral encephalitis in Asia, including India. Highly endemic states include West Bengal, Assam, Bihar, Karnataka, Tamil Nadu, Uttar Pradesh, Manipur and Goa. Outbreaks have been reported from different parts of the country. The outbreak of JE usually coincides with the monsoon and post monsoon period when the density of mosquitoes increases. The risk is highest in children aged 1-15 years, especially in the rural areas.

JE is transmitted by infective bites of female mosquitoes mainly belonging to *Culex tritaeniorhynchus* which prefers to breed in irrigated rice paddies. Other less common vectors belong to *Culex vishnui* and *Culex pseudovishnui* group. Epidemiological studies have shown that after the monsoon rains, mosquitoes breed prolifically.

JE virus is primarily zoonotic in its natural cycle and the human being is an accidental host. Humans become infected with JE virus coincidentally when living or travelling in close proximity to animals and birds infected with JE. Although most cases occur in the rural areas, JE virus is also found on the edge of the cities. Although the virus has occasionally been isolated from human peripheral blood, viremias are usually brief and titers low; as a result, humans are considered a dead-end host from which transmission does not normally occur. Pigs and wild birds are the reservoir of infection.

3. When to suspect JE and how to diagnose it?

JE should be suspected in any case presenting with acute onset of fever with CNS manifestation, especially during the monsoon season, in the areas where JE is endemic. History of recent travel to such area is also an important risk factor. The criteria set down for clinical diagnosis of JE are:
- Acute onset of fever, not more than 5-7 days' duration
- Change in mental status with/without new onset of seizures (excluding febrile seizures)
- Other early clinical findings include irritability, somnolence or abnormal behavior greater than that seen with usual febrile illness.

Important

In an epidemic situation, fever with altered sensorium persisting for more than two hours with a focal seizure or paralysis of any part of the body is encephalitis. Presence of rash on the body excludes JE.

Laboratory diagnosis

Several laboratory tests are available for JE virus detection, which include:
- Antibody detection: Hemagglutination Inhibition Test (HI), Compliment Fixation Test (CF), Enzyme-linked Immunosorbent assay (ELISA) for IgG (paired) and IgM (MAC) antibodies, etc.
- Antigen Detection: IFA, Immunoperoxidase, etc.
- Genome Detection—RTPCR
- Isolation—Tissue culture, infant mice, etc.

In view of the limitations associated with various tests, IgM ELISA is the method of choice, provided the samples are collected 3-5 days after the infection. In recent years, good quality IgM-capture ELISA kits are available. In the sentinel surveillance network, JE will be diagnosed by IgM-capture ELISA, and virus isolation will be done in National Reference Laboratory.

Diagnosis of JE is mainly done in a suspected case with any one of the following markers:
- Presence of IgM anti-JEV antibody, mainly in CSF. In an endemic region and during outbreak, presence of IgM antibody to JEV in serum is also considered as a confirmative test
- Fourfold difference in IgG antibody titer in paired sera
- Virus isolation from brain tissue
- Antigen detection by immunofluorescence
- Nucleic acid detection by PCR.

JEV cross reacts with other flaviviruses including dengue viruses. Therefore, to rule out false positivity in a suspected case, confirmatory testing is needed. Positive IgM-capture ELISA should be confirmed in the following situations:
1. Ongoing dengue or other flavivirus outbreaks
2. High vaccination coverage
3. In the areas where there are no epidemiological or entomololgical data supporting JE transmission.
4. A nonvalidated assay is used at the primary testing laboratory.

Attempts to isolate Japanese encephalitis virus from clinical specimens are usually unsuccessful, probably because of low viral titers and the rapid production of neutralizing antibodies. The diagnosis of JE is usually made serologically using IgM-capture enzyme-linked immunosorbent assay (ELISA). The hemagglutination inhibition test was used for many years, but it had various practical limitations, and as it required paired serum, could not provide an early diagnosis. In the 1980s, IgM- and IgG-capture enzyme-linked immunosorbent assays (ELISAs) were developed, which have become the accepted standards for the diagnosis of Japanese encephalitis. After the first 9-10 days of illness, the presence of anti-Japanese encephalitis virus

IgM in the CSF has a sensitivity and specificity of >95% for CNS infection with the virus (before this, false negatives may occur). The sensitivity for the detection of JE-specific IgM in the serum is approximately the same as for CSF. Antibodies begin to appear soon after the onset, but only about 70-75% of the patients have IgM antibody in specimens collected up to 4 days after onset. However, all the patients will have antibody 7-10 days after the onset. CSF is the preferred sample for the diagnosis of JE because if anti-JE IgM is detected in the CSF, this confirms infection of the central nervous system with JEV. Asymptomatic infection with JEV or vaccination with live attenuated JE vaccines may cause an antibody rise in the serum, but they do not lead to antibody production in the CSF. If the CSF and/or serum sample is taken too early in the illness, it may not be positive for JE IgM antibody. A second serum sample collected approximately one week after the first sample can be very helpful in accurate diagnosis, if the first one is IgM-negative. Even if the first serum sample is positive, a second sample can be useful because it will usually show an increased titer compared to the first sample, which aids in confirming an acute infection.

RT-PCR (Reverse transcriptase PCR)

PCR assays are not recommended for routine diagnosis. The short period of viremia in the infected humans may also limit the usefulness of PCR as a clinical diagnostic tool.

Detection of virus genome by RT-PCR is very specific for JE diagnosis; however, it is not sensitive. Virus is usually undetectable in a clinically ill JE case. Virus genome in CSF is usually found only in the fatal cases. However, PCR assays combined with sequencing can be useful for providing information about the molecular epidemiology and evolution of viruses. PCR testing is a function of the reference and specialized laboratories of the network. Quantitative PCR and loop mediated isothermal amplification (LAMP- RTPCR-based) can diagnose JE as early as in the first 3-5 days.

Virus isolation

All the arboviruses, including the JE virus, are high-risk pathogens and laboratory procedures that amplify or concentrate the agent are potentially high-risk activities. All the attempts at virus isolation must take account of these risks and appropriate laboratory biosafety practices observed and the staff should be vaccinated against JE.

Isolation of JE virus from routine clinical samples is very challenging but may occasionally be successful from CSF or from brain tissue samples of fatal cases. After isolation, the virus can be confirmed and identified using appropriate polyclonal or monoclonal antibodies, by indirect immunofluorescence, by RT-PCR using JEV-specific primers, or by nucleotide sequencing. Viral isolation can also be performed, but it is slow and technically difficult, and is often negative because the virus has cleared by the time the patients present to the hospital. Hence, negative result does not rule out JE.

Other test procedures

Plaque reduction neutralization test (PRNT)

It is possible to confirm JE ELISA results using the sensitive plaque reduction neutralization test (PRNT) method to differentiate JE antibody from other flaviviruses. The PRNT is a quantitative biological assay measuring neutralizing antibodies with the end-point determined by the neutralization of JE or other flavivirus plaques in cell monolayers, by the serum under test. This assay is considered more sensitive than ELISA for differentiating between different flaviviruses. However, PRNT is time-consuming to perform, has a long incubation period and is labor-intensive. It is recommended for use only in reference laboratories with experience in this assay and for samples which cannot be easily differentiated by ELISA method.

Specimen collection and handling

Blood and cerebrospinal fluid (CSF) are the most important specimens for detection of IgM antibodies to JEV. These samples should be collected as soon as possible after admission of the patient. For virological investigations, a minimum of 0.5 mL of CSF is required. CSF samples for virological testing should be sent to the designated laboratory as soon as possible. Before transport in the hospital laboratory, they should be held at 4°C for short-term storage (1 to 3 days) or at or below –20°C for longer term storage. If a –20°C freezer is not available, they should be stored in the freezer section of the refrigerator. If specimens have been frozen, they should be transported frozen. Repeated freezing and thawing of CSF should be avoided as this may lead to instability of IgM antibodies.

Serum samples received for IgM analysis should be tested as soon as possible after receipt in the laboratory. Short-term storage of serum (1–3 days) should be at 4°C. Longer term storage of serum should be at or below –20°C. Repeated freezing and thawing of serum should be avoided as this may lead to instability of IgM antibodies.

Imaging

- JE mainly affects thalmus, coupus striatum, brain stem and even spinal cord
- Leptomeningeal enhancement and low-density lesions are common CT findings
- MRI: Panda Sign—due to thalamic hyperdensity. However, its absence will not rule out JE.

4. What is the main reason for higher mortality in JE/AES and what is to be done?

High mortality in cases with JE/AES is mainly due to delay in diagnosis, lack of awareness about the condition, delay in starting optimum supportive management and delay in transferring the index case to higher centre.

Specific therapy for JE/AES is not available. Hence, lack of skilful applications of supportive and symptomatic measures is a prime factor for poor outcome.

The disease affects the central nervous system and can cause severe complications, seizures and even death. To reduce severe morbidity and mortality, it is important to identify early warning signs and refer patients to health facility and educate the health workers about the first line management at the grassroot level.

Addressing the following issues with optimum threshold will improve the prognosis:
1. Management of airways and breathing
2. Management of circulation
3. Control of convulsion and intracranial pressure
4. Control of temperature
5. Fluid and electrolytes and calories/nutrition
6. General management
7. Specific treatment of any for the treatable cause
8. Investigations, samples collection and transportation
9. Reporting of a case
10. Rehabilitation.

5. What is the common sequelae of complications of JE?

After the acute disease, neuronal deficits often persist. These may include spastic paralysis, wasting, fasciculation, extrapyramidal abnormalities and cranial nerve involvement. Severe weight loss, mental retardation, emotional instability, personality changes, speech disturbances are long-term sequelae. The frequency of sequelae is about 5–70%, out of which moderate to severe sequelae is found in 28–30% cases. Focal muscle wasting is one of the most important consistent sequelae.

6. What vaccines are available for JE and how to administer them?

JE is a vaccine preventable disease. Various vaccines used against JE are discussed here briefly.

Mouse brain derived inactivated purified vaccine: It is associated with high incidence of sometimes fatal complications, currently not available in India. This vaccine is prepared from either the Nakayama/Beijing strain of JE virus grown in mice brain, purified, inactivated by formalin and preserved with thimerosal.

The vaccine is given subcutaneously—0.5 mL in children 1–3 years, and 1 mL in older children.

Primary immunization consists of three doses given on 0, 7 and 30 days. In special circumstances, when time is short, a 0-, 7- and 14-day schedule may be used. Two doses 7 days apart provide only short-term immunity in 80% of vaccinees for 6 months and may be used in travelers for logistic reasons. The last dose should be given at least 10 days prior to travel to the endemic area. For long-term protection, regular boosters every 2–3 years are recommended. Common adverse reactions include fever, malaise, local tenderness and redness in 20% of the recipients. Acute neurologic events have been reported in 1–2.3 per million vaccinees. Allergic reactions, mainly Type I hypersensitivity reactions, including anaphylactic shock, have been reported at a frequency of 1–100 per 10,000 traveler vaccinees varying with different batches of the vaccine. The risk of reactions is higher in those with the history of hypersensitivity. All the vaccinees should be cautiously monitored for possible allergic reactions and asked to remain in the vicinity of medical facility for 10 days after vaccination. Owing to drawbacks (high cost, complicated dosing schedule, requirement of numerous doses and boosters, concerns about side-effects and reliance neurological tissue for production) and availability of better vaccines, production of this vaccine and availability has markedly declined. This vaccine was used in Japan and other parts of the world for a long time. To avoid reactogenicity and reduce cost, tissue culture vaccines are developed.

Tissue culture vaccines: These include:
1. Cell culture derived, inactivated JE vaccine based on Bejing P-3 strain (available only in China).
2. Cell culture derived, live attenuated vaccine based on SA 14-14-2 strain (this is only JE vaccine currently available in India). This vaccine is also being used in China, South Korea and Nepal.
   It is based on the genetically stable, neuroattenuated SA-14-14-2 strain of JE virus, which elicits broad immunity against heterologus JE viruses.
   Administration: 0.5 mL subcutaneously to children at 8 months of age and a second dose at the age of 2 years. In some areas, a booster at 7 years is also given. It should not be used as an outbreak vaccine. It can be administered to all the susceptible children up to 15 years and can be administered as a catch-up vaccination.
   The vaccine should be stored and shipped at 8C, protected from sunlight.
3. JE vaccines on the horizon: These include Chimeric vaccine, Inactivated SA 14-14-2 vaccine, and inactivated vero cell-derived JE vaccine—Being-1 JE strain.

JE vaccine should not be used as an "outbreak response vaccine". IAPCOI recommends that the government should implement universal immunization with this vaccine in all children in JE-endemic states. The SA-14-14-2 vaccine appears best suited for this purpose and can safely be coadministered with the measles vaccine at 9 months. Along with all infants, all susceptible children up to the age of 15 years should be administered catch-up vaccination. JE vaccine is also recommended for the travelers to JE-endemic areas, provided they are expected to stay for a minimum of 4 weeks in the rural areas in the JE season.

7. How to recognize Herpes Simplex Encephalitis (HSE)?

Viral encephalitis caused by HSE is the most common cause of sporadic viral encephalitis. A common presentation, like all other AES, will be history of fever, headache, vomiting, irritability, altered sensorium, confusion and seizures, etc. A preceding respiratory catarrh or labial herpes may or may not be present. Clinical presentation ranges from aseptic meningitis and fever to a severe rapidly progressive form involving altered consciousness. In adults, HSV-1 accounts for 95% of all the fatal cases of sporadic encephalitis and usually results from reactivation of the latent virus.

In HSE, the neurological findings are mainly related to the involvement of fronto-parietal lobes. This will include personality changes, confusion, and disorientation, and focal seizures. However, absence of herpes labialis, unilateral neurological findings or focal seizures will not exclude HSE. Less commonly, HSV-1 may produce brain stem encephalitis, and HSV-2 may produce a myelitis.

Typical findings on presentation include the following:
- Alteration of consciousness (97%)
- Fever (92%)
- Dysphasia (76%)
- Ataxia (40%)
- Seizures (38%)—Focal (28%); generalized (10%)
- Hemiparesis (38%)
- Cranial nerve defects (32%)
- Visual field loss (14%)
- Papilledema (14%).

CSF examination

CSF is often hemorrhagic in HSE.

CSF PCR for HSV 1 is optimally positive from 2–10 days of illness. It remains positive even 1 week after starting the antiviral therapy.

Imaging

CT scan of brain may be normal in first 4–6 days of illness, but MRI is rarely normal in a case of HSE.

Hyperdensities in temporal lobe are common CT findings in HSE. CT scans classically reveal hypodensity in the temporal lobes either unilaterally or bilaterally, with or without frontal lobe involvement. Hemorrhage is usually not observed. A gyral or patchy parenchymal pattern of enhancement is observed. Contrast enhancement generally occurs later in the disease process.

MRI findings in HSE include abnormal signal intensity in medial temporal lobe, cingulate gyrus, and orbital surface of frontal lobe. T2-weighted MRI reveals hyperintensity corresponding to edematous changes in the temporal lobes, inferior frontal lobes, and insula, with a predilection for the medial temporal lobes. Foci of hemorrhage occasionally can be observed on MRI.

EEG

EEG findings in HSE include periodic lateralized epileptiform discharges. Previously, these findings were considered pathognomic but are now regarded as non-specific. Normal EEG does not exclude HSE.

8. How to manage HSE?

Stabilization of the child, maintaining of airway, breathing and circulation is most important. Acyclovir is the drug of choice.

In any index case of AES, especially when sporadic, acyclovir should be started empirically, since HSE is the treatable cause of ASE. In such case, acyclovir should be stopped if an alternative diagnosis is made or HSV PCR in CSF and MRI is normal.

Dose of acyclovir

For children from the age of 3 months to 12 years: 500 mg/m^2 8-hourly
  Children >12 years of age: 10 mg/kg 8-hourly

Duration of acyclovir

Confirmed case: In a confirmed case, acyclovir should be given for 14–21 days intravenously, and minimum 21 days for those aged 3 months to 12 years. Dose reduction is required in the presence of existing renal failure.

Empiric use: In such case, acyclovir should be stopped if an alternative diagnosis is made or HSV PCR in CSF is negative on two occasions (24–48 hours apart) and MRI is not suggestive of HSE.

Further Reading

1. Consensus guidelines on evaluation and management of suspected acute viral encephalitis in children in India. Indian Pediatr. 2012;49:887-910.
2. Guidelines for prevention and control of JE. WHO: Geneva. Available from www.whoindia.org/Linkfilles/Communicable_Diseases_Guidelines_for_Prevention_and_control_ Japanese_Encephalitis.pdf.
3. Guidelines for Clinical Management of Acute Encephalitis Syndrome including Japanese Encephalitis. Government of India, 2009. Available from www.nvbdcp.
4. IAP Guide book on immunization. 2011;pp.137-9.
5. Japanese Encephalitis. Clinical care guidelines. PATH, November, 2006. Available from: www.path.org/vaccineresources/files PDF.

30

Upper Respiratory Infection

Nupur Ganguly

1. Which part of the respiratory tract is involved in URTI?

Upper respiratory tract infection (URTI) is the most common cause of office visit in our day-to-day practice, and it involves the nose, sinuses, pharynx and larynx giving rise to common cold, tonsillitis, pharyngitis, sinusitis, laryngitis, and otitis media.

2. What are the common organisms responsible for common cold? How do we manage?

Common cold occurs throughout the year, and has considerable disease burden. In common colds patient feels unwell, there is excessive nasal discharge and a sensation of chill that is oversensitivity to ambient temperature, which may be the reason why it is called cold. Usually, the infection starts in the nasal cavity (the typical common cold), however, it may start in the throat, the sinuses, the ears, or the bronchi, in which case the first symptom could be a sore throat, pain in the facial bones, earache, cough respectively followed by running nose.

Organism responsible for common cold are mainly viruses. Rhinoviruses, coronaviruses, respiratory syncytial viruses, influenza viruses, parainfluenza viruses, bocavirus, human metapneumovirus are common offenders. Coronaviruses are generally associated with more severe symptoms than the rhinoviruses.

Treatment

The management of the common cold is primarily symptomatic. Although, bacteria is often isolated from mucopurulent nasal discharge, they do not indicate nasal colonization. As per cochraine analysis database antibiotics do not reduce the duration of purulent rhinitis or prevent complication. Antihistamine and decongestant combination are found to have limited role in young children but in adults and older children they are beneficial in improving nasal symptoms and general recovery. Vitamin C and zinc has no role in common cold.

In influenza viral infections the neuraminidase inhibitors—oseltamivir and zanamivir have a modest effect on reducing the duration of symptoms provided the therapy is started early in the illness (within 48 hour of onset of symptoms). The difficulty of distinguishing influenza from other common cold pathogens limits the use of these agents. Antibiotics are not indicated in the treatment of the common cold.

3. **What is acute rhinosinusitis? What are the common causative organisms? How do you diagnose and treat?**

Sinusitis or rhinosinusitis

In children, acute bacterial rhinosinusitis usually follows a viral infection or allergic rhinitis. It is a common infection and rarely it may lead to life-threatening complications. As the signs and symptoms of acute bacterial rhinosinusitis are similar to those of viral upper respiratory tract infection, establishing an accurate diagnosis in children poses a clinical challenge.

Causative organisms are usually viral. Common bacterial organisms are *Streptococcus pneumoniae* accounts for 30-66% of episodes of acute bacterial rhinosinusitis and rest by *Haemophilus influenzae* (20-30%) and *Moraxella catarrhalis* (12-28%).

Diagnosis

The diagnosis of acute bacterial sinusitis in children is mainly clinical. But the common diagnostic problem is to differentiate clinically between viral URI from bacterial sinus infection. The finding of purulent secretion in the region of middle meatus is highly suggestive of bacterial sinusitis. As per the IDSA, AAP, AAFP, CDC guideline, diagnosis of acute bacterial sinusitis may be made in children with symptoms of acute rhinosinusitis (nasal obstruction or purulent discharge, facial fullness or pain, fever, or anosmia) who have any of the three following clinical presentations:
1. Persistent symptoms of viral URI (nasal discharge or daytime cough) lasting more than 10 days without clinical improvement.
2. Severe illness with high fever (>39°C) and purulent nasal discharge, or facial pain for more than 3 consecutive days at the beginning of illness.
3. Worsening symptoms or signs (new onset fever, headache or increase in nasal discharge) following typical URI that lasted 5-6 days and were initially improving.

The finding of purulent secretion in the region of middle meatus is highly suggestive of bacterial sinusitis. Other diagnostic modalities like sinus aspirate culture is not of practical use in day-to-day practice. Radiographic studies like plain film and CT scan may confirm the presence of sinus inflammation but cannot determine the etiology. According to American Academy of Pediatrics (AAP) guideline diagnosis is to be made solely on clinical criteria and laboratory help is to be sought only in those patients who do not recover or who worsen during the course of antimicrobial therapy. Routine use of CT scan for diagnosis of rhinosinusitis is not recommended.

Allergy should be considered in children showing watery rhinorrhea, sneezing, seasonal pattern and treated accordingly with antihistaminics and topical steroids.

Treatment

Nearly all cases of acute viral sinusitis resolve without antibiotics. In selecting initial antimicrobial therapy, priority should be given to drugs with activity against *S. pneumoniae* and *H. influenzae* and *Moraxella catarrhalis*.

Antibiotic use should be reserved for moderate symptoms not improving after 10 days, or that are worsening after 5-7 days, and severe symptoms as mentioned above.

First line therapy
- Amoxycillin 45 mg/kg/day in 2 divided doses.
- Amoxycillin high dose (90 mg/kg/day in 2 divided doses) for those at higher risk for penicillin resistant S. pneumoniae infection, in high risk individual (fever > 39°C, threat of suppurative complications), attending day-care center, less than 2 years of age, history of recent hospitalization, antibiotic use within the past month, and immunocompromised individual.

Second line therapy

It is indicated when standard therapy has failed and we need to cover beta lactamase producing *H. influenzae* and *Moraxella catarrhalis*.
- Amoxycillin-clavulanate 45 mg/kg/day used initially, may increase dose to 90 mg/kg/day cefdinir or cefpodoxime or cefuroxine.

For non-anaphylactic β-Lactam allergy
- Cefdinir 14 mg/kg/day in one 2 divided doses
- Cefpodoxime 10 mg/kg/day once daily
- Cefuroxine 30 mg/kg/day in 2 divided doses.

For severe β-Lactam allergy
- Clarithromycin 15 mg/kg/day in 2 divided doses
- Azythromycin 10 mg/kg/day
- Clindamycin 30–40 mg/kg/day in 4 divided doses.

Intramuscular ceftriaxone may be appropriate for patients who fail on a second course of antibiotic treatment.

Duration of treatment

Despite the potential benefits of short-course therapy including improved compliance, fewer adverse events, reduced risk of treatment failure and bacterial resistance, and reduced cost, traditional management of acute bacterial rhinosinusitis treatment is to be continued for 10 to 14 days. If the condition worsens after 48-72 hours of antibiotics, or failure to improve after 3-5 days of antibiotics one should re-evaluate the patient and switch to second line antibiotic. Direct sinus aspiration for culture may be necessary for workup of patients with severe or refractory sinusitis.

Adjuvant therapy

American Academy of Pediatrics (AAP) does not recommend use of antihistamines, decongestant, mucolytic agents, saline nasal irrigation and topical intranasal steroids. AAP also does not recommend antibiotic prophylaxis in children with recurrent episodes of acute bacterial sinusitis.

4. What is acute suppurative otitis media (ASOM), otitis media with effusion (OME) and chronic suppurative otitis media (CSOM)?

Acute suppurative otitis media (ASOM)

A diagnosis of ASOM require all the 3 following criteria :
1. A history of acute onset of signs and symptoms.
2. The presence of middle ear effusion, which is indicated by any of the following:
    a. Bulging tympanic membrane
    b. Limited or absent mobility of the tympanic membrane
    c. Air fluid level behind the tympanic membrane
    d. Otorrhea.
3. Signs and symptoms of middle ear inflammation as indicated by either:
    a. Distinct erythema of the tympanic membrane or
    b. Distinct otalgia (discomfort clearly referable to ear/ears that results in interference with or precludes normal activity or sleep).

Otitis media with effusion (OME)

OME is a condition where there is a presence of fluid in the middle ear for at least 8 weeks in the absence of signs and symptoms of acute infection.

The middle ear in OME is usually sterile though in about 30% of case the pathogens responsible for AOM are also found. The significance of these pathogens are not clear at present whether they are indicative of past or recent infection.

Chronic suppurative otitis media (CSOM)

CSOM consists of persistent middle-ear infection with discharge through a tympanic membrane perforation. The disease is initiated by an episode of AOM with rupture of the membrane. The mastoid air cells are invariably involved. The most common etiologic organisms are *P. aeruginosa* and *S. aureus;* however, the typical AOM bacterial pathogens may also be the present.

5. What is the management of ASOM in different age groups?

Management of acute otitis media varies with different age group. In children above 2 years and above with less severe symptoms can be observed without giving antibiotics. The management in different age groups is given below in Table 1.

Table 1: Management of ASOM in different age groups

Age	Certain diagnosis	Uncertain diagnosis
Less than 6 months	Antibiotic is recommended	Either with certain or uncertain diagnosis
6 month–2 year	Antibacterial therapy	Antibiotic if severe illness
>2 year	Antibiotic in severe illness Observaztion in less severe illness	Observation option

During observation, analgesics and antipyretics (Oral ibuprofen/acetaminophen) may be used after assessment of pain. Topical benzocaine may be used in (grater than 5 years of age). Principles of therapy are same as for acute bacterial sinusitis as shown in Table 2.

Intramuscular (IM) ceftriaxone may be used who are unable to tolerate oral antibiotic and in case of poor compliance.

The duration of treatment of AOM is preferably 10 days. Studies comparing shorter with longer durations of treatment suggest that short-course treatment will often prove inadequate in children below 2 year of age. Thus, for most episodes in children, treatment that provides tissue concentrations of an antimicrobial for at least 10 days would seem advisable. Treatment for shorter periods of 3–5 days, may be appropriate for older children with mild episodes who improve quickly, however, in these cases, simple observation without antimicrobial therapy may often be the preferred intervention. Treatment for longer than 10 days may be required for children who are very young or are having severe episodes or whose previous experience with otitis media has been problematic.

6. What are the complications of ASOM?

Most complications of ASOM consist of the spread of infection to adjoining or near by structures or the development of chronicity or both. The complications of AOM may be classified as either intratemporal or intracranial.

Table 2: Principles of therapy of ASOM

Organism	First line	Second line
S. pneumoniae	Amoxycillin 40–45 mg/kg/24 h the drug of choice	Amoxycillin 80–90 mg/kg/24 hours
Drug resistant Streptococcus pneumoniae	Amoxycillin + Clavulanate	Cefuroxime Cefpodoxime
H. influenzae (H flu)	Amoxycillin + Clavulanate	Azithromycin, Clarithromycin
M. cattarhalis	Amoxycillin + Clavulanate	Azithromycin, Clarithromycin

Intratemporal complications

Direct but limited extension of AOM leads to complications within the temporal bone. These complications include dermatitis, tympanic membrane perforation, chronic suppurative OM (CSOM), mastoiditis, hearing loss, facial nerve paralysis, cholesteatoma formation, and labyrinthitis.

Infectious dermatitis

This is an infection of the skin of the external auditory canal resulting from contamination by purulent discharge from the middle ear. The skin is often erythematous, edematous, and tender. Management consists of proper hygiene combined with systemic antimicrobials and ototopical drops as appropriate for treating AOM and tube otorrhea.

Tympanic membrane perforation

Rupture of the tympanic membrane can occur with episodes of either AOM or OME. Although, damage to the tympanic membrane from these episodes generally heals spontaneously, chronic perforations can develop in a small number of cases and require further surgical intervention in the future.

Chronic suppurative otitis media (CSOM)

CSOM treatment is guided by the results of microbiologic investigation. If an associated cholesteatoma is not present, parenteral antimicrobial treatment combined with aural cleaning will be adequate, but in refractory cases, tympanomastoidectomy may be required.

Acute mastoiditis

Initially all cases of AOM are accompanied by mastoiditis by virtue of the associated inflammation of the mastoid air cells. However, early in the course of the disease, no signs or symptoms of mastoid infection are present, and the inflammatory process is reversible, along with the AOM, in response to antimicrobial treatment. Spread of the infection to the overlying periosteum, but without involvement of bone, constitutes acute mastoiditis with periosteitis. In such cases, signs of mastoiditis are usually present, including inflammation in the postauricular area, often with displacement of the pinna inferiorly and anteriorly. Treatment with myringotomy and parenteral antibiotics, if instituted promptly, usually provides satisfactory resolution.

Intracranial complications

Meningitis, epidural abscess, subdural abscess, focal encephalitis, brain abscess, sigmoid sinus thrombosis (also called *lateral sinus thrombosis*), and otitic hydrocephalus each may develop as a complication of acute or chronic middle-ear or mastoid infection, through direct extension, hematogenous spread, or thrombophlebitis. Bony destruction adjacent to the dura is often involved, and a cholesteatoma may be present. In a child with middle-ear or mastoid infection, the presence of any systemic symptom, such as high spiking fevers, headache, lethargy of extreme degree, a finding of meningismus or of any central nervous system sign on physical examination should prompt suspicion of an intracranial complication.

7. What is the management of OME?

In the management of otitis media with effusion (OME) primarily it has to be distinguished from acute otitis media by pneumatic otoscopy as the primary diagnostic method. However, tympanometry may be used to confirm the diagnosis of OME (presence of effusion with immobility of tympanic membrane) without signs or symptoms of acute infection. Repeated examination with hearing assessment is required monthly to detect the resolution of the effusion as most cases resolve without treatment within 3 months. If middle ear effusion (MEE) persists for longer than 3 months, consideration of surgical management with tympanostomy tubes is to given as antihistamines and decongestants are ineffective for OME, and they should not be used for treatment. Antimicrobials and corticosteroids do not have long-term efficacy and should not be used for routine management. At a minimum, children with OME persisting more than 3 more months require close monitoring of their hearing levels with skilled audiologic evaluation; frequent assessment of developmental milestones, including speech and language.

8. What are the common organism of croup syndrome?

Croup (Laryngotracheobronchitis) is the most common form of URTI. It is the infection of the glottic and subglottic region. Viruses are the most common causative organism, parainfluenza, rhinovirus, respiratory synsitial virus and Influenza virus. However, when the infection involves the structure above the cord it is known as epiglottitis. The common organism for epiglottitis is H Flu. Some form of laryngotracheobronchitis is associated with bacterial superinfection occurring 5–7 days following the onset of infection.

Further Reading

1. IDSA Releases Guidelines for Management of Acute Bacterial Rhinosinusitis.
2. Johnson D. Croup. Clinical Evid. 2005;14:310-27.
3. Lieberthal AS, Carroll AE, Chonmaitree T, Ganiats TG, et al. American Academy of Pediatrics. Clinical Practice Guideline. The Diagnosis and Management of Acute Otitis Media.
4. Puhakka T, Makela MJ, Alanen A, et al. Sinusitis in the common cold. J allergy Clinical Immunol. 1998;102:403-8.
5. Ronald B, Turner F, Hayden G. The common cold. Nelson Textbook of Pediatrics 19th edition. 1434-5.

31. Community Acquired Pneumonia

Upendra Kinjawadekar, Jaydeep Choudhury

1. What are the organisms responsible for CAP in different age groups?

Community acquired pneumonia (CAP) is an acute infection of the pulmonary parenchyma in a previously healthy child, acquired outside of a hospital setting. The patient should not have been hospitalized within 14 days prior to the onset of symptoms or has been hospitalized less than 4 days prior to the onset of symptoms.

Etiological agents

In a recent study from India, bacterial etiology was demonstrated in 16% of the population, viruses in 38%, *Mycoplasma* in 24% and *Chlamydia pneumoniae* in 11% of the cases. Mixed infection was present in 8%.

Age is a good predictor of the likely pathogen of pneumonia and can help narrow down the list of etiological agents. While Gram negative agents are common under 3 months of age, *Streptococcus pneumoniae* is common at all ages, thereafter *H. influenzae* is a common organism upto 2 years of age. *Staphylococcus* though not very common, is an important formidable enemy. Table 1 gives the probable agents at various age groups in order of common prevalence.

2. Does the etiology differ by age?

The etiology differs in various age groups as shown in Table 1.

Table 1: Etiological agents at various age groups

Age	Microbial agent
0–3 months of age	Gram Negative organisms Group B *Streptococcus* *Streptococcus pyogenes* *Chlamydia* Viruses
3 months–5 years of age	*Streptococcus pneumoniae* *H. influenzae* Viruses *Staphylococcus* *S. pyogenes* *Mycoplasma pneumoniae*

Contd...

Contd...

>5 years of age	S. pneumoniae Chlamydia pneumoniae Viruses Staphylococcus S. pyogenes H. influenzae Mycoplasma pneumoniae

3. What are the common clinical presentations?

Clinical features

Symptoms

Children with suspected pneumonia can present with the following symptoms:
- Fever
- Cough, may or may not be productive
- Chest pain and/or abdominal pain
- Difficulty in breathing (dyspnea)
- Rapid breathing (tachypnea)
- Constitutional symptoms: Malaise, lethargy, refusal to take feeds, headache, nausea/vomiting.

Signs

Rapid respiration identifies children who have a very high probability of having pneumonia and are therefore candidates for antibiotic therapy. The WHO algorithm for children presenting with cough and/or difficulty in breathing proposes rapid breathing as the most critical sign to identify pneumonia.

The cut off values for fast breathing are shown in Table 2.

Table 2: Cut off values for fast breathing	
Age< 2 months	60 or more;
2 months upto 12 months	50 or more;
12 months upto 5 years	40 or more breaths/minute

Some authors recommend that the cutoff rates should be lowered by about 5 breaths per minute for severely malnourished cases. Respiratory rate should ideally be counted for full 60 seconds when the child is awake and not crying. Inconsistencies in respiratory rate measurement requires repeated observation.

The presence of lower chest in drawing indicates pneumonia of greater severity.

The presence of grunt, crackles, bronchial breathing is suggestive of pneumonia, but are not so common.

Often, there may be presence of signs of the complications of pneumonia like para-pneumonic effusions/empyema, pneumothorax. Clinical differentiation of viral and bacterial pneumonias is difficult.

4. What are the various modalities of laboratory diagnosis and how far they are helpful?

Pneumonia is diagnosed clinically. X-ray and blood counts are not needed most of the times.
   i. Radiology
       Not a very reliable diagnostic tool due to wide inter- and intra-observer error in reading radiographs.
   ii. Acute phase reactants
       Like Total leucocyte count (TLC), differential leucocyte count (DLC), C-Reactive protein (CRP) are not diagnostic but may be useful to monitor the response to treatment. A normal test may be more useful in excluding the diagnosis as compared to confirmation on the basis of a positive test.
   iii. Microbiological tests are of no use routinely.

5. What are the indications for chest X-ray in either primary care or hospital care?

- For diagnosis of child under 5 years with fever of 39°C of unknown origin,
- If complications suspected, (For example, pleural effusion as suggested by diminished air entry)
- Ambiguous features
- Unresponsive to treatment after 48 hours of treatment/deteriorates.

6. How to assess severity for management in OPD, hospital and ICU?

The severity has to be assessed to decide the level of facility at which to treat the child with pneumonia and also to determine the choice of treatment including antibiotics as shown in Table 3.

Table 3: Severity assessment of pneumonia

Age group	Mild	Severe
Infants	RR < 70 breaths/ min Mild recession Taking full feeds	RR > 70 breaths/ min Moderate to severe recession Nasal flaring Cyanosis Intermittent apnea Grunting respiration Not feeding
Older children upto 5 years	RR < 50 breaths/ min Mild breathlessness No vomiting	RR > 50 breaths/ min Severe difficulty in breathing Nasal flaring Cyanosis Intermittent apnea Grunting respiration Signs of dehydration

7. What are the indications for admission to hospital in pneumonia among children?

- Mild to moderate cases do not need admission
- Infants less than 3 months of age are best treated as inpatients
- Oxygen saturation < 92% or cyanosis
- Respiratory rate > 70 breaths /minute
- Difficulty in breathing
- Intermittent apnea, grunting
- Not feeding
- Signs of dehydration
- Family not able to provide appropriate observation or supervision.

8. What are the indications for transfer to pediatric intensive care unit (PICU)?

Transfer to PICU should be considered in the following circumstances:
- Failure to maintain Oxygen saturation (SaO_2) >92% in inspired air-oxygen mixture (FiO_2) >0.6
- Peripheral circulatory failure
- Rising respiratory and pulse rates with clinical evidence of severe respiratory distress and exhaustion with or without raised $PaCO_2$
- Recurrent apnea or slow irregular breathing.

9. How to treat CAP? How long the treatment should be continued?

The components of management are:
A. Oxygen as indicated by pulse oxymetry and/ or clinical signs of hypoxia,
B. Supportive therapy, and
C. Antibiotic

Using antibiotics for CAP—General principles

Empirical therapy should be based on knowing the most likely pathogen in each community. *S. pneumoniae* is an important causative agent for community acquired pneumonia at all ages. Because it is difficult to distinguish between bacterial, viral, and mixed infections, most children with community acquired pneumonia are treated with antibiotics as shown in Tables 4 and 5. Selection of antibiotic is dictated by the age of the child and epidemiological factors, and sometimes the results of the chest radiography.

For *Staphylococcal* infection ceftriaxone and cloxacilin or cefuroxime with aminoglycoside or amoxyclav with aminoglycoside is used. Vancomycin and linezolid are kept as reserve drugs and can be used with ceftriaxone.

Table 4: Antibiotic therapy in CAP

Setting	Domiciliary		
AGE	First Line	Second Line	Suspected Staphylococcal ds
Upto 3 month	Usually Severe, treated as inpatients		
3mo- 5yrs	Amoxycillin	Co-amoxy clavulinic acid OR Chloramphenicol OR Cefuroxime	Amoxycillin+Cloxacillin OR Cefuroxime OR Co-amoxy clavulinic acid
>5 years	Amoxycillin	Macrolide OR Co-amoxy-clavulinic acid OR Chloramphenicol	Amoxycillin+Cloxacillin OR Cefuroxime OR Co-amoxy clavulinic acid

Table 5: Antibiotic therapy in severe and very severe pneumonia

Treat as In-patient		
Age	First Line	Second Line
0–3 month	Inj third gen Cephalosporins: Cefotaxime/Ceftriaxone ± Aminoglycoside	Co-amoxy clavulinic acid + Aminoglycoside
3 month– 5 years	Inj Ampicillin OR Inj Chloramphenicol OR Inj Ampicillin + Inj Chloramphenicol (<2 years of age) OR Inj Co-amoxyclavulinic acid	Inj Co-amoxy clavulinic acid OR Inj third Gen Cephalosporins: Cefotaxime/Ceftriaxone
>5 years	Inj Ampicillin OR Inj Chloremphenicol OR Inj Co-amoxyclavulinic acid OR Macrolides (if Mycoplasma suspected)	Inj Co-amoxy clavulinic acid OR Inj third Gen Cephalosporins: Cefotaxime/Ceftriaxone AND Macrolides

10. How long treatment has to be continued?

Domiciliary cases: Total of 5–7 days.

Admitted cases: Total 7 days. Switch to oral as soon as patient can accept orally. However, if on second line therapy, then use IV antibiotics for 7–10 days. If suspected or confirmed *Staphylococcal* disease, treat for 2 weeks at least in uncomplicated cases and for 4–6 weeks for those with complications like empyema, metastatic abscesses, etc.

At the end of the treatment, X-ray is not needed in every case except when:
- The response is delayed or incomplete, or
- There were any ambiguous signs in initial film, or

- There are any associated complications, or
- Children with lobar collapse or ongoing symptoms.

11. What are the complications of CAP? How to manage empyema?

Clinically, the fever and tachypnea worsens and X-ray shows same or worsening picture. In such cases, it may be due to the following causes:
- Inappropriate choice of antibiotic therapy
- Two underlying organism
- Inadequate therapy (dose and duration)
- Non compliance of the patient
- Resistant organism
- Development of complication—effusion
- Underlying disease
   i. TB.
   ii. Fungal.
   iii. Foreign body.
   iv. Congenital malformation of lung.
   v. HIV and other immunodeficiency state.

Recurrent and persistent pneumonia

Recurrent—Two episodes of pneumonia in one year or more than three episodes at any time with radiographic clearance between two episodes.

Persistent—Persistence of symptoms and radiographic abnormalities of more than one month.

Recurrence may involve same lung, different lung and same site or the new site of the same or other lung. Hence, recurrent pneumonia is a symptom of underlying comorbid situation rather than a disease itself.

Recurrent opacity in the same lobe may be due to:
- Foreign body aspiration
- TB lymph node pressing the bronchus
- Vascular ring
- Congenital anomaly like cyst, aberrant bronchus, fistula, etc.

Recurrent pneumonia involving different lobe may be due to:
- Asthma
- CV shunt
- Cystic fibrosis
- Ciliary dyskinesia
- Immunodeficiency.

In case of recurrent and persistent pneumonia, X- ray (Both AP and lateral views) are indicated. Detailed investigations are required which include broncoscopy, bronchoalveolar lavage, CT scan of thorax, aortogram and immunodeficiency work up, etc as per the individual case scenario.

Further Reading

1. Jadavji T, Law B, Label MH, et al. A practical guide for the diagnosis and treatment of pediatric pneumonia. Can Med Assu J. 1996;156:S703-11.
2. Macintosh K. Community acquired pneumonia in children. N Eng J Med. 2002;346:429-37.

32 Infective Endocarditis

Dhritobrata Das

1. Which patients are susceptible to develop bacterial endocarditis?

Endocarditis is unusual in healthy individuals with normal heart. Conditions which increase the risk of endocarditis are:
a. Congenital heart disease
b. Rheumatic heart disease
c. Artificial heart valves
d. Previous history of endocarditis
e. Immunocompromised individuals
f. Intravenous drug abusers
g. Prolonged intravenous catheters

2. What are the common bacterial agents causing infective endocarditis in children?

Most of the cases of infective endocarditis are caused by a relatively small number of organisms. Leading this group is Streptococci (commonest *Streptococcus viridians*, rarely beta-hemolytic *Pneumococcus*, *Enterococcus* etc.) followed closely by Staphylococci (commonest *Staphylococcus aureus*, rarely coagulase negative staphylococcus). Gram negative organisms like *Pseudomonas sp.*, *Salmonella sp.*, HACEK group (*Haemophilus, Actinobacillus, Cardiobacterium, Eikenella, Kingella*) and *Neisseria sp.* are rare causes of infective endocarditis. Fungal endocarditis is on the rise due to increased use of prosthetic devices and prolonged intravenous catheters and is commonly caused by *Candida sp.*

3. What are the different clinical manifestations of infective endocarditis?

Clinical features

Nonspecific features

Fever is the most common nonspecific feature. It is continuous to start with and may be high or low grade depending upon the organism involved. Fever is often associated with other nonspecific symptoms like myalgia, arthralgia, fatigue, weakness, anorexia, weight loss and sweating.

Cardiac features

Cardiac manifestations may be appearance of a new murmur or change in the character of previous murmur. Sometimes tachycardia and breathing difficulty may be the presentation. Heart failure in endocarditis results from hemodynamic alterations due to damaged valves and associated myocarditis. Endocarditis usually affects left sided (mitral and aortic) valves and the resulting damage can cause severe regurgitation with left ventricular volume overload and features of congestive heart failure. Extension of endocarditis from valve into surrounding tissue may form abscess and rarely can rupture into pericardial cavity causing pericarditis. Rare instances also include embolism into coronary circulation resulting in myocardial infarction and conduction abnormalities.

Nocardiac features

Neurological manifestations are the commonest, occurring in more than one third of patients. Embolization to central nervous system may cause stroke or diffuse cerebral vasculitis. Other neurologic complications include aseptic or purulent meningitis, intracranial hemorrhage due to hemorrhagic infarcts or ruptured mycotic aneurysms, seizures and encephalopathy. Renal involvement is more common in patients with staphylococcal infections and may present with hematuria, glomerulonephritis or renal infarction. Anemia and splenomegaly are also common features. Splenomegaly is usually painless, but splenic infarcts may cause pain. Classic peripheral manifestations like Osler's nodes, subungual splinter hemorrhages, Roth's spots, Janeway lesions are late manifestations and found rarely if the disease is not treated timely.

Neonatal endocarditis

Infective endocarditis in neonates with prolonged hospitalization is on the rise. The signs are usually nonspecific, particularly in the preterm neonates. Many infants have feeding difficulties, respiratory distress and tachycardia. Fever is seldom present. Neonates may present with septicemia, hypotension, congestive cardiac failure, or a changing murmur. Neurological signs and symptoms such as seizures, hemiparesis and apnea occur in many infants. Septic embolisms are common in neonates and cause focuses of infection outside the heart, such as osteomyelitis, meningitis, and pneumonia.

4. **What is the ideal number and timing of blood culture to diagnose endocarditis?**

Bacteremia in patients with infective endocarditis is usually continuous. It is therefore not necessary to collect the blood sample at any particular phase of the febrile cycle. Three blood cultures from separate venipuncture sites at one hour interval before starting antibiotic are considered adequate.

5. What are the investigations for endocarditis?

Blood tests: Complete blood count, ESR, CRP and blood culture.
Urine: Routine examination (To look for hematuria).
Imaging: Chest X-ray, ECG, Echocardiography.

Complete blood count often shows anemia and raised white cell count (predominantly polymorphonuclear leukocytosis). Acute phase reactants like erythrocyte sedimentation rate and C-reactive protein are usually elevated.

Circulating immune complex titer and rheumatoid factor concentration are commonly increased in endocarditis.

Microscopic hematuria is very common. Hematuria with red cell casts, proteinuria and renal insufficiency suggest glomerulonephritis. Chest X-ray may reveal pulmonary infarct and ECG may rarely be useful if there is myocardial infarct or conduction anomaly.

6. What is Duke Criteria?

Modified Duke Criteria for Diagnosis of Infective Endocarditis

Pathological criterion
Positive histology or microbiology of pathological material obtained at autopsy or cardiac surgery (valve tissue, vegetations, embolic fragments or intracardiac abscess content)

Major Criteria

I. **Positive blood culture for infective endocarditis**
   A. Typical microorganism consistent with endocarditis from two separate blood cultures as noted below:
      Viridans streptococci, *Streptococcus bovis*, HACEK group, Community-acquired *Staphylococcus aureus* or enterococci, in the absence of a primary focus
   B. Microorganisms consistent with endocarditis from persistently positive blood cultures defined as:
      Two positive cultures of blood samples drawn >12 hours apart or all of three/a majority of four or more separate cultures of blood (with first and last sample drawn >1 hour apart).

II. **Evidence of endocardial involvement**
   A. Positive echocardiogram for endocarditis defined as:
      Oscillating intracardiac mass on valve or supporting structures in the path of regurgitant jets or on implanted material, in the absence of an alternative anatomic explanation, abscess, new partial dehiscence of prosthetic valve or new valvular regurgitation (worsening or changing of pre-existing murmur not sufficient).

Minor Criteria

I. **Predisposition:** Predisposing cardiac condition or intravenous drug use
II. **Fever:** Temperature greater than 38.0°C

Infective Endocarditis

III. Vascular phenomena: Major arterial embolization, septic pulmonary infarcts, mycotic aneurysm, intracranial hemorrhage, conjunctival hemorrhages and Janeway lesions

IV. Immunologic phenomena: Glomerulonephritis, Osler's nodes, Roth's spots, rheumatoid factor

V. Microbiological evidence: Positive blood culture but does not meet a major criterion as noted above or serological evidence of active infection with organism consistent with endocarditis.

Diagnosis

I. Definite
   A. Pathologic criterion, or
   B. Two major criteria, or
   C. One major and three minor criteria, or
   D. Five minor criteria

II. Possible
   A. One major and one minor criteria, or
   B. Three minor criteria

III. Rejected
   A. Firm alternative diagnosis, or
   B. Resolution of syndrome after ≤4 days of antimicrobial therapy, or
   C. No pathologic evidence at surgery or autopsy after ≤4 days of antimicrobial therapy, or
   D. Does not meet definite or possible criteria.

7. What empirical antibiotic should be started in endocarditis? How the treatment should be modified according to the culture reports and duration of treatment?

Empiric therapy should have a combination of antibiotics which will cover both *Streptococcus* and *Staphylococcus*. The final antibiotic regimen will depend upon the organism isolated and its sensitivity pattern.

Penicillin G or ampicillin or ceftriaxone for 4 weeks results in almost universal recovery in streptococcal infections. In patients with prosthetic valves, the duration of therapy should be extended to at least 6 weeks. When there is a relative resistance to penicillin, combination with an aminoglycoside is recommended for first two weeks. *Staphylococcus* is usually resistant to penicillin G and ampicillin as they produce β-lactamase. For endocarditis due to methicillin-susceptible *Staphylococcus aureus*, therapy should include semisynthetic β-lactamase-resistant penicillin, such as nafcillin or oxacillin, given for a minimum of 6 weeks. There is some evidence that combination with an aminoglycoside might result in earlier sterilization of the blood and faster resolution of fever, but this does not appear to change the outcome with respect to mortality. Patients with methicillin-resistant strains should be treated with vancomycin for a minimum of 6 weeks, with or without gentamicin for the first 3 to 5 days of therapy. In patients with endocarditis involving a prosthetic valve, rifampicin should be added for the entire duration of therapy, with the duration of the aminoglycoside treatment being extended to 2 weeks. Enterococcal infection is rare in children. In patients with endocarditis on native valves caused by susceptible strains, a combination of penicillin G or ampicillin, together with gentamicin, should be given for 4 to 6 weeks. When prosthetic material is infected, a minimum duration of 6 weeks is recommended. First-line antifungal therapy remains amphotericin B, although it does not penetrate vegetations well. Antimycotic therapy should continue for at least 6 weeks in case of fungal endocarditis.

8. **What is the current recommendation for prophylaxis of infective endocarditis?**

American Heart Association Infective Endocarditis Prophylaxis Recommendations

Antibiotic prophylaxis with dental procedures is reasonable only for patients with cardiac conditions associated with the highest risk of adverse outcomes from endocarditis, including:
• Prosthetic cardiac valve or prosthetic material used in valve repair
• Previous endocarditis
• Congenital heart disease only in the following categories:
   – Unrepaired cyanotic congenital heart disease, including those with palliative shunts and conduits
   – Completely repaired congenital heart disease with prosthetic material or device, whether placed by surgery or catheter intervention, during the first six months after the procedure*
   – Repaired congenital heart disease with residual defects at the site or adjacent to the site of a prosthetic patch or prosthetic device (which inhibit endothelialization)
• Cardiac transplantation recipients with cardiac valvular disease.

Procedures for which prophylaxis is reasonable (only in patients with above listed high risk cardiac conditions): • All dental procedures that involve manipulation of gingival tissue or the periapical region of teeth or perforation of oral mucosa • Invasive procedure of the respiratory tract that involves incision or biopsy of respiratory mucosa • Procedures involving infected skin, skin structures, or musculoskeletal tissue   Antibiotic prophylaxis solely to prevent infective endocarditis is not recommended for gastrointestinal or genitourinary tract procedure.

Further Reading

1. Baddour LM, Sullam PM, Bayer AS. The pathogenesis of infective endocarditis. In: Sussman M, ed. Molecular Medical Microbiology. San Diego, California: Academic Press; 2001; 999-1020.
2. Baddour LM, Wilson WR, Bayer AS, et al. Infective endocarditis: diagnosis, antimicrobial therapy, and management of complications: a statement for healthcare professionals from the Committee on Rheumatic Fever, Endocarditis, and Kawasaki Disease, Council on Cardiovascular Disease in the Young, and the Councils on Clinical Cardiology, Stroke, and Cardiovascular Surgery and

Anesthesia, American Heart Association: endorsed by the Infectious Diseases Society of America.Circulation. 2005;111(23):e394-434.
3. Baltimore RS. Infective endocarditis. In Jenson HB, Baltimore RS, eds. Pediatric Infectious diseases: principles and practice. Norwalk: Appleton and Lange, 1995.
4. Berkowitz FE. Infective endocarditis in childhood. St Louis: CV Mosby. 1995: 961-86.
5. Choudhury R, Grover A, Varma J, Khattri HN, Anand IS, Bidwai PS, et al. Active infective endocarditis observed in an Indian hospital 1981-1991. Am J Cardiol. 1992;70:1453-8.
6. Durack DT, Lukes AS, Bright VK. New criteria for diagnosis of infective endocarditis: utilization of specific echocardiographic findings. Duke Endocarditis Service. An J Med. 1994;96:200-9.
7. Durack DT. Prevention of infective endocarditis. N Engl J Med. 1995;332:38-44.
8. Saiman L, Prince A, Gersony WM. Pediatric infective endocarditis in the modern era. J Pediatr. 1993;122:847-53.
9. Stockhelm JA, Chadwick EG, Kessler S, et al. Are the Duke Criteria Superior to the Beth Israel Criteria for the diagnosis of infective endocarditis in children? Clin Infect Dis 1998;27:1451-6.
10. Van Hare GF, Ben-Shacher G, Liebman J, et al. Infective endocarditis in infants and children during the past 10 years: a decade of change. Am Heart J. 1984;107:1235-40.

33

Acute Gastroenteritis

Devdeep Mukherjee

1. What is the etiology of AGE (Aute Gastroenteritis)?

Pathogens vary between developed and developing countries. Bacterial and viral infections cause most infective diarrhea in developing countries. Viruses account for upto 40% of cases.

The organisms

Bacteria

   i. *E.coli*—It is the commonest cause being identified as enteropathogenic (EPEC), enterotoxigenic (ETEC), enteroaggregative (EAEC), enteroinvasive (EIEC), enterohemorrhagic (EHEC) or Shiga Toxin (STEC). ETEC causes most traveler's diarrhea. EHEC causes hemorrhagic colitis and hemolytic uremic syndrome in outbreaks. ETEC and rotavirus are the leading causes of dehydrating diarrheal disease among infants starting complementary feeding.
  ii. *Shigella*—It accounts for highest incidence in age 1 to 4 and causes 10% of all diarrheal episodes under the age of 5 worldwide. It is important cause of diarrheal deaths in 3-5 million children aged less than five years in developing countries. The emergence of pandemic strains with multiple antimicrobial resistance and severe illness is a matter of concern. It requires small inoculums, so direct person-to person transmission is much more common than with any other bacterial enteric infection. It rarely causes bacteremia.
 iii. *Salmonella species*—Acute non typhoidal Salmonellosis usually results from ingestion of contaminated meat, dairy, or poultry products. It requires a relatively large inoculum, so person-to-person transmission is rare. It is remarkably resistant to drying, often transmitted via commercially prepared dry or processed food and eggs. Spread from distant geographic areas by fruits and vegetables can occur. It is more common and severe in immunocompromised hosts.
  iv. *Campylobacter jejuni*—It is hyperendemic in developing countries, most frequent in the first year of life and in young adult years. Its reservoir include chickens and household dogs. Occasionally, associated is mesenteric lymphadenitis which causes profusely

tender abdomen mimicking appendicitis. Complications like toxic megacolon and colonic hemorrhage are common if anti-motility agents are used for it.

v. *Vibrios cholera* has major role in epidemics. Seafood poisoning is by *Vibrio parahaemolyticus*.

vi. *Clostridium difficile*—It is the most common cause of pseudomembranous colitis, during or following a course of antibiotics. Almost all antibiotics have been implicated but Clindamycin is the most identified. Newborn infants may be colonized with toxigenic *C. difficile* and yet remain well. It is spread easily from patient to patient within general ward.

vii. *Yersinia*—It occurs in colder countries. It affects lymphoid tissue in lamina propria mimicking appendicitis.

viii. *Other bacteria*—*Aeromonas* and *Plesiomonas shigelloides*.

Viruses

i. *Rotavirus*—It is the single most important cause of dehydrating diarrhea in children younger than 2 years who require hospitalization worldwide, accounting for about 3.5 million cases per year and as many as 110,000 hospital admissions for diarrhea according to surveillance published in Morbidity and mortality weekly report (MMWR) 2008. Bhan MK and associates found that in India 50% of all children hospitalized with rotavirus by age 5 were hospitalized by the age of 6 months, 75% by the age of 9 months, and almost 100% by the age of 2 years. Rotavirus was most prevalent in 31% children between 7 and 12 months of age, 20% in 1 and 2 years of age and 13% in <7 months of age. It is transmitted by feco-oral spread with secondary spread via respiratory route.

ii. *Norwalk virus*—It is responsible for outbreaks of short lived gastroenteritis in older children and adults.

iii. *Enteric adenoviruses and Astroviruses*—These are emerging as significant causes of diarrheal disease in developed countries. Enteric adenoviruses account for 5-20% of hospitalizations for acute diarrhea. They have a longer incubation period of 8-10 days and diarrhea lasts longer for 5-12 days. Astroviruses and caliciviruses each account for 3-5% hospitalizations for acute diarrhea. Cytomegalovirus has emerged particularly in both acquired and iatrogenic immunodeficiency.

iv. *Severe measles*—This infection is often accompanied by severe diarrhea.

v. *Other viruses*—This includes Torovirus, enteric Coronaviruses, and Picorna viruses.

Parasites

i. *Giardia lamblia*—It is the most frequent amongst parasites with prevalence upto 30% in developing countries in young children. It

may be carried asymptomatically. It multiplies in small bowel but rarely invades the mucosa. Its disease pattern is opposite to the usual acute diarrhea, with an insidious onset over 5 to 10 days.
  ii. *Cryptosporidia*—It is often an acute onset but tends to be more chronic.
  iii. Other important diarrheal gut parasites include *Isospora belli, Strongyloides stercoralis, Trichuris trichiura,* and *Entamoeba histolytica* and *Cyclospora.* They have a variable importance, depending on geographic location and immune status of the child.
  iv. *Nonpathogenic isolates*—It includes *Entamoeba coli, Endolimax nana, Iodamoeba butschlii,* and *Blastocystis hominis.*
  v. *Giardia* and *Cryptosporidium* species and *Entamoeba histolytica* may cause a protracted illness. Parasitic diarrhea may be a significant contributing factor to persistent enteric disease and malnutrition. *Giardia* can cause intermittent or persistent diarrhea with fat malabsorption.

Conditions predisposing to infective diarrhea

  i. *Sickle cell disease*—It predisposes to *Salmonella* species diarrhea.
  ii. *AIDS*—It predisposes to *Mycobacterium avium,* in addition to the other bacteria, Cytomegalovirus and Rotavirus viruses and protozoa *Cryptosporidium* species, *Isospora belli, Giardia lamblia, Entamoeba histolytica, Cyclospora* species and *Microsporidia.*
  iii. *Liver diseases or malignancy*—It predisposes to *Plesiomonas* species.
  iv. *Close animal contact*—Like dogs and cats predispose to *Campylobacter* and turtles to *Salmonella* species.
  v. *Traveler's diarrhea*—It is mostly caused by *E. coli* but may be caused by *Shigella, Salmonella, Campylobacter and* Rotavirus.
  vi. Intestinal dysmotility, malnutrition, achlorhydria, hemolytic anemia (especially sickle cell disease), immunosuppression and malaria predispose to *Salmonella* species.
  vii. Agammaglobulinemia, chronic pancreatitis, achlorhydria, cystic fibrosis predisposes to *Giardia* species.

2. **What is acute bacillary dysentery and which organisms are responsible for it?**

It is characterized by marked inflammation of the intestine, especially of the colon, with abdominal pain, tenesmus, and frequent stools often containing blood and mucus. It is caused mainly by bacteria of the genus *Shigella, Salmonella, Campylobacter species.* and *Aeromonas.* It is most common in the tropics, the subtropics, and East Asia and can be fatal, especially among children. It can erupt at any place where sanitation is poor and large groups of people, including carriers of the disease, are crowded together.

The disease is spread through the feces of carriers who have the bacteria in their intestines, such individuals may have diarrhea or dysentery or may seem perfectly well inspite of carrying the disease. Infection may come after eating or drinking from anything contaminated with bacteria from the feces of these carriers. Even touching something contaminated and then touching the mouth can cause infection. Flies also spread the disease.

Attacks of bacillary dysentery are always acute after the incubation period of a few days. Temperature may rise as high as 40°C (104°F), sometimes with symptoms of dehydration, shock, and delirium. Bowel movements may be as many as 30 to 40 times a day. Running its normal course, without special medicines, it is usually over within a few weeks from its outset, although an attack in a child may be more serious and last longer.

The greatest threat of dysentery is from deficient fluid volume and electrolyte imbalance, which must be corrected by the intravenous administration of fluids and electrolytes lost in the watery stools.

Although the usual dysenteric illness may last a few weeks if not treated with special medicines, symptoms of intestinal ulceration, diarrhea, and painful spasms in evacuation may in a few cases continue for a longer time.

3. What is the pathophysiology of diarrhea in *Cholera*, rotavirus and invasive bacteria like *Shigella*?

Vibrio cholerae

Vibrio cholerae is a highly motile Gram-negative bacterium with a single-sheathed flagellum. In the course of cholera pathogenesis, *V. cholerae* expresses a transcriptional activator ToxT, which subsequently transactivates expressions of two crucial virulence factors: toxin-coregulated pilus and cholera toxin (CT). These factors are responsible for intestinal colonization of *V. cholerae* and induction of fluid secretion, respectively. In intestinal epithelial cells, CT binds to GM1 ganglioside receptors on the apical membrane and undergoes retrograde vesicular trafficking to endoplasmic reticulum, where it exploits endoplasmic reticulum associated protein degradation systems to release a catalytic A1 subunit of CT (CT A1) into cytoplasm. CT A1, in turn, catalyzes ADP ribosylation of α subunits of stimulatory G proteins, leading to a persistent activation of adenylate cyclase and an elevation of intracellular cAMP. Increased intracellular cAMP in human intestinal epithelial cells account for pathogenesis of profuse diarrhea and severe fluid loss in cholera.

Rotavirus

The process leading to diarrhea is initiated when Rotavirus binds to and infects enterocytes in the small intestine. Binding is mediated by sequential interaction with a series of sialic acid-containing and non sialylated receptor molecules. The virus is internalized by an unknown mechanism, and the outer capsid is lost, activating the virion-associated transcriptase and viral macromolecular synthesis. Viral proteins and RNAs concentrate in cytoplasmic structures called viroplasms, where RNA replication and packaging takes place. Intracellular events, probably involving NSP4 (viral protein), cause release of Ca^{2+} from the endoplasmic reticulum. The increase in intracellular Ca^{2+} concentration, triggering a number of cellular processes, including disruption of the microvillar cytoskeletal network, lowered expression of disaccharidases and other enzymes at the apical surface, general inhibition of the Na^+ solute cotransport systems, and necrosis. NSP4 appears to be released specifically by a Ca^{2+} dependent, nonclassical secretion pathway prior to cell lysis. These events lead to a malabsorption component of the diarrhea through reduction in absorptive capacity of the epithelium, reduced activity of Na^+ solute cotransporters, and reduction of digestive enzyme expression on the epithelial surface. The secretory component of rotavirus diarrhea appears to be secondary to virus-induced functional changes at the villus epithelium.

Shigella

A type III secretion system (T3SS) encoded on a large plasmid is a key virulence factor of *Shigella flexneri*. The T3SS determines the interactions of *S. flexneri* with intestinal cells by consecutively translocating two sets of effector proteins into the target cells. *Shigella* passes the epithelial cell barrier by transcytosis through the microfold (M) cells and encounters resident macrophages. The bacteria evade degradation in macrophages by inducing an apoptosis like cell death, which is accompanied by proinflammatory signaling. Free bacteria invade the epithelial cells from the basolateral side, move into the circulation by vectorial actin polymerization and spread to adjacent cells. Proinflammatory signaling by macrophages and epithelial cells further activates the innate immune response involving NK cells and attracts polymorphonuclear (PMN) leukocytes. The influx of PMN disintegrated the epithelial cell lining, which initially exacerbates the infection and tissue destruction by facilitating the invasion of more bacteria. Ultimately, PMN phagocytose and kill *Shigella*, thus contributing to the resolution of infection. Thus, *S. flexneri* controls invasion into epithelial cells, intra- and intercellular spread, macrophage cell death, as well as host inflammatory responses. Some of the translocated effector proteins show novel biochemical activities by which they intercept host cell signal transduction pathways.

4. **What are the various possible laboratory investigations in AGE, are they of any help in management?**

Microbiological investigations are generally not needed. Blood in the stool, fever, or persistence of the diarrhea may call for laboratory tests of an etiologic agent but WHO recommendations limit laboratory exploration primarily to treatment failures.

Stool test

Microscopy especially for polymorphs and guaiac test. Although a fresh stool sample is preferable, several well-saturated rectal swabs can be utilized. Dysentery and fever have a high predictive value but low sensitivity for a bacterial pathogen. Stool polymorphonuclear cells have a high sensitivity (> 80%) and lower predictive value (60%) for bacterial pathogens.

Stool culture

It remains critical for testing antibiotic resistance and serotype-sub-typing in bacterial outbreaks. Considering rapid emergence of resistance in *Shigella* culture should be mandatory when suspected. Enteric viruses however cannot be grown in routine laboratory.

Overall stool culture yields 1.5% to 5.8% for enteric pathogens. So, it is often considered having high cost per relative yield as most diarrheal illnesses are self-limiting and provide little information directly relevant to clinical care. But this information may have great public health importance to detect and control outbreaks. The yield can be improved by proper selection of target organism and its growth media based on clinical and epidemiologic setting. Fresh stool on first day of illness before antimicrobials and specimens with evidence of an inflammatory process gives better yield. Samples submitted in hospitalized patient after more than 3 days usually give poor yield except in immunosuppressed conditions. Evidence of an inflammatory response is often not present in non invasive toxin-mediated infections such as those due to *Shiga* toxigenic *Escherichia coli* or enterotoxic *E. coli*.

Organism specific diagnosis helps to prevent unnecessary procedures and treatment: Considering differential diagnosis of non infectious conditions in protracted and atypical cases, contain spread by food handlers and health care workers, monitor complications like HUS (*E. coli* 0157:H7), emergence of resistant organism (e.g. *Salmonella, Shigella*) and establish area specific sensitivity pattern, and thus avoid overtreatment with wide spectrum antimicrobials.

Cysts in the stool

These are excreted episodically; at least three stool specimens must be tested if *Giardiasis* is suspected. *Amebic* cysts are found in many pediatric stools, the majority of infections do not cause symptoms.

Stools for pH or reducing substances

There is no value in routinely testing it. They are often positive when lactose intolerance is clinically insignificant.

Clostridium difficile toxin assay

In stool, culture can be done.

Immunoassays

These are available for Group A rotaviruses, enteric adenoviruses, and astrovirus and neutrophil marker lactoferrin.

New methods

Enzyme immunoassay (EIA) and DNA probe nonculture techniques are rapidly being developed and hold promise for improved sensitivity.

Additional diagnostic evaluations

Like blood cell counts, blood cultures, urinalysis, abdominal radio/sonography, anoscopy, and endoscopy may be considered for selected cases in which disease severity or clinical and epidemiological features mandate such testing.

Serum electrolytes testing

Rarely, change the management. These values are often misinterpreted, leading to inappropriate treatment.

5. What are the indications of antibiotics in AGE? Which antibiotics are to be used and for what duration?

Antimicrobials are not usually indicated on outdoor basis even in suspected bacterial cause because majority of acute diarrheas are self-limited, their duration is not shortened by use of antimicrobials.

Use of antimicrobials should be made on individual basis and selected according to local sensitivity pattern in following cases:

i. Organisms needing antimicrobial the most are *Shigella* and *V. cholerae*.
ii. Organisms needing antimicrobials in selected circumstances are *E. coli* (EPEC if protracted; ETEC with continued severe diarrhea despite rehydration and supportive), *Campylobacter* in compromised hosts, *Yersinia* in sickle cell disease, *Salmonella* in febrile very young or positive blood cultures.
iii. Outbreaks of Shigellosis, Cryptosporidiosis, or Giardiasis to eliminate carriage and control outbreak.
iv. All severely malnourished children should receive broad spectrum antimicrobial treatment.
v. Treatment for amoebiasis should be given in dysentery if trophozoites of *E. histolytica* are seen in the stool or two different antimicrobials usually effective for *Shigella* in the area have been given without clinical improvement.
vi. Giardiasis should be treated only if cysts or trophozoites of *G. duodenalis* are seen in persistent diarrhea.
vii. Persistent diarrhea with diagnosed infections in intestines or outside it (pneumonia, sepsis, urinary tract infection and otitis media).

viii. Special needs of individual children (e.g., prematurity, immunocompromised or underlying disorders).

ix. Systemic sepsis, serious non-intestinal infections such as pneumonia.

Antibiotics may even prolong illness. Antimicrobials can increase susceptibility to other infections like resistant *Salmonella species*; carrier status in Salmonella infection; risk of Hemolytic-uremic syndrome (HUS) in Enterohemorrhagic *E. coli* (CHEC). Use of Metronidazole or Vancomycin considering *C. difficile* diarrhea in hospitals increase colonization of Vancomycin-resistant enterococci.

6. What is low osmolarity ORS? How to use them in AGE?

Oral rehydration solution with the WHO-recommended new improved hypo-osmolar (245 mOsm/L) electrolyte concentration (sodium and glucose each 75 mmol/L) is to be used universally.

It is safe and efficacious in cholera and non-cholera diarrhea and diarrhea in severely malnourished too. It lowers need of intravenous fluid rescue, reduces vomiting and has similar rates of hyponatremia as compared to standard ORS. Diarrhea associated electrolyte disturbances are all adequately treated by it. It also stimulates child's appetite due to improved water and potassium balance.

7. What are the roles of probiotics, zinc and antispasmodics in AGE?

Probiotics

Lactobacillus GG and *Saccharomyces boulardi* are consistently effective as adjunctive therapy at dose of 10^{10} CFU/day, especially in young infants with viral diarrhea when started early in illness. Probiotics can assist treatment of *C.difficile* diarrhea, shorten the duration of Rotavirus and prevent antibiotic-associated diarrheal disease. The improvements have been modest but reproducible. But in developing countries, it has not achieved a consensus acceptance due to high prevalence of bacterial diarrhea where it is less effective; cost factors and safety issues related to immunosuppression. There is no evidence to support prebiotics.

Zinc

Zinc deficiency is common (30–50%) in developing countries and associated with impaired electrolyte and water absorption; decreased brush border enzymes and decreased immunity. Intestinal zinc losses during diarrhea aggravate pre-existing deficiency. Supplementation either in prevention or in treatment of acute diarrhea in developing countries has shown a decrease in duration and severity of acute diarrhea, and reduces recurrence in next 2 to 3 months. WHO, UNICEF and IAP National Task Force recommend zinc supplementation starting during the illness (14 days of 10 mg zinc in 2 to 6 months of age and 20 mg in older ones).

Intestinal motility reducers

Loperamide, Diphenoxylate+Atropine and opoid products alter intestinal motility but do not reduce fluid loss. They are banned due to risk of paralytic ileus, drowziness, protraction of Shigellosis, toxic megacolon in *Clostridia* and HUS in *E.coli* infections.

Further Reading

1. Bhatnagar S, et al. IAP Guidelines—2006 on Management of Acute Diarrhea. Indian Pediatrics. 2007;44:380.
2. Estimation of the burden of diarrheal diseases in India, 2005. National Institute of Cholera and Enteric Diseases, Kolkata.
3. Global Burden Disease Death Estimates 2008, Department of measurement and health information April-2011 WHO.
4. Guarino A, et al. ESPGHAN-ESPID-based Guidelines for the Management of Acute Gastroenteritis in Children in Europe. Journal of Pediatric Gastroenterology and Nutrition. 2008;46:S81-S184.
5. Guerrant RL, et al. Practice Guidelines for the Management of Infectious Diarrhea—Infectious Diseases Society of America Guideline. Clinical Infectious Diseases. 2001;32:331-50.
6. Jain V, Parashar UD, Glass RI, Bhan MK. Epidemiology of rotavirus in India. Indian J Pediatr. Sep 2001;68(9):855-62.
7. Kosek M, Bern C, Guerrant RL. The global burden of diarrheal disease, as estimated from studies published between 1992-2000. Bulletin of the WHO, 2003;81(3):197-204.
8. Northrup RS, Flanigan TP. Gastroenteritis. Pediatrics in Review 1994;15:461.
9. The Rational Use of Drugs in the Management of Acute Diarrhea in Children. Geneva, World Health Organization, 1990.
10. The Selection of Fluids and Food for Home Therapy to Prevent Dehydration from Diarrhea: Guidelines for Developing a National Policy. WHO document WHO/CDD/93.44.
11. The treatment of diarrhea. A Manual for Physicians and Other Senior Health Workers-4th rev. WHO, 2005.

34 Urinary Tract Infection

Jayati Sengupta, Kheya Ghosh Uttam

1. How to recognize simple and complicated urinary tract infection?

The symptoms of urinary tract infection (UTI) in young children are nonspecific and diagnosis requires a high index of suspicion. Unexplained fever, which persists beyond 48 hours, may be the only symptom in infants. All infants with unexplained fever, lethargy, vomiting, poor feeding, failure to thrive and children with dysuria, urinary frequency, suprapubic or loin pain, hematuria, cloudy or offensive urine, should have a urinary examination performed prior to starting antibiotics.

Patients with features of systemic toxicity are considered as having complicated UTI. The presence of temperature >39°C, systemic toxicity, persistent vomiting, dehydration and renal angle tenderness is considered as complicated UTI. Neonates often present with features of sepsis including lethargy, temperature instability, hyperbilirubinemia and shock.

UTI in adolescents are often limited to the lower tracts. Symptoms include dysuria, frequency, urgency and suprapubic pain. Renal parenchymal involvement is indicated by fever, chills, rigors and flank pain.

The distinction between simple and complicated UTI has implications for therapy. Children less than 3 months of age and those with complicated UTI should be hospitalized and treated with parenteral antibiotics. Children with simple UTI and those above 3 months of age are treated with oral antibiotics.

2. What are the diagnostic tests?

A clean catch midstream urine sample after local cleansing is preferred. However, this may be difficult to obtain in small children. Bag urines have a high false positive rate. An aseptically obtained catheter urine sample or a suprapubic aspirate with ultrasound guidance may be indicated if there is a suspicion of false positive results. The urine should be transported to the lab rapidly and plated into culture plates within 4 hours.

The definitive diagnosis of an UTI is based on demonstrating a pure growth on culture of urine, colony count varying according to the method of collection as below.
  i. *Midstream clean catch:* Colony count of $>10^5$/mL of a single species.
  ii. *Suprapubic aspirate:* Urinary pathogen in any number.
  iii. *Catheter specimen:* $\geq 50 \times 10^3$ CFU/mL.

However, we need to be fairly certain that this was not a contaminated sample (i.e., was collected appropriately) and plated within 4 hours of collection.

Since these two factors cannot always be definitely ascertained, co-existence of clinical clues and/or abnormalities on dipstick testing or urine microscopy may help to differentiate a true UTI from a contaminated or poorly preserved sample. Dipsticks are not freely available in our country; however, a urine microscopy can prove extremely useful (although not diagnostic) and must be requested in every patient.

Rapid diagnostic dipsticks impregnated with nitrite and/or leukocyte-esterase positivity can give a clue while waiting for formal urine report, however, these are more useful for excluding UTI when both are negative, positive result indicating need for further investigation.

Urine microscopy can also support the diagnosis of an UTI, with 80 to 90% of children with symptomatic UTIs having urine leukocyte counts (pus cells) >10/ml of uncentrifuged midstream urine. Leukocyturia can also be seen in nonurinary systemic inflammations or infections, glomerulonephritis and periurethral inflammatory disorders. The sensitivity and specificity of various screening tests is shown in Table 1.

Table 1: Sensitivity and specificity of components of urinalysis

Test	Sensitivity (%)	Specificity (%)
Leukocyte esterase	83	78
Nitrite	53	98
Microscopy: Leukocyturia	73	81
Microscopy: Bacteriuria	81	83
Leukocyte esterase + nitrite + microscopy positive	99.8	70

3. How to approach a case of asymptomatic bateriuria?

Asymptomatic bacteriuria is the presence of significant bacteriuria in absence of symptoms of UTI. Asymptomatic bacteriuria is a benign condition, does not cause renal injury and requires no treatment. The organism isolated in most instances is *E. coli*, of low virulence. Eradication of these organisms is often followed by symptomatic infection with more virulent strains. Therapy of asymptomatic bacteriuria or antibiotic prophylaxis is not required. The presence of asymptomatic bacteriuria in a patient previously treated for UTI should not be considered as recurrent UTI.

4. What are the risk factors and management of recurrent UTI?

Recurrent UTI after the first episode is observed in 30–50% children, more commonly infants. Most recurrences occur within 3 months of the initial episode. Recurrent UTI is defined as recurrence of symptoms with significant bacteriuria in a patient who has recovered clinically, following treatment and

occurs more commonly in girls. While *E. coli* is the commonest organism isolated, *Proteus* sp., *Klebsiella* and *Enterobacter* species are often seen. Predisposing risk factors for recurrent UTI in children are as follows:
1. Female gender
2. Age below 6 months
3. Obstructive uropathy
4. Severe (grade III–V) VUR
5. Repeated pyelonephritis
6. Voiding dysfunction
7. Constipation
8. Repeated catheterization in neurogenic bladder

Interventions that have been associated with a decrease in incidence of UTI include relief of constipation and voiding dysfunction. Breastfeeding is believed to confer protection from UTI in infants. Antibacterial prophylaxis is indicated in children with recurrences, even in the absence of vesicoureteral (VUR).

It is emphasized that patients with recurrent UTI at any age should undergo detailed imaging with ultrasonography, micturating urethrogram (MCU) and dimercaptosuccinic acid (DMSA) scintigraphy. Patients with recurrent UTI and/or VUR should be evaluated for bowel and bladder dysfunction. Long-term, low dose, antibacterial prophylaxis is used to prevent recurrent, febrile UTI. Since the risk of recurrent UTI and renal scarring is low after 4–5 years of age, it is advised that prophylaxis be discontinued in children older than 5 years with normal bowel and urinary habits, even if mild to moderate reflux persists.

5. What is the treatment for simple and complicated UTI?

The antibiotics recommended by the IAP consensus guidelines on UTI framed by the Indian Pediatric Nephrology Group (IPNG) in 2001 are reproduced in Table 2.

Sick children and those in whom the clinical suspicion of UTI is high, should be started on a "best guess" antibiotic selected keeping in mind common urinary tract pathogens (*E. coli*, *Klebsiella*, *Proteus* or *Pseudomonas*). The selection should also be based on known common bacterial sensitivities of the region. Once the results of the urine examination are available, the antibiotic may be optimized according to the culture and sensitivity reports.

The definite indications for IV therapy are small infants, very toxic or septic patients, those with known complicated structural anomalies of the urinary tract, those with vomiting, or those not improving with oral antibiotics. All others may be treated with oral drugs. Some authorities advocate different choice and duration of antibiotic according to whether the child has clinical suggestion of infection affecting the upper or lower urinary tract. However, such differentiation is not fulproof and all patients with a definite UTI should be treated with a course of antibiotics for 7–10 days. Supportive treatment

Table 2. Recommended antibiotics with doses in consensus guideline by Indian Pediatric Nephrology Group in 2001

Parenteral			Oral		
Medication	mg/kg/day	Doses/day	Medication	mg/kg/day	Doses/day
Ampicillin	100	3	Amoxycillin	30–35	3
Gentamicin	5–6	2	Cotrimoxazole	6–10 (trimethoprim)	2
Amikacin	15–20	2	Cephalexin	50–70	3
Cefotaxime	100–150	3	Co-amoxyclav	30–35 (amoxycillin)	2–3
Ceftriaxone	75–100	1–2	Cefaclor	40	3
			Ciprofloxacin	10–20	2
			Cefixime	8–10	2

with fluids, frequent voiding, antipyretics and nutrition should be continued side by side.

In most settings, the 3rd generation cephalosporins should be firstline for parenteral therapy, as they are inexpensive, safe, effective and readily available. Aminoglycosides have been used traditionally, but they have a narrow therapeutic range, renal and ear toxicities often go undetected, and monitoring of serial creatinine levels and drug levels are necessary for their safe utilization, but rarely practical. There is evidence that single daily doses of aminoglycosides may be less toxic but as effective.

Oral therapy may be started with co-amoxyclav or cefixime. The place of quinolones in pediatric practice is still controversial and they should only be used if the urine sensitivity results allow no other safe choice. Nitrofurantoin and cotrimoxazole are better reserved for use as prophylactic agents. Nalidixic acid does not reach good therapeutic levels in renal parenchyma and therefore, is not recommended.

Follow-up urine examination to ascertain clearance of infection is not routinely recommended in patients who have become asymptomatic after treatment, but may be necessary if there is no or partial improvement.

6. What are the recent guidelines for antimicrobial prophylaxis of UTI?

Conventionally, the use of prophylactic antibiotics have been advocated:
  i. In the first UTI until investigations are complete
  ii. Vesicoureteric reflux
  iii. UTI in infants in diapers (iv) scarred kidneys with UTI (v) recurrent UTIs
  vi. Bladder voiding dysfunction

The drugs recommended for prophylaxis of UTI by the IPNG are shown in Table 3.

Urinary Tract Infection

Table 3: Drugs recommended for prophylaxis of UTI by the IPNG

Drug	mg/kg/day	Remarks
Cotrimoxazole	1–2 (trimethoprim)	Avoid in infants <3 months age and G-6PD deficiency.
Nitrofurantoin	1–2	Gastrointestinal upset; avoid in infant <3 months of age, G-6PD deficiency and renal insufficiency.
Cephalexin	10	Drug of choice in first 3–6 months of life.

The dose is usually given at bedtime to ensure good concentrations in the bladder urine overnight when drinking and bladder voiding is infrequent. The duration of treatment varies according to the underlying condition. The drugs are chosen such that they reach good concentration in urine, are non-toxic on long-term use and do not promote growth of aggressive or resistant bacteria.

The use of "routine" prophylaxis has become controversial as (i) poor compliance is well-recognized, and (ii) systematic reviews indicated that they were not useful in preventing UTI recurrence or renal scars. Therefore, there is a suggestion that the focus of management should shift to rapid detection and treatment of acute UTI as and when it occurs. On the contrary, anecdotal reports describe development of scars more frequently in patients where compliance to prophylaxis is poor. This issue is still not fully clear, particularly in patients with differing underlying etiologies, and even more so in our country where the alternative recommendation of high index of suspicion, rapid diagnosis and prompt and rapid therapy of UTI is not a reality in many patients. Further long-term local studies considering the different underlying causations of UTI are required before a definite answer to this dilemma can be reached.

7. How to follow-up a child with first UTI?

Even a single confirmed UTI should be taken seriously, especially in young children, due to the potential for renal parenchymal damage. UTI can be the first indication of an underlying structural or functional urinary tract anomaly. Some of these anomalies such as posterior urethral valves, ureteroceles, stones and bladder voiding problems require early intervention and treatment. Therefore, some methods to exclude such abnormalities are indicated in every patient. What should constitute these methods remains controversial.

The current Indian guidelines for management of pediatric UTI include the performance of an ultrasound scan (USS) in all children after documented UTI, and a MCUG and/or DMSA based on age and risk as shown in Flow chart 1. The aim of such investigation is to detect underlying structural anomalies of the renal tract, and to detect or prevent renal parenchymal scarring.

As per current guidelines, all children with the first UTI should undergo radiological evaluation. Due to unavailability of routine antenatal scans in

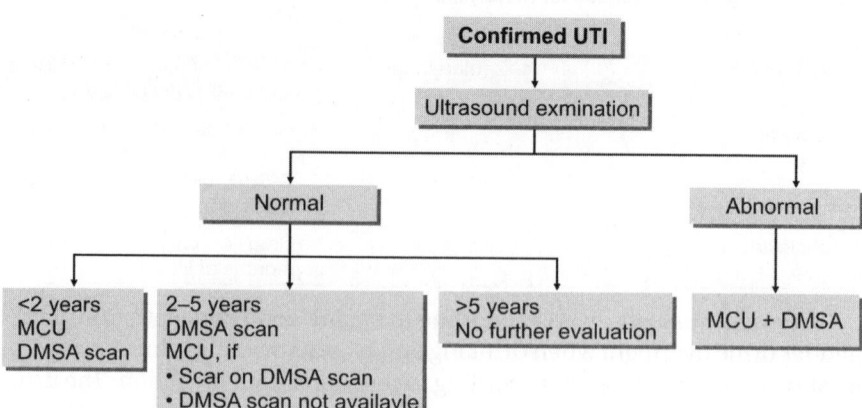

Flow chart 1: Guidelines for follow-up investigations after UTI

our country, it is still recommended that all infants with UTI be screened by ultrasonography, followed by MCU and DMSA scintigraphy. Since older patients (1–5 years old) with significant reflux and scars or urinary tract anomalies are likely to show abnormalities on ultrasonography or scintigraphy, a MCU is advised in patients having abnormalities on either of the above investigations. Children older than 5 years are screened by ultrasonography and further evaluated only if this is abnormal. The detection of significant scarring, high grade VUR or obstructive uropathy might enable interventions that prevent progressive kidney damage on the long-term.

Infants with the first UTI need to be evaluated with a micturating cystourethrography. Vesicoureteric reflux (VUR) is initially managed with antibiotic prophylaxis. The prophylaxis is continued till 1year of age in patients with VUR grades I and II, and to 5 years in those with higher grades of reflux or until it resolves. Patients and their families are counseled about the need for early recognition and therapy of UTI. Children with VUR should be followed up with serial ultrasonography and direct radionuclide cystograms every 2 years, while awaiting resolution. Prophylactic antibiotic therapy is initiated in children below 1 year of age, until appropriate imaging of the urinary tract is completed.

Further Reading

1. Consensus guidelines on management of urinary tract infection in children. Indian Pediatr. 2001;38:1106-15.
2. Coulthard MG, Lambert HJ, Keir MJ. Do systemic symptoms predict the risk of kidney scarring after urinary tract infection? Arch Dis Child. 2009;94:278-81.
3. Hansson S, Jodal U. Urinary tract infection. In : Avner ED, Harmon WE, Maude P (Eds). Pediatric Nephrology 5th Edition. 2004.p.1007-26.
4. National Collaborating Centre for Women's and Children's Health, UK. Urinary tract infection in children - diagnosis, treatment and long-term management. Clinical Guideline. http://www.nice.org.uk/CG54. (Accessed August, 2007).

35

Enteric Fever

Monjori Mitra

1. What is the epidemiology of typhoid fever?

Typhoid fever is a systemic infection caused by *Salmonella enterica serotype typhi* (*S. typhi*). It is an important public health problem more common in children and young adults than in older patients. In 2000, it was estimated that over 2.16 million episodes of typhoid occurred worldwide, resulting in 216000 deaths, and more than 90% of this morbidity and mortality occurred in Asia. This is most prevalent in impoverished areas that are overcrowded with poor access to sanitation.

In Asia, a large population-based prospective study confirmed the high incidence of typhoid fever in the region, particularly among children and adolescents, but also demonstrated that substantial variation in incidence occurs between surveillance sites in the same region. Simultaneously, *S. paratyphi A* was responsible for a growing proportion of enteric fever in a number of Asian countries, sometimes accounting for 50% of *Salmonella* bloodstream isolates among patients with enteric fever. This trend raises important concerns about the impact of typhoid fever vaccine on enteric fever rates. In Latin America, there is evidence that typhoid fever incidence has decreased in parallel with both economic transition and with water and sanitation measures introduced to control cholera during the last pandemic. Though improved water quality and sanitation constitute ultimate solutions to this problem, vaccination in high-risk areas is a potential control strategy recommended by WHO for the short-to-intermediate term.

2. How typhoid fever is transmitted?

Salmonella typhi lives only in humans. Persons with typhoid fever carry the bacteria in their bloodstream and intestinal tract. In addition, a small number of persons, called carriers, recover from typhoid fever but continue to carry the bacteria.

Typhoid is transmitted mainly by feco-oral route. The bacilli are excreted for varying periods in feces and urine of cases and carriers. There is no evidence that the bacilli are excreted in sputum. Typhoid infection can spread through contaminated drinking water or food. Large epidemics is usually related to fecal contamination of water supplies.

Vehicle transmission

The major vehicles of infection are water and food, contaminated by feces or urine of infected patients or carriers. Paratyphoid fever is seldom conveyed by water unless the infecting dose is large; it is generally transmitted by contaminated foods, water, ice (if unboiled water used), raw vegetables, salads and shellfish are important sources for travellers.

Direct contact

the disease commonly occurs in association with poor standards of hygiene in food preparation and handling. A small proportion of typhoid cases may occur due to direct transmission of infection through contaminated hands. The hands may be contaminated while handling patients, their excreta or infected linen. Transmission by flies is also a possibility in endemic areas.

3. What are the clinical features and complications of typhoid fever?

The incubation period of typhoid fever is usually 7–14 days, but depends on the infecting dose and ranges between 3 and 30 days. The clinical presentation varies from a mild illness with low-grade fever, malaise, and slight dry cough to a severe clinical picture with abdominal discomfort and multiple complications.

Many factors influence the severity and overall clinical outcome of the infection. They include the duration of illness before the initiation of appropriate therapy, choice of antimicrobial treatment, age, previous exposure or vaccination history, virulence of the bacterial strain, quantity of inoculum ingested, and several host factors such as age, gastric acidity, and immunologic status.

The majority of patients with typhoid fever present with abdominal pain, fever, and chills.

Classic reports in preantibiotic era described the characteristic stages of typhoid fever in untreated individuals. In the first week of illness, rising ("stepwise") fever and bacteremia develop. While chills are typical, frank rigors are rare. Relative bradycardia or pulse temperature dissociation may be observed. In the second week of illness, abdominal pain develops and 'rose spots' (faint salmon-colored macules on the trunk and abdomen) may be seen. During the third week of illness, hepatosplenomegaly, intestinal bleeding, and perforation due to ileocecal lymphatic hyperplasia of the Peyer's patches may occur, together with secondary bacteremia and peritonitis. Septic shock or an altered level of consciousness may develop. In the absence of acute complications or death from overwhelming sepsis, symptoms gradually resolve over weeks to months.

Constipation occurs with approximately equal frequency but diarrhea may be more common, particularly in young children. Among 552 patients with culture-confirmed typhoid fever in Bangladesh, abdominal tenderness or distension (57%) and rectal bleeding (9%) were equally distributed across age groups. Headache is a frequent symptom reported in 44 to 94% of cases. Cough is not rare and has been observed in approximately 20 to 45%; arthralgias and myalgias occur in about 20%.

The clinical features in the below Table 1 were observed in a study in India.

Table 1: Clinical features

Clinical findings	%
Fever >38.4°C	100
Headache	67.8
Constipation/diarrhea	55.9
Poor appetite	35.7
Abdominal pain	63.3
Splenomegaly	24.7
Hepatomegaly	66.9

Complications

Although altered liver function is found in many patients with enteric fever, clinically significant hepatitis, jaundice, and cholecystitis are relatively rare and may be associated with higher rates of adverse outcome.

Intestinal perforation generally occurs more frequently among adults than children and is associated with high mortality rates. Among 105 adults with typhoid fever in India, this complication was observed in 10% of patients. In the Bangladesh study, intestinal perforation was observed in 3% of overall patients, and in 25% of patients over 31 years old.

Intestinal perforation may be preceded by a marked increase in abdominal pain (usually in the right lower quadrant), tenderness, vomiting, and features of peritonitis.

Rare complications include toxic myocarditis, which may manifest as arrhythmias, sinoatrial block, or cardiogenic shock.

Patients with severe typhoid fever may develop, 'typhoid encephalopathy,' with altered consciousness, delirium and confusion, myelitis, acute cerebellar ataxia, chorea, deafness, and Guillain-Barré's syndrome. Although case fatality rates may be higher with neurologic manifestations, recovery usually occurs with no sequelae.

Other reported complications include fatal bone marrow necrosis, disseminated intravascular coagulation (DIC), hemolytic-uremic syndrome, pyelonephritis, nephrotic syndrome, meningitis, endocarditis, parotitis, orchitis, and suppurative lymphadenitis.

4. **What are the laboratory investigations for diagnosis of typhoid fever at different phases of illness?**

The mainstay of the diagnosis of typhoid fever is a positive result of blood culture. Blood cultures are positive in 40 to 80 percent of patients, depending upon the series and culture techniques used. The diagnosis can also be made by culture of stool, urine, rose spots, or duodenal contents (via string capsule).

However, the sensitivity of blood cultures in diagnosing typhoid fever in many parts of the developing world is limited because widespread liberal antibiotic use may render bacteriologic confirmation difficult.

Bone marrow cultures may be positive in as many as 50% of patients after as many as five days of antibiotics. Although bone marrow cultures may increase the likelihood of bacteriologic confirmation of typhoid, collection of the specimens is difficult and relatively invasive, and hence not routinely practiced.

S. typhi isolates should be screened for resistance to nalidixic acid, or have formal sensitivity testing for the clinically used fluoroquinolones. Organisms with nalidixic acid resistance should be anticipated to have reduced susceptibility to fluoroquinolones, even if the laboratory reports fluoroquinolone sensitivity.

Patients with typhoid fever frequently have anemia and either leukopenia or leukocytosis; leukopenia with left shift is typically seen in adults while leukocytosis is more common in children. If observed in the third week of illness, leukocytosis should prompt suspicion for intestinal perforation. Thrombocytopenia may be a marker of severe illness and may accompany DIC.

Liver function test results may be deranged, but significant hepatic dysfunction is rare. In an outbreak in 34 patients, abnormal liver function tests were observed in all but one patient. In some patients, the clinical and laboratory picture may be suggestive of acute viral hepatitis.

Cerebrospinal fluid studies are usually normal or reveal a mild pleocytosis (<35 cells/mm^3), even in patients with neuropsychiatric symptoms.

5. **What is the importance of Widal test? What is the role of newer serological tests?**

Serologic tests such as the Widal test are of limited clinical utility in endemic areas because positive results may represent previous infection. Positive results have been reported in 46 to 94% of cases. As many false-positive and false-negative results occur, diagnosis of typhoid fever by Widal test alone is prone to error.

Other relatively newer diagnostic tests using monoclonal antibodies have been developed that directly detect *S. typhi* specific antigens in the serum or *S. typhi* Vi(virulence) antigen in the urine.

A nested polymerase chain reaction analysis using *H1-d* primers has been used to amplify specific genes of *S. typhi* in the blood of patients, it is a promising means of making a rapid diagnosis, especially given the low level of bacteremia in enteric fever.

Newer serologic assays, Typhidot, using enzyme-linked immunosorbent assay (ELISA) and dipstick techniques perform somewhat better than the Widal test, but sensitivity and specificity are not adequate for routine diagnostic use. An ELISA for antibodies to the capsular polysaccharide Vi antigen is useful for detection of carriers, but not for the diagnosis of acute illness.

Despite these innovations, the mainstay of diagnosis of typhoid remains clinical in much of the developing world, and several diagnostic algorithms have been evaluated in endemic areas.

6. What is the treatment for typhoid fever? What is MDR typhoid and how it should be managed?

Treatment of typhoid fever has been complicated by the development and rapid dissemination of typhoidal organisms resistant to ampicillin, trimethoprim-sulfamethoxazole, and chloramphenicol, the first line antibiotics. Resitence to these three above mentioned antibiotics is known as MDR typhoid. In recent years, development of creeping resistance to fluoroquinolones has resulted in more challenges. Table 2 shows the treatment of typhoid.

Table 2: Treatment of typhoid

Susceptibility	Optimal therapy			Alternative effective drugs		
	Antibiotic	Daily dose (mg/kg/day)	Days	Antibiotic	Daily dose (mg/kg/day)	Days
Uncomplicated Typhoid Fever						
Fully sensitive	Chloramphenicol	50–75	14–21	Fluoroquinolone, e.g. ofloxacin or ciprofloxacin	15	5–7*
	Amoxycillin	75–100	14			
Multidrug-resistant	Fluoroquinol one	15	5–7	Azithromycin	20	7
	or					
	Cefixime	15–20	7–14	Cefixime	15–20	7–14
Quinolone-resistant[†]	Azithromycin	10–20	7	Cefixime		
	or					
	Ceftriaxone	75	10–14		20	7–14
Severe typhoid fever						
Fully sensitive	Ampicillin	100	14	Fluoroquinolone, e.g., ofloxacin or ciprofloxacin**	15	10–14
	or					
	Ceftriaxone	60–75	10–14			
Multidrug-resistant	Fluoroquinolone	15	10–14	Ceftriaxone	60	10–14
				or		
				Cefotaxime	80	10–14
Quinolone-resistant	Ceftriaxone	60–75	10–14	Azithromycin	20	7
				Gatifloxacin	10	7

* A 3-day course is also effective, particularly for epidemic containment.
† The optimum treatment for quinolone-resistant typhoid fever has not been determined. Azithromycin, 3rd-generation cephalosporins, or high-dose fluoroquinolones for 10–14 days is effective.
** That DCGI doesn't approve use of quinolones below 14 years hence other drugs may be used in Indian children below 14 years.

Multidrug-resistant (MDR) strains have caused numerous outbreaks in the Indian subcontinent, Southeast Asia, Mexico, the Arabian Gulf, and Africa. A study from India has reported the "reemergence" of sensitivity to older drugs: 67% of 60 *S. typhi* blood isolates and 80% of 20 *S. paratyphi* blood isolates from 2001 through 2004 were sensitive to chloramphenicol.

Resistance patterns have led to a shift toward the third generation cephalosporins, azithromycin, and fluoroquinolones as empiric therapy for typhoid fever while awaiting the results of antimicrobial susceptibilities. A report of 113 *S. typhi* strains collected in India from 1987–2006 demonstrated possible 'MIC creep' for ceftriaxone, though no frank resistance. A gradual increase in ceftriaxone MIC has been observed in five-year increments: 0.047 mcg/mL, 0.098 mcg/mL, 0.211 mcg/mL, and 0.365 mcg/mL for ceftriaxone Minimum inhibitory concentration (MIC).

With the development of fluoroquinolones resistance, third generation cephalosporins were used in treatment but sporadic reports of resistance to these antibiotics also followed. Recently, azithromycin is being used as an alternative agent for treatment of uncomplicated typhoid fever. Aztreonam and imipenem are also potential third line drugs used recently in complicated cases.

7. What is the management for relapse typhoid?

Relapse was considered present with the recurrence of clinical disease, culture-proven infection with *Salmonella typhi* and *paratyphi* isolates (as described above), and with an antibiogram identical to the original isolates, within eight weeks of cessation of successful therapy of the initial infection. The rate of relapse in nalidixic acid resistance *S. typhi* (NARST) infection is shown in Table 3.

Table 3: Rate of relapse in NARST infection

Drug	Dosage	Fever clearance time (Median or Mean)	Rate of Treatment Failure	Relapse Rate
Ofloxacin high dose	10 mg/kg bid × 7d	8.2d	36%	<1%; insufficient data
Azithromycin	10–20mg/kg od × 7d	4.4d	9%	<1%; insufficient data
Cefixime	10mg/kg bid × 7d	5.8d	27%	9%
Ceftriaxone	60–75mg/kg qd × 10–14d	6.1d	9%	5%

The relapse rate also varies with the antibiotic used for the initial treatment, though insufficient data, but it shows least rate of relapse with azithromycin and ofloxacin high dose.

Treatment of MDR enteric fever with quinolones may be predicted to better eradicate *Salmonella* from the Reticuloendothelial system (RES) than treatment with first-line antimicrobials. Infection for greater than 14 days prior to therapy may lead to a greater immune system activation, thereby allowing improved *Salmonella* clearance from the RES. Likewise, as this organism is shed through the stool, it is possible that constipation may lead to a higher load of organism within the body, whereas, diarrhea could be predicted to cause the opposite effect.

Despite appropriate therapy, 2–4% of infected children may experience relapse after initial clinical response to treatment. The same therapy should be repeated with proper dose and duration after sending culture. In case, the empiric antibiotic is not sensitive then it should be changed to appropriate sensitive antibiotic and the total duration should be based on the antibiotic type.

Further Reading

1. Ackers ML, Puhr ND, Tauxe RV, Mintz ED. Laboratory-based surveillance of *Salmonella serotype Typhi* infections in the United States: antimicrobial resistance on the rise. JAMA; 2000;283:2668.
2. Aggarwal A, Ghosh A, Gomber S, Mitra M, Parikh AO. Efficacy and safety of azithromycin for uncomplicated typhoid fever: an open label non-comparative study. Indian Pediatr. 2011 Jul;48(7):553–6.
3. Ahmad K, Khan LH, Roshan B, Bhutta ZA, Factors associated with typhoid relapse in the era of multiple drug resistant strains J Infect devctries, 2011; 5(10):727–31.
4. Beaulieu AA, Boggild AK. Enteric fever in two vaccinated travelers to Latin America. CMAJ; 2011;183:1740.
5. Butler T, Islam A, Kabir I, Jones PK. Patterns of morbidity and mortality in typhoid fever dependent on age and gender: review of 552 hospitalized patients with diarrhea. Rev Infect Dis; 1991;13:85.
6. Connor BA, Schwartz E. Typhoid and paratyphoid fever in travelers. Lancet Infect Dis; 2005;5:623.
7. Crump JA, Mintz ED. Global trends in typhoid and paratyphoid Fever. Clin Infect Dis; 2010;50:241.
8. Edelman R, Levine MM. Summary of an international workshop on typhoid fever. Rev Infect Dis; 1986;8:329.
9. El-Newihi HM, Alamy ME, Reynolds TB. Salmonella hepatitis: analysis of 27 cases and comparison with acute viral hepatitis. Hepatology; 1996;24:516.
10. Gasem MH, Dolmans WM, Isbandrio BB, et al. Culture of *Salmonella typhi* and *Salmonella paratyphi* from blood and bone marrow in suspected typhoid fever. Trop Geogr Med; 1995;47:164.
11. Gilman RH, Terminel M, Levine MM, et al. Relative efficacy of blood, urine, rectal swab, bone-marrow, and rose-spot cultures for recovery of *Salmonella typhi* in typhoid fever. Lancet; 1975;1:1211.
12. Gotuzzo E, Echevarría J, Carrillo C, et al. Randomized comparison of aztreonam and chloramphenicol in treatment of typhoid fever. Antimicrob Agents Chemother; 1994;38:558.
13. Gotuzzo E, Frisancho O, Sanchez J, et al. Association between the acquired immunodeficiency syndrome and infection with *Salmonella typhi* or *Salmonella paratyphi* in an endemic typhoid area. Arch Intern Med; 1991;151:381.

14. Hoffman SL, Punjabi NH, Rockhill RC, et al. Duodenal string-capsule culture compared with bone-marrow, blood, and rectal-swab cultures for diagnosing typhoid and paratyphoid fever. J Infect Dis; 1984;149:157.
15. House D, Wain J, Ho VA, et al. Serology of typhoid fever in an area of endemicity and its relevance to diagnosis. J clinmicrobiol; 2001;39:1002.
16. Klotz SA, Jorgensen JH, Buckwold FJ, Craven PC. Typhoid fever. An epidemic with remarkably few clinical signs and symptoms. Arch Intern Med; 1984;144:533.
17. Kumar Y, Sharma A, Mani KR. Re-emergence of susceptibility to conventionally used drugs among strains of *Salmonella Typhi* in central west India. J Infect devctries, 2011;5:227.
18. Lakshmi V, Ashok R, Susmita J, Shailaja VV. Changing trends in the antibiograms of *Salmonella* isolates at a tertiary care hospital in Hyderabad. Indian J Med Microbiol 2006;24:45.
19. Lanata CF, Levine MM, Ristori C, et al. Vi serology in detection of chronic *Salmonella typhi* carriers in an endemic area. Lancet 1983;2:441.
20. Lin FY, Becke JM, Groves C, et al. Restaurant-associated outbreak of typhoid fever in Maryland: Identification of carrier facilitated by measurement of serum Vi antibodies. J clinmicrobiol 1988;26:1194.
21. Lutterloh E, Likaka A, Sejvar J, et al. Multidrug-resistant typhoid fever with neurologic findings on the Malawi-Mozambique border. Clin Infect Dis; 2012;54:1100.
22. Merselis JG JR, Kaye D, Connolly CS, Hook EW. Quantitative bacteriology of the typhoid carrier state. Am j trop med hyg 1964;13:425.
23. Misra S, Diaz PS, Rowley AH. Characteristics of typhoid fever in children and adolescents in a major metropolitan area in the United States. Clin Infect Dis; 1997;24:998.
24. Nath G, Maurya P. Drug resistance patterns in *Salmonella enterica* subspecies enterica serotype *typhi* strains isolated over a period of two decades, with special reference to ciprofloxacin and ceftriaxone. Int J Antimicrob Agents; 2010;35:482.
25. Neil KP, Sodha SV, Lukwago L, et al. A large outbreak of typhoid fever associated with a high rate of intestinal perforation in Kasese District, Uganda, 2008-2009. Clin Infect Dis; 2012;54:1091.
26. Ostergaard L, Huniche B, Andersen PL. Relative bradycardia in infectious diseases. J Infect; 1996;33:185.
27. Parry CM, Hien TT, Dougan G, et al. Typhoid fever. N Engl J Med 2002;347:1770.
28. Parry CM, Thuy CT, Dongol S, et al. Suitable disk antimicrobial susceptibility breakpoints defining Salmonella entericaserovartyphi isolates with reduced susceptibility to fluoroquinolones. Antimicrob Agents Chemother; 2010;54:5201.
29. Punjabi NH, Hoffman SL, Edman DC, et al. Treatment of severe typhoid fever in children with high dose dexamethasone. Pediatr Infect Dis J 1988;7:598.
30. Rastegarlari A, Validi N, Ghaffarzadeh K, Shamshiri AR. In vitro activity of cefixime versus ceftizoxime against *Salmonella typhi*. Patholbiol (Paris) 1997;45:415.
31. Rowe B, Ward LR, Threlfall EJ. Multidrug-resistant *Salmonella typhi*: A worldwide epidemic. Clin Infect Dis 1997;24 Suppl 1:S106.
32. Shukla S, Patel B, Chitnis DS. 100 years of Widal test & its reappraisal in an endemic area. Indian J Med Res; 1997;105:53.
33. Stuart BM, Pullen RL. Typhoid; clinical analysis of 360 cases. Arch Intern Med (Chic) 1946;78:629.
34. Threlfall EJ, Ward LR. Decreased susceptibility to ciprofloxacin in *Salmonella enterica* serotype *typhi*, United Kingdom. Emerg Infect Dis 2001;7:448.
35. Tran TH, Bethell DB, Nguyen TT, et al. Short course of ofloxacin for treatment of

multidrug-resistant typhoid. Clin Infect Dis 1995;20:917.
36. Vinh H, Wain J, Vo TN, et al. Two or three days of ofloxacin treatment for uncomplicated multidrug-resistant typhoid fever in children. Antimicrob Agents Chemother 1996;40:958.
37. Vollaard AM, Ali S, Widjaja S, et al. Identification of typhoid fever and paratyphoid fever cases at presentation in outpatient clinics in Jakarta, Indonesia. Trans R Soc Trop Med Hyg 2005;99:440.
38. Watson KC. Laboratory and clinical investigation of recovery of *Salmonella typhi* from blood. J clinmicrobiol 1978;7:122.
39. World Health Organization. Background document: The diagnosis, treatment and prevention of typhoid fever, 2003. Available from: http://whqlibdoc.who.int/hq/2003/WHO_V&B_03.07.pdf.

36 Intra-abdominal Infections

Suhas V Prabhu

1. What are intra-abdominal infections?

The abdomen contains a number of organs like the liver, spleen, stomach, intestines, etc. Infection can occur in any of these. However, the term intra-abdominal infection generally refers to infections within the abdomen but outside the solid organs and the retroperitoneal space i.e. infection in the peritoneal cavity either in the whole space or parts of it.

2. How do you recognize them?

Peritoneal infections generally occur by spread from other abdominal organs such as intestinal perforation, appendicitis, ruptured hepatic abscess, and so on. Direct incursion of microbes from the outside environment may occur by a penetrating injury or after abdominal surgery. In such cases, peritonitis is a definite consequence of the primary pathology and is so recognized. Infection without such a definite pre-existing cause is called primary peritonitis where the infection is carried via the bloodstream or ascending from the genital tract (in females). This is more difficult to recognize than secondary peritonitis. The vast majority of cases of primary peritonitis occur in children with a pre-existing ascites due to nephrotic syndrome or cirrhosis. Depression of the immunity in these cases is an important factor leading to peritonitis.

The symptoms of peritonitis are fever, restlessness, marked anorexia, nausea and vomiting, abdominal pain and tenderness, and diarrhea or constipation. Signs on local examination are distension of the abdomen, decreased or absent bowel sounds and rebound tenderness on touch. Digital rectal examination may reveal a boggy pouch of Douglas and marked tenderness. Imaging such as plain X-ray abdomen in erect position, abdominal ultrasound or computerized tomography is useful in the diagnosis if peritonitis is secondary to intra-abdominal pathology like intestinal perforation, hepatic abscess, etc. or if the collection is localized. In primary peritonitis, symptomatology may be blunted and high index of suspicion is required. Confirmation can be made by paracentesis and finding an exudative fluid or presence of organisms.

3. What are the different types of intra-abdominal infections?

When the infection is generalized within the entire peritoneal space it is called peritonitis. If however, it is localized to small areas or parts of the peritoneal cavity (natural cul-de-sacs like the sub-diaphragmatic space or the para-colic gutter or in other areas by formation of peritoneal adhesions), the result is a peritoneal abscess.

From bacterial etiology point of view, primary and secondary bacterial peritonitis are completely different. Primary peritonitis is generally due to a single microorganism usually *Streptococcus pneumoniae* but its incidence is declining and being replaced by other causative gram positive organisms like group A Streptococci, Enterococci and Staphylococci. Gram negative organisms like *E. coli, Enterobacter, Klebsiella,* or *Acinetobacter* account for about half the cases.

Secondary peritonitis is often polymicrobial, especially if it is following the rupture of a hollow viscus. Multiple gram-negative organisms primarily from the family Enterobacteriaceae (*E. coli, Klebsiella, Enterobacter*) and anerobes (*Clostridium perfringens, B. fragilis* and *Bifidobacterium sp.*) are involved.

4. How to assess the severity of the infection?

The severity of the case is reflected by the rapidity of increase and degree of local and systemic symptoms. Usually, the patient is toxic with high fever but a sub-normal temperature is an ominous sign. Signs of sepsis are generally seen with tachycardia, bounding pulses and oliguria but in severe cases, there may be hypotension and shock. Severity will also be reflected in the height of the polymorphonuclear leukocytosis, bandemia and acute phase reactants like C-reactive protein. In severe cases these may be absent, especially in moribund or immunocompromised cases.

5. When and what empiric antibiotic therapy is indicated?

Intravenous antibiotic therapy in full doses should be started as soon as peritonitis is suspected, even though diagnosis may be delayed for want of investigations like imaging. In a patient of nephrotic syndrome who has primary peritonitis, as a gram positive organism like *Strep pneumoniae* is the commonest organism, the antibiotic of choice is Ceftriaxone with possible addition of an aminoglycoside.

In secondary peritonitis or abscesses, polymicrobial coverage with multiple antibiotics is called for. Coverage should include gram positive as well as gram negative organisms and a usual first line therapeutic combination is a 3rd generation cephalosporin with an aminoglycoside. Anerobic coverage needs to be added in the form of an imidazole like metronidazole or clindamycin. Higher antibiotics like βlactam-βlactam inhibitor combinations (cefoperazone-sulbactam or piperacillin-tazobactam), fluoroquinolones (ofloxacin or ciprofloxacin), aztreonam or carbapenems (meropenem or imipenem) may be empirically started in children who have already received the first-line antibiotics listed above before they developed the peritonitis.

6. How do you follow-up following antibiotic therapy?

Improvement on treatment can be judged by regression of signs of sepsis, relief of pain, resumption of normal bowel movements and return of appetite. Follow-up examination is done daily for reduction in abnormality of vital signs, distension of abdomen and tenderness on palpation. Auscultation will show return of normal peristalsis. Successful resolution of the infection will be suggested by decreasing trend in white cell counts and acute phase reactants.

7. How long it should be treated?

Parenteral antibiotic therapy is usually continued until the patient is non-toxic, almost afebrile and there is absence of pain or tenderness in the abdomen. Additionally, parenteral antibiotics may need to be given longer in view of poor bowel movements and vomiting precluding oral therapy. Once the fever and symptoms have regressed, patient can be switched to oral therapy with appropriate antibiotics either chosen empirically or on the basis of bacterial culture results. Total duration of antibiotic therapy is usually at least 3 weeks. Longer treatment up to 6 weeks may be required in patients with unusual organisms, complications or resistant bugs.

Further Reading

1. Alwadhi RK, Mathew JL, Rath B. Clinical profile of children with nephrotic syndrome not on glucorticoid therapy, but presenting with infection. J Pediatr Child Health. 2004;40:28-32.
2. Gulati S, Kher V, Gupta A, Arora P, Rai PK, Sharma RK. Spectrum of infections in Indian children with nephrotic syndrome. Pediatr Nephrol. 1995;(9):431-4.
3. Gupta S, Muralidharan S, Gokulnath, Srinivasa H. Epidemiology of culture isolates from peritoneal dialysis peritonitis patients in southern India using an automated blood culture system to culture peritoneal dialysate. Nephrology (Carlton). 2011;16:63-7.
4. Khournis IP, Kuti JL, Nicolau DP. Intra-abdominal infections: considerations for the use of carbapenems. Expert Opin Pharmacother. 2007;8:167-82.
5. Levison ME, Bush LM. Peritonitis and Intraperitoneal Abscesses. Mandell, Douglas & Bennett's Principles and Practice of Infectious Diseases. 7th Ed. Churchill Livingstone. In Mandell BL, Bennet JE, Dolin R (Eds). 2010.p.1011-32.
6. Prasad N, Gulati S, Gupta A, Sharma RK, Kumar A, Kumar R, et. al. Continuous peritoneal dialysis in children: a single centre experience in a developing country. Pediatr. Nephrol. 2006;21:403-7.
7. Runyon BA. The evolution of ascetic fluid analysis in the diagnosis of spontaneous bacterial peritonitis. Am J Gastroenterol. 2003;98:1675-7.

37

Bone and Joint Infections

Narendra Rathi

1. What are the pathophysiologies of osteomyelitis and septic arthritis?

Hematogenous osteomyelitis generally begins in the metaphysis. Trauma or emboli cause occlusion of slow the flowing sinusoidal vessels, leading to the formation of nidus for infection. The sluggish flow of blood is the main factor predisposing to infarction secondary to thrombosis. Bacteria settling in this avascular area initiates infection, which spreads through Volkmann canals and Haversian systems and ultimately spreads laterally through cortex elevating or rupturing periosteum. In young infants and neonates, particularly in the hip, where epiphysial growth plate is traversed by nutrient vessels terminating in the distal ossification center, septic thrombophlebitis of a nutrient vessel can lead to growth discrepancies. As the capsule of the joint extends to metaphysis, rupture of infection through the cortex leads to the development of septic arthritis. In the newborns, osteomyelitis in long tubular bones is accompanied by contiguous septic arthritis in 50-70% of the cases. Other peculiarities of neonatal osteomyelitis are multifocal involvement and presence of antecedent infection in 50% cases, usually nosocomial. Puncture wound osteomyelitis, osteomyelitis caused by spread of infection from a contiguous focus and orthopedic fixator device osteomyelitis are examples of nonhematogenous osteomyelitis.

In septic arthritis, organisms can spread to joint space by hematogenous route, direct inoculation or extension of contiguous focus of infection. During transient bacteremia, bacteria are delivered to highly vascular synovial membrane (vascularity of synovial membrane is comparable to that of brain).

2. What are the various etiologies in different age groups?

The various etiologies in different age groups are shown in Table 1.

Table 1: Etiology of bone and joint infections

S. No.	Situation	Organism
1.	Most common cause	*Staphylococcus aureus*, Group A *Streptococcus*, *Streptococcus pneumoniae*
2.	Less common causes	*Haemophilus influenzae* (below 5 years of age)
3.	Culture negative osteoarticular disease	*Kingella kingae*
4.	Sickle cell disease	*Salmonella* sp.
5.	Illicit drug users	*Pseudomonas aeruginosa*
6.	Paranasal, sinus, mastoid osteoarticular disease	*Bacteroides* sp.
7.	Spread from contiguous infectious foci, distal extremity compromised by vascular insufficiency or neuropathy	Polymicrobial
8.	Neonatal period	*Neisseria gonorrhaeae*, Gram-negative enteric bacteria
9.	Chronic monoarticular disease with granulomatous reaction	*Brucella*, *Mycobacteria*, *Nocardia*

3. **What are the common differential diagnoses of the bone and joint infections?**

    1. Fracture and trauma
    2. Rheumatic fever
    3. Septicemia
    4. Cellulitis
    5. Ewing's sarcoma
    6. Leukemia
    7. Bone infarction of sickle cell disease or Gaucher's disease
    8. Reflex neurovascular dystrophy
    9. Toxic synovitis
    10. Infective endocarditis.

4. **What are the various investigations of osteomyelitis and septic arthritis?**

1. Complete blood count, CRP, ESR—Leucocytosis along with raised CRP and ESR are suggestive.
2. Gram stain and culture of bone, subperiosteal aspirate and joint fluid— Overall such cultures provide bacteriological diagnosis in 66 to 76% of the cases, while blood cultures yield an organism in about half the cases. Subperiosteal needle aspiration can be done if point tenderness is localized. There is a risk of causing epiphyseal damage and subsequent

length discrepancy in invasive bone aspiration. Joint fluid should be collected in heparinized syringe and identification of organism in joint fluid forms the primary criterion for the diagnosis of septic arthritis.
3. Blood culture.
4. Plain radiograph—In osteomyelitis, radiological changes occur in three stages. The first stage, occurring three days after the symptom onset, is the formation of small area of localized, deep soft tissue swelling in the metaphyseal region. Hence, in early stages, looking at the soft tissue rather than the bone is more important. In the second stage, during 3–7 days, swelling of muscles with obliteration of interposed translucent fat planes is noted. The third stage of visible bone destruction comes during 10–21 days after the onset of symptoms in the form of subperiosteal bone resorption, areas of bone destruction and periosteal new bone formation. Various findings in septic arthritis of hip are swelling of joint capsule displacing fat lines, obturator sign and raised femoral portion of Shenton line.
5. MRI—This is imaging modality of choice having sensitivity of near 100% and has an advantage of delineating pus collections that might need surgical drainage.
6. CT scan—Occasionally used as it provides excellent definition of cortical bone and high spatial resolution and is specially useful in detecting sequestrum and subperiosteal abscesses.
7. Scintigraphy—Radionuclide scanning using Technetium-99m is most commonly used and has an advantage of detecting multifocal disease and high sensitivity to the tune of 95% with the exception of CA-MRSA and neonates.
8. Ultrasound—Helpful for evaluating septic arthritis of hip.

5. What is the treatment of bone and joint infections and for how long should it be treated?

Immobilization, antimicrobial therapy and surgical procedures are various modalities.

Immobilization is useful for pain relief and prevention of pathological fractures. Surgical therapy is needed for soft tissue, subperiosteal and intramedullary abscesses, removal of sequestra and drainage of septic arthritis. Antimicrobial therapy should begin with drugs having potent activity against the most common pathogens, i.e. *S. aureus* and Group-A *Streptococcus*. The antimicrobial agents can get modified subsequently depending on microbiological diagnosis. In the areas where >90% *S. aureus* isolates are methicillin-susceptible, initial choice of cloxacillin or injectable first generation cephalosporine, cephazatin nafcillin, oxacillin or cefuroxime and in areas where CA-MRSA is common, initial choice of vancomycin or clindamycin is reasonable. Addition of third generation cephalosporin to the above antibiotics empirically for younger children can be considered to include *H. influenzae* also. Third generation cephalosporin or chloramphenicol for salmonella, ceftazidime and aminoglycoside for *P. aeruginosa* or for enteric gram-negative organisms and clindamycin for suspected anerobic infections are recommended. Sequential use of the intravenous and oral routes of administration is now accepted. Intravenous antibiotics are continued till the patient is afebrile, local signs and symptoms are considerably reduced and the patient is able to maintain caloric and fluid balance by oral route. Oral antibiotics are used in higher doses than for the treatment of other infections except clindamycin. In most cases, clinical improvement is noted in 3–7 days of initiation of antimicrobials. Monitoring of the therapy is done by serial acute phase reactants, although ESR and CRP increase during the first three days of the therapy. CRP returns to normal in 7–10 days and slower decline in it's level is associated with more extensive radiological damage. Failure of ESR to decrease during the second week of the therapy may indicate the need for surgical drainage or development of chronic osteomyelitis. The minimum duration of antimicrobial therapy is three weeks but conservative and individualized approach to continue antibiotics till ESR and CRP are back to normal usually requires 4–6 weeks.

Further Reading

1. Kaplan SL. Osteomyelitis in children. Infect Dis Clin N Am 2005, 19. pp. 787-97.
2. Krogstad P. Osteomyelitis, In Feigin & Cherry's textbook of Pediatric Infectious Diseases, 6th ed, 2009, Saunders Elseviour, pp. 725-42.
3. Verdier I, Gayet A, Ploton C, Taylor P. Contribution of a broad range PCR to diagnosis of osteoarticular infections. Ped Infect Dis J. 2005, 24. pp. 692-6.

38

Skin and Soft Tissue Infections

Sandipan Dhar

1. What are common bacterial skin infections and their management?

Furunculosis

This is an acute, usually necrotic infection of a hair follicle with *S. aureus*. A furuncle presents initially as a small, follicular, inflammatory nodule, soon becoming pustular and then necrotic and healing after discharge of a necrotic core to leave a violaceous macule and ultimately a permanent scar. Tenderness is a constant feature. Lesions may be single or multiple and tend to appear in crops. The sites involved are the face and neck, the arms, wrists and fingers, the buttocks and the anogenital region.

Impetigo

Impetigo is a contagious superficial pyogenic infection of the skin. Two main clinical forms are recognized, nonbullous and bullous impetigo. Bullous impetigo is caused by *staphylococci*, the nonbullous form may be caused by staphylococci or streptococci or both organisms together. The nonbullous form presents as a thin walled vesicle on an erythematous base. However, the vesicle ruptures rapidly and so may be missed. The exuding serum dries to form yellowish brown crusts. The face and the limbs are commonly involved.

Ecthyma

Ecthyma is a pyogenic infection of the skin characterized by the formation of adherent crusts beneath which ulceration occurs. It begins as small bullae or pustules on an erythematous base which is soon surrounded by a hard crust of dried exudate. The base may become indurated and a red edematous areola is often present. The crust is removed with difficulty, to reveal a purulent irregular ulcer. Healing occurs after a few weeks, with scarring. The buttocks, thighs and legs are most commonly affected.

Cellulitis and erysipelas

The term cellulitis is applied to inflammation of subcutaneous tissue. Erysipelas is a bacterial infection of the dermis and upper subcutaneous tissue. The two have similar bacteriology with streptococcal antigens being demonstrated in both lesions. Erythema, heat swelling and pain or tenderness are constant features. In erysipelas, the edge of the lesion is well-demarcated and raised, but in cellulitis it is diffuse. The leg is most commonly involved followed by the face without effective treatment.

Management

For furunculosis, impetigo, ecthyma either oral cloxacillin, amoxycillin and clavulenic acid combinations or erythromycin is to be given for 7–10 days. Topical mupirocin or fucidic acid cream can be applied over surrounding skin to prevent contamination.

For erysipelas and cellulitis either cefadroxil, erythromycin may be chosen. In severe cases IV benzyl penicillin at a dose of 600-1200 mg 6 hourly is preferred and continud for 10 days. To combat long-term carriage state of *S. aureus* (particularly in atopics) twice daily application of mupirocin cream inside nostril, external auditory meatus and perianal area for at least 6 months has been found to be very effective.

2. **What are the clinical feature, differential diagnosis and management of acute lymphangitis?**

Acute lymphangitis is a streptococcal infection of lymphatic vessels of the subcutaneous tissue, seen as erythematous, linear streaks of varying width, extending from the local lesion towards the regional lymph nodes. The latter are tender and enlarged. There may be associated low-grade to high-grade fever.

Differential diagnosis

Lymphangiitis needs to be differentiated from thrombophlebitis. In cases of thrombophlebitis, the red streak of inflamed vein corresponds to the course of a superficial vein and often a part of vein is visible as bluish line as continuation of the red line.

Management

Either cefadroxil, cefixime, erythromycin may be chosen to treat acute lymphangitis. In severe cases IV benzyl penicillin at a dose of 600–1200 mg 6 hourly is preferred and continud for 10–14 days.

3. **What are the various manifestations of cutaneous tuberculosis and how they are managed?**

Lupus vulgaris

This is a progressive form of cutaneous tuberculosis which occurs usually on the head or neck. The skin of and around the nose is frequently involved. The lesions consist of one or a few well demarcated, reddish-brown patches containing deep seated nodules, each about 1 mm in diameter. The disease is very chronic, with slow peripheral extension of the lesions. In the course of time the affected areas become atrophic, with contraction of the tissue. Characteristically new lesions may appear in areas of atrophy.

Scrofuloderma

Scrofuloderma represents a direct intension to the skin of an underlying tuberculous infection, present most commonly in a lymph node or a bone. The lesion first manifests itself as a blue-red, painless sweling that breaks open and then forms an ulcer with irregular, undermined blue borders. Numerous fistulae may intercommunicate beneath ridges of a bluish skin. Progression and scarring produce irregular adherent masses, densely fibrous places and fluctuant or discharging in others. After healing, characteristic puckered scarring marks the site of the infection.

Tuberculosis verrucosa cutis

This type of cutaneous tuberculosis results from inoculation in a person who has moderate or high degree of immunity. Laboratorist laborers and manual workers are often the victims and is secondary to trauma and commonly lower limbs are affected.

The clinical features are variable but large warty lesions of long duration affecting the hands or feet should arouse suspicion. Initially, the lesions are dull red, deep-seated papule or nodule which slowly enlarge and become warty over the period. These lesions sometimes become worse during summer season and may become crusted. On healing, there are atrophic scars left behind.

Management

Multidrug therapy has eased the treatment of cutaneous tuberculosis and the outcome is very good. The total duration of treatment is essentially 6 months, which is divided into—initial 2 months intensive phase and continuation phase for 4-7 months. During intensive phase, drugs used are isoniazide (5 mg/kg/day), rifampicin (10 mg/kg/day), pyrazinamide (30 mg/kg/day) and ethambutol (15 µg/kg/day). For cutaneous tuberculosis without any systemic involvement, four months' continuation phase is adequate. However, if there is underlying systemic involvement, the duration may need to be prolonged. Associated malnutrition, if any, needs to be treated simultaneously.

4. What are the clinical manifestations and management of molluscum contagiosum?

This condition caused by poxviridae is characterized by the appearance of umbilicated skin nodules. The incubation period varies from 14 days to 6 months. The individual lesion is a shiny, pearly, white hemispherical, umbilicated papule, which may show a central pore. It grows to a diameter of 5-10 mm in 6-12 weeks. The lesions spread frequently and are sometimes present in large number. After trauma or spontaneously after several months, inflammatory changes result in suppuration, crusting and virtual destruction of the base. The most common sites affected are the limbs. It may also affect the scalp, face, oral mucous membrane or any other part of the body. Most cases are self-limiting in 6–9 months.

Management

Lesions are treated by chemical cautery by 50–60% trichloracetic acid, phenol, cantharidin or silver nitrate. The caustic is applied with either a needle or a tooth pick. Other options are electrodesiccation, cryotherapy or application of currently available imiquimod, an immunomodulator.

5. What are common fungal skin infections and their management?

Tinea corporis and tinea faciei

Tinea corporis is a dermatophyte infection of the glabrous skin typically occurring on exposed areas. Lesions are circular, sharply marginated with a raised edge. Single lesions occur or there may be multiple plaques. The degree of inflammation is variable. In inflammatory lesions, pustules or vesicles may dominate. Central resolution is common but not complete and the central skin may show post-inflammatory pigmentation, a change of texture or residual erythematous dermal nodules.

Tinea faciei is infection of the glabrous skin of the face with a dermatophyte fungus. Complaints of itching, burning and exacerbation after sun exposure are common. Lesions may be simple papular lesions or flat patches of erythema. Sometimes annular or circinate lesions, indurated lesions with raised margins may be seen.

Management

For a single patch, topical antifungals are enough. Various topical antifungals used are clotrimazole (1%), miconazole (2%), xiconazole (1%), ketoconazole (2%), terbinafine (1%), butenafine (1%) and ciclopirox olamine (1%). Once or twice a day application for 2–3 weeks is recommended.

Systemic antifungals are required for extensive or persistent infection, infection over scalp and nails. Griseofulvin is the drug of choice for tinea capitis and is also fairly effective for other types of dermatophytosis. Ultramicronized form of griseofulvin has enhanced bioavailability and lower dosage schedule. It is given in a dose of 5–10 mg/kg of body weight/day. For skin infections 4–6 weeks and for scalp infection 6–8 months courses are required.

In case of intolerance to griseofulvin other drugs which can be given are terbinafine 250 mg/day for older children and adolescents for 14 days. Ketoconazole 4–7 mg/kg/day for 2–4 weeks, fluconazole 50 mg weekly for 4–6 weeks, itraconozole 100 mg daily for 10–14 days are alternative drugs.

For kerion, along with antifungals oral antistaphylococcal antibiotics for 7–10 days and systemic corticosteroids for 7–14 days are to be given. Local application of clotrimazole or miconazole gel or lotion for 3-4 weeks prevents the spread of fungal spores to others.

Tinea pedis and tinea manum

Tinea pedis is a fungal infection of the toe with predilection for web space involvement. It is commonly seen in adolescents and sometimes in prepubertal children. While in some cases scaling and fissuring predominate.

In others vesicopustular lesions, erythema and masceration are found. The infection starts and may remain in between and along toes. However, the lesions can spread over the dorsal and plantar surfaces as well. Patients complain of intense itching and at times burning sensation. Similarly, involvement of palm is known as tinea manum.

Diagnosis

Diagnosis is confirmed by KOH preparation and culture of fungus.

Treatment

It is carried out by topical clotrimazole, miconazole, ketoconazole or recently available terbinafine creams in mild cases and in severe cases oral antifungals like griseofulvin, fluconazole or lately available terbinafine preparations.

Pityriasis versicolor

This is a mild chronic infection of the skin caused by *Malassezia* yeasts and characterized by discrete or concrescent scaly discolored or depigmented areas mainly on the upper trunk. The primary lesion is a sharply demarcated macule characterized by a fine branny scaling. The eruption shows large confluent areas, scattered oval patches and outlying macules. The upper trunk is most commonly affected followed by the upper arms, the neck and the abdomen.

Treatment

Topical application of 2.5% selenium sulfide solution once a week for 3-4 weeks, then once a month for 3-4 months is effective. Other agents are topical crotrimazole, ketocanazole, miconazole, terbinafine. For extensive and persistent lesions various systemic antifungals which can be used are oral ketoconazole 200-200 mg/day for 5-7 days, fluconazole 50-100 mg single dose or itraconazole 100-200 mg/daily for 5-7 days.

6. What are common parasitic skin infections?

Common parasitis infections in pediatric age group are scabies, pediculosis of scalp, body and pubis.

7. What is the management of scabies in children?

Permethrin (5%) cream is the treatment of choice in infants and children. It is safe even in infants as young as 2 months of age. It is to be applied in adults and young children from neck to toes and in infants from head to toes including palms and soles. It is to be left on for 6-8 hours in infants and 12-14 hours in children. If necessary, it may be repeated after two weeks.

Gamma benzene hexachloride (1%) is the most widely used antiscabetic because of its efficacy and it is being cheaper than permethrin. There are occasional reports of neurotoxicities which are almost exclusively due to its inappropriate, prolonged or repetitive use or accidental ingestion by infants/ young children. It is not recommended in infants and small children and cannot be applied over head and face. A second application after one week is a must. The current breakthrough in the treatment of scabies has been oral ivermectin. It is considered to be safe in children above 2 years of age. Two doses of 200 µg/kg of body weight at one week interval has been recommended.

8. **How are pediculosis capitis and corporis managed?**

Pediculosis capitis (head louse infestation)

it is caused by infestation of the scalp with pediculus humanus capitis. Head louse is brown in color and lays about 50-150 ova (nits) during an average adult life of approximately 16 days and it measures 1-2 mm in length. They moult 3 times to develop into an adult over a period of almost 2 weeks. Head louse infestation commonly affects females with long hair. The nits are firmly attached to the hair and can slide along the hair but cannot be shed off like scales and the nits are grayish white, oval in shape and about 0.5 mm in length. The transmission is through close contact, sharing of headgear, combs and hairbrushes. In head louse itching is the predominant symptom and secondary infection with enlargement of occipital lymph glands is the common presentation. Diagnosis is definitive when crawling lice can be seen on a naked eye but microscopic identification of the louse or the stuck on nits on the hair shafts is confirmatory. Exudation, crusting, excoriations and red papules on the neck in females should arouse suspicion of pediculosis capitis.

Treatment consists of treating the associated secondary infection if any. Treatment of pediculosis consists of application of gamma benzene hexachloride (1%) or malathion (0.5%) or permethrin (1%). Gamma benzene hexachloride and malathion both should be applied at night and should be left on for 10-12 hours and washed off in the morning. Permethrin should also be applied for 30-45 minutes and washed off. Repeat application after a week is desirable. To prevent reinfection, ensure that all family contacts and close friends are also treated.

Pediculosis corporis (Body louse infestation)

It is generally seen among the poor, homeless or mentally retarded subjects. Body lice generally thrive in conditions of poverty, war and natural disaster.

The body louse is about 4 mm in length and lives in the seams of cloths and lays about 270-300 ova during an average of 18 days of adult life. Nits incubate for 8-10 days and nymphs mature into adults over about 2 weeks.

Severe itching, excoriations, blood crusts and blood stained cloths are the presentation of body louse infestation. In chronic cases hyperpigmentation and lichenification can also be seen. The diagnosis can be made by high degree of suspicion and demonstration or lice or nits from the seams of clothing. Treatment consists of proper hygiene, laundering and ironing of cloths and application of insecticides to clothing. Application of permethrin or gamma benzene hexachloride to body hair may be helpful.

Further Reading

1. Committee on School Health & Committee on Infectious Diseases 2001-2002. The 2002 national guideline on the management of scabies. American Academy of Pediatrics - Medical Specialty Society. National Guideline Clearinghouse. Available from: www.guideline.gov.
2. K Karthikeyan, DM Thappa, B Jeevankumar. Pattern of Pediatric Dermatoses in a Referral Center in South India. Indian Pediatrics. 2004;41:373-7.
3. KS Negi, SD Kandpal, D Parsad. Pattern of Skin Diseases in Children in Garhwal Region of Uttar Pradesh. Indian Pediatrics. 2001;38:77-80.
4. MJ Sladden, GA Johnston. More common skin infections in children. BMJ. 2005;330:1194-8.
5. R Sarkar, AJ Kanwar. Three Common Dermatological Disorders in Children (Scabies, Pediculosis and Dermatophytoses). Indian Pediatrics. 2001;38:995-1008.
6. MJ Sladden, GA Johnston, Common skin infections in children. BMJ 2004;329:95-9.
7. Practice Guidelines Committee. University of Texas at Austin School of Nursing, Family Nurse Practitioner Program - Academic Institution. Recommendations for the treatment of pediculosis capitis (head lice) in children. National Guideline Clearinghouse. Available from: www.guideline.gov.

39 Tuberculosis

Sangeeta Sharma

1. When to suspect pulmonary tuberculosis?

Pulmonary tuberculosis should be suspected in a child if the following symptoms are present and it becomes all the more likely in the presence of following high risk factors.

Symptoms
- Fever (usually moderate grade with/without an evening rise) and/or cough with expectoration for at least 2 weeks duration
- Hemoptysis
- Breathlessness, wheeze
- Chest pain
- Fatigue, lethargy
- Loss of weight (>5% of the highest weight recorded in the past 3 months) or no weight gain
- Anorexia
- History of contact [with an adult having active tuberculosis (TB) within the last 2 years]
- Symptoms related to the site of involvement for EPTB.

High-Risk Factors for Active TB
- Extremes of age: Infants and adolescents
- Poor immune status due to malnutrition, human immunodeficiency virus (HIV) infection, any chronic debilitating disease, diabetes
- Drugs: steroids, chemotherapeutics or immunosuppressive medications
- Overcrowding, poor unsanitary living conditions, immigration.

2. What bacteriological test can be done in Pediatric TB?

Bacteriological test can be classified as conventional and newer rapid techniques.

Conventional methods

Direct Smear

Smears made from sputum, induced sputum, body secretions or aspirates on a clean slide and stained with Ziehl-Neelsen stain for detecting AFB. Use of fluorescent dyes like Auramine O, etc. can improve the sensitivity of this test.

Conventional culture techniques

Two types of solid media have traditionally been used:
1. an egg-based medium (Lowenstein Jensen) and
2. an agar-based medium (Middle brook 7H10 and 7H11).

The growth of mycobacteria takes 6-8 weeks for the colonies to appear and another 6-8 weeks for the drug sensitivity testing (DST). Sensitivity of culture methods in detecting mycobacteria is greater than direct smears.

In our study, out of a total of 1,098 cases of PTB, sputum/induced sputum/GA was possible in only 818 patients. Out of these, 414 and 404 were smear positive and negative respectively, while it could not be done in 280 patients. Sputum positivity increased with age. Smear positivity was highest (59%, 325/551) in 11-14 years age group followed by 6-10 years age group (34.7%; 68/196) and 0-5 years age group (29.6%; 21/71) for both new and retreatment cases combined. It increased significantly from the age group of 6-10 years to 11-14 years (or 3.42; 95% CI 2.0-5.86), whereas the increase was insignificant from 0-5 years to 6-10 years (or 1.26; 95% CI 0.70-2.28) stressing the fact that it was worth sending specimens like gastric lavage (GL), induced sputum and "a deeply coughed up sputum after proper instructions" for microbiological examination for all PTB suspects. Also, simple measures like neutralization of GL within 1 hour of collection, liquefaction, decontamination and concentration of sputum, as was done in our study, increased bacterial yield appreciably. These procedures can be safely and effectively performed even for very small children.

Newer techniques

Rapid detection of mycobacterium isolates

this can be done by lipid analysis, specific gene probes, PCR-RFLP methods or ribosomal RNA sequencing. Advances in knowledge about the complete genomic structure of tubercle bacillus has helped to develop gene probes and gene amplification methods for identification and detection of tubercle bacillus, either from the culture specimen or directly from the clinical specimens. These rapid molecular techniques help in the fast detection of drug resistance also. While the gene probes can help in rapid identification of isolates, gene amplification methods (PCR as well as isothermal, real-time PCR) developed for the diagnosis of TB is not only highly sensitive, especially in culture negative specimens, but also in children with paucibacillary forms of the disease. With these molecular methods and gene probes, drug-resistant mutants to the drugs like rifampicin can be detected with reasonable certainty within 90 minutes using the latest GeneXpert, while combined rifampicin and isoniazid resistance and, more recently, probes to other first-line and reserve drugs can detect resistance within few hours using Line probe assays. These gene probes, gene amplification methods and *in situ* approaches offer unmatched sensitivity and specificity to enhance the diagnosis of TB in the future. At present, they are used only for drug-resistant TB.

Newer rapid growth techniques

Liquid culture techniques for the detection of early growth (5-14 days as compared to 2-8 weeks with conventional methods) have been developed, which can help in obtaining the culture and sensitivity reports relatively early.

Rapid methods are based on the principles of bacillary growth linked to the detection of radioactivity, immunofluorescence and colorimetry, and include the following:

- BACTEC system, which is an automated radiometric culture method, can detect the growth of mycobacteria more quickly than other conventional culture methods which use solid media. The system uses a liquid medium containing radio-labeled palmitic acid with radioactive carbon (^{14}C). Growth of mycobacteria within the system is measured as a daily growth index that detects the production of ^{14}CO by the living metabolizing organisms. Disadvantages are radioactive exposure of technicians involved in the procedure
- Septicheck which is a biphasic broth-based system based on the principle of growth detection by colorimetry
- Mycobacterial growth indicator tubes (MGIT) based on the principle of growth detection by immunofluorescence. This is being widely used nowadays because there is no risk of radioactivity.

Polymerase chain reaction

Polymerase chain reaction (PCR) is a promising tool for rapid diagnosis of TB but has the disadvantages of cost, standardization of technique, contamination and false positivity.

3. **What is the current status of BCG test, serodiagnosis, interferon gamma assay?**

- **BCG test**
  Has no role; therefore, not recommended.
- **Enzyme-linked immunosorbent assay (ELISA)**
  Using A60 or 38kDa antigen is one of the commonest tests used. Several recent studies have been conducted in children using ELISA to detect antibodies to various purified or complex antigens of MTB but none of these serodiagnostic tests has adequate sensitivity, specificity or reproducibility under various clinical conditions to be useful for routinely diagnosing TB in children; therefore not recommended.

Interferon gamma radioimmunoassay (IGRA): These antigen-based tests are used to identify interferon producing peripheral mononuclear cells in the patients of TB, namely IGRA, called QuantiFERON-Gold and enzyme-linked immunospot (ELISPOT) using CFP-10 and ESAT-6 antigen specific to Mycobacterium tuberculosis (MTB). These are used to measure the patient's immune reactivity to MTB. These are used for initial and serial testing of persons with the risk of latent tubercular infection (LTBI) in the developed countries, where the incidence prevalence of TB is low. Sensitivity is comparable to the routinely used Mantoux test, being slightly more sensitive than the Mantoux test with results not influenced by the BCG vaccination; thus may be helpful in identifying true infections due to MTB but it does not diagnose the disease. Use of IGRAs is more difficult in the field due to quality assurance issues and it is not more user-friendly as is claimed. Recent studies in zinc-deficient patients have shown inferior results with IGRA. Similarly, in HIV patients also, IGRAs do not perform better. Elispot assays show it to be inferior to TST with reproducibility less than 70% in some recent studies. Thus, IGRAs are not superior over tuberculin skin test (TST) as an adjunct test. WHO recommends that it should not be used in high-burden countries, while it can be used as a screening tool in developed countries for homeless populations and immigrants. In India, Pediatric TB guidelines recommend that IGRAs should not be used for the diagnosis of active TB and names Quantiferon 'Gold'/'Platinum' are misleading. Hence, their use in diagnostics should be dissuaded.

4. **What are the different treatment categories and regimens for childhood tuberculosis?**

Different antitubercular drugs have different activities, i.e. some are bactericidal or bacteriostatic. Their action also differs in their sterilizing activity, bactericidal activity and prevention of emergence of resistance. Hence, there are different treatment categories and regimens for childhood tuberculosis. Rifampicin and isoniazid are active against all four subpopulations. Pyrazinamide has a very potent bactericidal activity against intracellular organisms, especially those inside the macrophages in an acidic environment. Clinical studies indicate that its maximum effect during the initial phase of the therapy rather than throughout the full course of treatment and contributes to an early sterilization. Ethambutol is an oral drug and safe to use in children, making it easier and cheaper to administer than injectable streptomycin. Recent recommendation is that it should be used for all age groups including the cases of TBM except in the cases of optic neuritis. Therefore, rifampicin, isoniazid, pyrazinamide form the backbone of all initial modern short-course chemotherapy regimens given in intensive initial phase to eradicate most of the tubercle bacilli quickly. Most of the currently recommended WHO and RNTCP regimens include an initial intensive phase of 2 months with four drugs (rifampicin, isoniazid, pyrazinamide and ethambutol), followed by a continuation phase containing two drugs (rifampicin and isoniazid) for all the new patients. Isoniazid and rifampin are most commonly used drugs in the continuation phase because they kill bacilli and eliminate the several logs that remain. Further, recent recommendation is to prolong the continuation phase to 10 months for patients with meningeal (TBM), miliary or bone-joint and spinal TB with total treatment duration of 12 months.

Daily versus intermittent therapy

Prolonged treatment of minimum 6-8 months, number of adverse drug reactions associated with daily therapy and cost of therapy are important factors for noncompliance contributing toward the treatment failure. The scientific basis of intermittent chemotherapy is the long generation time (18–21 hours) of the tubercle bacilli called "Lag Phase", after a culture of MTB is exposed to a particular anti-tubercular drug. It is of variable duration depending on the type of drug used and the length of exposure to that drug. This forms the basis of intermittent therapy. But the intermittent therapy should always be given under direct observation and the patient actually swallows the drugs in front of a treatment supervisor, as even a single dose cannot be missed. Thus, self-administered intermittent therapy should be strongly discouraged.

Directly observed treatment short-course (DOTS) strategy

Under directly observed treatment short-course (DOTS) strategy of WHO and RNTCP endorsed by the Government of India, thrice weekly regimens are given in patient-wise boxes (PWB) under direct observation. Recently, daily DOTS therapy has been recommended for children for all age groups and for all cases but this is awaiting implementation by RNTCP. Though there is utility of Category III regimen in some pediatric TB cases, in view of evidence of a relatively high INH resistance in India and increasing evidence of safety of Ethambutol in the doses used under RNTCP, Category III has been abolished. Hence, there are only two treatment categories—one for treating 'new' cases and another for treating 'previously treated cases' (Table 1).

The revised recommended dosages given according to the child's weight as mg/kg are shown in Table 2.

Patients with TBM are prescribed anti-tubercular drugs along with decongestive measures and steroids.

Recent WHO (2010) and RNTCP (2012) recommendations

- Recently, daily DOTS therapy has been recommended for children for all age groups and for all cases, but this is awaiting implementation by RNTCP. Following are the daily doses (mg per kg of body weight per day): Rifampicin 10–12 mg/kg (max 600 mg/day), isoniazid 10 mg/kg (max 300 mg/day), ethambutol 20–25 mg/kg (max 1500 mg/day), PZA 30–35 mg/kg (max 2000 mg/day) and streptomycin 15 mg/kg (max 1 g/day). Currently, only a select group of seriously ill admitted patients is given daily supervised therapy during their stay in the hospital using daily drug dosages. After discharge, these patients are put on thrice weekly DOT regimen (with suitable modification to thrice weekly dosages)
- Recommended dosages for children have recently been increased for isoniazid, rifampicin, pyrazinamide and ethambutol (Table 2). Previous experience suggests that these drugs are well tolerated with very low risk of toxicity when used in the revised dosages, at least in HIV-uninfected children
- Six weight bands have been recommended instead of the existing four, with a patient wise box (PWB) for each weight band. This is to ensure that no child gets either underdosed or overdosed and to keep a sufficiently

Table 1: Revised national tuberculosis program treatment categories and regimens for children

Category of treatment	Type of patients	Tuberculosis treatment regimens	
		Intensive phase	Continuation phase
New	New sputum smear-positive pulmonary tuberculosis (PTB) New sputum smear-negative PTB New extrapulmonary tuberculosis (EPTB)	$2\,H_3R_3Z_3E_3$***	$4\,H_3R_3$
Retreatment	Relapse Failure Treatment after default	$2\,S_3H_3R_3Z_3E_3$*** $+1\,H_3R_3Z_3E_3$	$5\,H_3R_3E_3$

*In children, PTB includes all forms of PTB including primary complex. EPTB includes lymph node TB, skin TB, pleurisy, pleural effusion, TB meningitis (TBM), miliary TB, disseminated TB, TB pericarditis, TB peritonitis and intestinal TB, spinal TB with or without neurological complications, genitourinary TB and bone-joint TB.
***Prefix indicates month and subscript indicates thrice weekly.

Table 2: Pediatric dosages as mg/kg

Drugs	RNTCP 2012 (Thrice a week)	WHO (2010) (Daily)	Major adverse effects
Isoniazid	15 (12–17)	10 (10–15)	Peripheral neuropathy, hepatotoxicity
Rifampicin	15 (12–17)	10 (10–20)	Hepatotoxicity, gastritis, flu like illness
Pyrazinamide	35 (30–40)	35 (30–40)	Arthralgia, hepatotoxicity
Ethambutol	30 (25–30)	30 (15–25)	Ocular toxicity
Streptomycin	15–25	15 (12–18)	Tinnitus, renal toxicity

narrow range to avoid large fluctuations at the ends of the weight band. It has also been decided to create generic boxes for each of the weight bands instead of the current practice of having to combine the boxes which significantly increases the pill burden in children with body weight of >18 kgs
- Weight gain in response to anti-TB therapy can be such that the child moves to another weight band during the therapy requiring a higher dosage
- Children with suspected or confirmed TBM, miliary TB and osteoarticular (OA) TB and spinal TB should be treated with a four-drug regimen (HRZE) for 2 months, followed by a two-drug regimen (HR) for 10 months; the total duration of treatment being 12 months
- Tablets of fixed-dose drug combinations have several advantages over individual drugs including the less likelihood of prescription errors and lesser pill burden.

Indian data on directly observed treatment short-course (DOTS) strategy

Directly observed treatment short-course appears to be highly efficacious treatment strategy for pediatric PTB and EPTB as has been shown by our studies.

In our study on retrospective analysis of DOTS strategy for treatment of 1,098 patients of pediatric Pulmonary TB, the cure rate was 92.4% (302/327) and 92% (80/87) for new and retreatment cases ($\chi^2 = 0.02$, $p = 0.901$) but the treatment completion rate was significantly higher for new cases (97%; 636/656) than retreatment cases (53.6%; 15/28) ($\chi^2 = 100.8$, $p < 0.001$). Overall success rate was 95.4% and 82.6% for new and retreatment cases respectively ($\chi^2 = 30.35$, $p < 0.001$). There was an overall 3% default rate, 1.9% failure rate and 1% death rate in the study.

For extrapulmonary TB, retrospective analysis of 669 children of lymph node TB treated with DOTS strategy over 9½ years showed that the overall treatment completion rate was 94.9% and the default rate was 2.2% with a failure rate of 2.5%, death rate was 0.3%, while overall treatment completion rate was 94.3%, 4.7% default rate, 0.9% failure rate and no deaths for 106 children of tubercular pleurisy.

5. What is the current preventive therapy of pulmonary tuberculosis?

TB preventive therapy

The revised recommended dose of INH for chemoprophylaxis is 10 mg/kg instead of previously recommended 5 mg/kg administered daily for 6 months. TB preventive therapy should be provided to:

a. All asymptomatic contacts (under 6 years of age) of a smear positive case, after ruling out active disease and irrespective of their BCG or nutritional status.
b. All HIV-infected children who either had a known exposure to an infectious TB case or are Tuberculin skin test (TST) positive but have no active TB disease.
c. All TST positive children who are receiving immunosuppressive therapy (e.g. children with nephrotic syndrome, acute leukemia, etc.).
d. A child born to the mother who was diagnosed to have TB in pregnancy, should receive prophylaxis for 6 months, provided congenital TB has been ruled out. BCG vaccination can be given at birth even if INH chemoprophylaxis is planned.

6. What are the different forms of neurotuberculosis and how to diagnose them?

Neurotuberculosis can be of two forms:

1. Tubercular meningitis (TBM) is an outcome of poor immunity and is frequently seen in very young children or infants. It usually develops within the first year of infection. Fever, convulsions, altered sensorium, neurological deficit with signs of meningeal irritation and raised intracranial tension confirmed by abnormal CSF cytology, biochemistry, Ziehl-Neelsen (ZN) staining and ADA (adenosine deaminase) levels and, in some cases, by CT scan or MRI spectroscopy.
2. Tuberculoma presenting as space occupying lesion of the head is mostly seen in older children. It may present:

- as a focal seizure in supra-tentorial cortical lesion or
- with symptoms and signs of raised intracranial tension
- with multiple localizing signs
- hydrocephalus in posterior fossa lesion
- It may sometimes also be seen as a part of TB meningitis.

Diagnosis

1. In TBM, CSF is clear or opalescent, usually with a moderate cell count (under 500 cells/mm^3) and lymphocytosis. Biochemical investigations reveal elevation of proteins and mild reduction in glucose. This typical CSF picture may, however, not always be seen. Furthermore, this CSF picture can also be mimicked by partially treated pyogenic meningitis, necessitating reassessment after 48-72 hours of broad spectrum potent antibiotics treatment with evaluation of improvement in clinical status as well as in CSF.
2. Efforts should be made to establish the diagnosis with other supportive investigations like TST and chest skiagrams. Bacteriological diagnosis from appropriate samples including CSF is diagnostic. Many a times concomitant TB lesions elsewhere in the body (say, pulmonary) coexist and can clinch the diagnosis. Mycobacterial culture from CSF should also be attempted, although CSF culture has poor sensitivity (16%) but specificity is high (90%). CSF abnormalities in TBM may take variable time up to few months to return to normal.
3. Neuroimaging may reveal one or more of the following findings: basal meningeal enhancement; hydrocephalus with or without peri-ventricular ooze; tuberculoma(s); and/or infarcts seen in different areas, especially in basal ganglia. This is the most important diagnostic modality. Normal CT scan does not rule out TBM and, in case of strong clinical suspicion of diagnosis, a repeat follow-up CT scan after a few days may show newly developing lesions.
4. Besides routine CSF examination, CSF ADA (adenosine deaminase) is high in TBM with a cut-off point between 7 and 11.3 IU/L for diagnosis.
5. CSF antigen and PCR tests are neither routinely available nor reproducible. They are, therefore, not recommended. CSF antibody tests have poor sensitivity and specificity and, hence, are not useful.
6. Differentiation between tuberculoma and neurocysticercosis (NCC) is difficult in cortical lesion. A ring enhancing lesion is not pathognomonic of tuberculoma. A larger lesion >20 mm with peri-lesional oedema, disc lesion or ring lesion with thicker rim with central nodule favors tuberculoma while multiple, smaller, thin rim with minimal peri-lesional oedema, epicentric nodule favors NCC. MR spectroscopy may help in the diagnosis of tuberculoma as it shows lipid peak.

7. **Which lymph nodes are involved in tuberculous lymphadenitis?**

In our experience, lymph node TB (71.1%) is the commonest form of EPTB for all ages followed by pleurisy 11.2%, bones-joint TB and abdominal TB in

6.4% cases each and 1.9% cases each of neuro TB and miliary or disseminated TB respectively. Out of total 669 cases of lymph node TB, cervical tuberculous lymphadenitis (88.2%) was the commonest site for all ages followed by axillary lymphadenitis in 3.3%. TB lymphadenitis of other sites was seen in only 57 (8.5%) cases.

8. **What are the sites and types of abdominal tuberculosis and how to diagnose them?**

Abdominal tuberculosis

It may present as:
- localized disease such as mesenteric lymphadenopathy
- intestinal disease
- peritoneal involvement or
- systemic disseminated disease presenting as hepatosplenomegaly
- large matted lymph node mass.

Establishing the diagnosis of abdominal tuberculosis may be clinically evident but should be confirmed by ultrasound or ultrasound-guided biopsy.

1. There are no standard guidelines for sonography diagnosis of abdominal tuberculosis.

   However, corroborative evidence includes: echogenic thickened mesentery with lymph nodes > 10 mm in size; thickened, dilated and matted bowel loops; thickened omentum, and ascites. None of these findings, however, is specific to TB alone. In our experience, we have diagnosed ovarian cancer in adolescent girls showing slow or no response to ATT as it can also mimic abdominal tuberculosis. This must be kept in mind when treating the adolescent girls with short history, showing slow or no response to ATT.

2. Barium follow-through examination may be suggestive of intestinal disease but is not confirmatory.

3. Exudative peritoneal disease presents as ascites that is often clinically evident. The ascitic tap should always be done and the fluid tapped is an exudate, typically shows lymphocytic predominance with high proteins (>3g/dL).

9. **What is the role of corticosteroids in the treatment of tuberculosis?**

Corticosteroids are given as 1 mg/kg body weight and tapered gradually over 6–8 weeks for the following indications:
- Tuberculous meningitis—Steroid is helpful in reducing vasculitis, inflammation and intracranial pressure to prevent long-term neurologic sequelae in patients with TBM
- Pericarditis and pericardial effusion
- Conditions causing severe respiratory distress or fall in oxygen saturation, e.g. miliary TB with alveolar-capillary block, endobronchial TB causing localized obstruction and emphysema, mediastinal lymph nodal compression

- Massive pleural effusions, peritonitis occasionally
- To suppress severe drug-related hypersensitivity reactions

But under RNTCP, corticosteroids are given only for TBM and pericardial effusion.

10. When to suspect MDR tuberculosis and how to approach?

Drug resistance is an emerging problem in children. With the resurgence of TB, Multidrug resistant (MDR), bacilli strains resistant to rifampicin and isoniazid and Extreme-drug resistant (XDR), strains resistant to rifampicin, isoniazid plus injectable aminoglycoside and fluoroquinolone strain are being increasingly found in children. Nonadherence, dependency on parents for finances and medicines and poor compliance result in treatment failure and drug resistance. Various other contributing factors, like poor drug prescription, use of substandard drugs, poor case management, HIV epidemic and, in addition, population shift are contributing to this problem.

Resistance can be primary, if the source of infection has resistant MDR-TB but can be secondary resistance in a child who has taken irregular ATT in the past, remains smear positive on category I or category II retreatment regimen with sputum AFB positive at 5 months or more (failure) or there is a fall and rise phenomenon, i.e. initially sputum smear becomes negative (or less positive) and later becomes persistently positive.

In all the suspected cases, patients should be managed in a specialized unit. Bacteriological studies are mandatory on samples from sputum, induced sputum, gastric lavage (GL), bronchoalveolar lavage (BAL), histopathology samples, fluid aspirates wherever available. Prompt diagnosis of drug resistance is made by specialized newer rapid investigations like MGIT/BACTEC culture and, most recently, GeneXpert or Line probe assay from a standardized WHO-accredited laboratory. At present, one intermediate reference laboratory (IRL) has been set up in every state while there are four national reference laboratories (NRLs) in the country. Blood sugar and HIV testing is to done in all the suspected cases. These patients are prescribed reserve drugs in adequate doses, which are very toxic, less effective and costly. Therefore, reserved drugs should be given as a daily regimen under direct observation until completion of full course of therapy, minimum of 2 years as DOTS-Plus. DOTS-Plus is being implemented in a phased manner with three types of PWB been made available for 16–25, 26–45 and more than 45 kg, three weight bands.

Dual infection with HIV, the lethal combination must be kept in mind when treating TB, especially in cases of failure and suspected drug resistance. Thus, HIV testing should always be done. Anti-tubercular treatment and highly active antiretroviral therapy (HAART) should be started simultaneously in patients with dual infection. Other chronic debilitating diseases, diabetes, drug addiction, malignancy, use of steroids and chemotherapeutic agents should also be ruled out.

Further Reading

1. Graham SM. Treatment of tuberculosis in children: Revised WHO Guidelines; Paediatr Respir Rev. 2011;12:22-6.
2. Sharma S. Childhood tuberculosis. In: Arora VK, Arora R (Eds). Issues in practical approach to tuberculosis management, 1st edition. Delhi: Jaypee Brothers Medical Publishers Pvt Ltd; 2006. pp.39-55.
3. Sharma S. Drug-resistant tuberculosis in children. In: Ganguly N, Ghosh TK (Eds). Typhoid, Tuberculosis and Malaria, 1st edition. Kolkata: An IAP ID Chapter Publication; 2005.
4. Sharma S, Sarin R, Khalid UK, et al. Clinical profile and treatment outcome of tubercular pleurisy in pediatric age group using DOTS strategy. Indian J Tuberc. 2009;56:191-200.
5. Sharma S, Sarin R, Khalid UK, et al. Clinical profile and treatment outcome of tuberculous lymphadenitis in children using DOTS strategy. Indian J Tuberc. 2010;57(1):4-11.
6. Sharma S, Sarin R, Khalid UK, et al. The DOTS strategy for treatment of pediatric pulmonary tuberculosis in South Delhi, India. Int J Tuberc Lung Dis. 2008;12(1):74-80.
7. World Health Organization. Treatment of tuberculosis in children; WHO/HTM/TB/2010:13.

40 Congenital Infections

Anand K Shandilya

1. When should one suspect a congenital infection in a neonate?

Congenital infections are those infections which are transmitted to the fetus in utero. Perinatal infections are acquired in the intrapartum or postpartum period. These infections, when they occur in immunocompetent children, or adults, are generally benign. In the neonate, the immune system is not developed, so they can have devastating consequences.

Viral infection of the fetus follows maternal secondary viremia or viral replication in the placenta. Those viruses that reach the fetus early in gestation are more virulent. Those infections to which the mother does not have immunity have a virulent course.

Congenital infections can have clinical manifestations that are apparent antenatally by ultrasonography or when the infant is born, whereas perinatal infections may not become clinically apparent until after the first few days or weeks of life. A high index of suspicion for congenital infection and awareness of the prominent features of the most common congenital infections help to facilitate early diagnosis.

The spectrum of congenital infections varies from mild to life-threatening. The timing of the exposure, inoculum size, immune status, and virulence of the etiologic agent influence the expression of the disease. Infection may result in early spontaneous abortion, congenital malformations, intrauterine growth restriction, premature birth, stillbirth, acute or delayed disease in the neonatal period, or asymptomatic persistent infection with sequelae later in life. In some cases, no apparent effects are seen in the newborn infant.

The timing of the infection during gestation affects the outcome. First-trimester infection may alter embryogenesis, with resulting congenital malformations (congenital rubella). Third-trimester infection often results in active infection at the time of delivery (toxoplasmosis, syphilis). Infections that occur late in gestation may lead to a delay in clinical manifestations until some time after birth (syphilis).

Clinical features that raise the suspicion of a congenital infection are intrauterine growth restriction, microcephaly, hydrocephalus, intracranial calcifications, chorioretinitis, cataracts, myocarditis, hydrops fetalis, skin manifestations, pneumonia and hepatosplenomegaly. Prolonged direct hyperbilirubinemia, anemia and thrombocytopenia may also indicate a congenital infection.

Late sequelae in the form of sensorineural hearing loss, visual disturbances, seizures and neurodevelopmental anomalies may be seen.

Most cases of congenital Cytomegalovirus infection are not associated with any illness. Congenital Varicella, neonatal Herpes, congenital Rubella and perinatally acquired HIV have a high morbidity. Congenital Parvovirus B19 infections are usually asymptomatic. Hepatitis B and C viruses lead to chronic infections. Lymphocytic choriomeningitis virus infection in the first trimester presents as chorioretinitis, macro or microcephaly and intracranial calcifications.

Localization of infections to a particular organ or system or some typical features may suggest the type of infection and help focus on the work up. Central nervous system infections are commonly seen in Herpes Simplex Virus and Enteroviral infections. Sepsis is seen in Enterovirus, Herpes simplex and respiratory Syncytial Virus infections. Cardiac insufficiency due to anemia is the hallmark of Parvovirus B19 infection. Direct cardiac damage is seen in Coxsackie B, Echovirus and Enterovirus myocarditis. Pneumonia is seen in Respiratory Syncytial Virus, Parainfluenza, Influenza A, Adenovirus, Enterovirus, Cytomegalovirus, Rubella and Herpes Simplex Virus infections. Ocular and hearing abnormalities are noted in Cytomegalovirus and Rubella infections.

2. What are the screening tests for congenital infections?

When congenital or perinatal infections are suspected clinically, the diagnosis of each of the possible infectious agents should be considered separately and the most appropriate and rapid diagnostic test requested in order to implement therapy as quickly as possible. Asymptomatic infants generally are not screened for congenital infections. Useless information is often obtained when the diagnosis is attempted by drawing a single serum sample which is sent for measurement of TORCH titers. These antibodies are acquired by passive transmission to the fetus and merely reflect the maternal serological status. These tests are difficult to interpret. Hence, general screening is discouraged. Testing for specific pathogens should be based on clinical presentation.

The initial evaluation of a newborn with clinical findings compatible with intrauterine infection may include:

Review of Maternal history (evidence of rubella immunity, syphilis serology, history of Herpes simplex virus, exposure to cats, etc.):
- Assessment of physical stigmata consistent with various intrauterine infections
- Complete blood count and platelet count
- Liver function tests
- Radiographs of long bones
- Ophthalmologic evaluation
- Audiologic evaluation
- Neuroimaging
- Lumbar puncture

Congenital Infections

Table 1: Clinical manifestations suggestive of specific congenital infections in the neonate

Congenital Infection	Clinical Manifestations
Congenital Cytomegalovirus	Periventricular intracranial calcifications Microcephaly Thrombocytopenia
Congenital Herpes Simplex Virus	Mucocutaneous vesicles in crops or scarring CSF pleocytosis Thrombocytopenia Elevated liver transaminases Conjunctivitis or keratoconjuctivitis
Congenital Rubella	Cataracts, congenital glaucoma, pigmentary retinopathy Congenital heart disease (Most commonly PDA or PS) Radiolucent bone disease Sensorineural hearing loss
Congenital Syphilis	Skeletal abnormalities (Osteochondritis and Periostitis) Pseudoparalysis Persistent rhinitis Maculopapular rash (particularly on palms and soles or in diaper area)
Congenital Toxoplasmosis	Intracranial calcifications (Diffuse) Hydrocephalus Chorioretinitis Unexplained mononuclear CSF pleocytosis or elevated CSF protein

The results of the initial evaluation may help to determine whether evaluation for a specific pathogen (or pathogens) is warranted. Findings that are more prominent in particular infections may prompt evaluation for a specific pathogen.

Clinical manifestations which are suggestive of specific congenital infections in the neonate are shown in Table 1.

3. What are the various clinical manifestations of Congenital Rubella Syndrome (CRS)?

Classically, congenital rubella syndrome (CRS) is characterized by the constellation of cataracts, sensorineural hearing loss and congenital heart disease.

The most commonly described anomalies with CRS are the following:

Ophthalmologic: Unilateral or bilateral cataracts occur in 1/3rd of infants. Salt and pepper retinopathy may also be seen. Other ocular defects are microphthalmia and glaucoma.

Cardiac defects: Approximately one-half of children infected during the first two months of gestation have congenital heart disease. The lesions that are commonly seen are patent ductus arteriosus and branch pulmonary artery stenosis. Other lesions, including pulmonary valvular stenosis, aortic valve stenosis, ventricular septal defect, tetralogy of Fallot, and coarctation of the aorta have been reported.

Auditory: Nearly 2/3rd of children with intrauterine rubella infection have deafness, which is usually bilateral and sensorineural.

Central nervous system (CNS): Meningoencephalitis is present in 10–20% of infants with CRS and may persist for up to 12 months. Microcephaly (27%), behavioral disorders, electroencephalographic abnormalities and hypotonia may be seen.

Neonatal manifestations of CRS include low birth weight or intrauterine growth restriction, interstitial pneumonitis, dermatoglyphic abnormalities, hepatosplenomegaly, thrombocytopenic purpura and radiographic bone lucencies. Neonatal deaths or spontaneous abortions may also be noted. Leukopenia, neutropenia and mild thrombocytopenia are the common laboratory findings.

Mild forms of the disease can be associated with few or no obvious clinical manifestations at birth.

The onset of some of the abnormalities of CRS may be delayed for months to years. Psychomotor retardation may be seen later in infancy and childhood. Many additional rare complications have been described including myocarditis, chronic progressive panencephalitis, hepatitis, hypogammaglobulinemia, thymic hypoplasia, cryptorchidism, and polycystic kidney disease. Progressive rubella panencephalitis (PRP) has also been recognized rarely after CRS. Postnatal growth retardation and short stature have been reported in some cases. Late onset manifestations like PRP, diabetes mellitus (20%), thyroid dysfunction (5%), glaucoma, visual abnormalities associated with retinopathy may be seen.

4. **What should be done if a pregnant lady is exposed to rubella? What are the risk factors associated with it at different times of gestation?**

If a pregnant woman is exposed to Rubella, it poses a potential risk to the fetus.

For the pregnant woman exposed to rubella, obtain a blood sample for rubella IgG antibody testing and save a frozen aliquot for later testing. If the result is positive, it indicates that the mother is immune. If the result is negative, obtain a 2nd specimen after 2 to 3 weeks and test concurrently with the saved specimen. If both are negative, obtain a 3rd specimen 6 weeks after exposure and test concurrently with the saved specimen. If the 2nd or 3rd specimens test positive, it indicates seroconversion in the mother and implies recent infection. If both the 2nd and 3rd specimens test negative, it indicates that there is no infection.

If the mother tests positive, counsel her about the risks and benefits of termination of pregnancy. If termination is not possible due to maternal preferences, then consider immunoglobulin in a dose of 0.55 mL/kg intramuscular. Immunoglobulin prophylaxis may reduce the risk but does not guarantee the prevention of fetal infection.

The most important risk factor for severe congenital defects is the stage of gestation at the time of infection and the extent of chronic viremia. Maternal infection during the first 8 weeks of gestation results in the most severe and widespread defects in the neonate.

Risk for congenital defects has been estimated at 90% for maternal infection before 11 weeks of gestation, 33% at 11-12 weeks, 11% at 13-14 weeks and 24% at 15-16 weeks of gestation. Defects occurring after 16 weeks of gestation are uncommon, even if fetal infection occurs.

Causes of cellular and tissue damage in the infected fetus may include tissue necrosis due to vascular insufficiency, decreased cellular multiplication time, chromosomal breaks and production of a protein inhibitor causing mitotic arrests in certain cell types.

The most distinctive feature of congenital rubella is the chronicity. Once the fetus is infected early in gestation, the virus persists in fetal tissue until well beyond delivery. Persistence suggests the possibility of ongoing damage and reactivation, most notably in the brain.

5. What are the different routes by which a neonate acquires congenital CMV infection?

The incidence of congenital CMV infection ranges from 0.2% to 2.2% of all live births. Vertical transmission can occur at any time in gestation or in the perinatal period and is usually asymptomatic, especially for women who are seropositive before pregnancy. The risk for fetal infection is greatest with maternal primary CMV infection (30%) and less likely with recurrent infection (<1%).

Perinatal transmission is common, accounting for an incidence of 10-60% through the first 6 months of life. CMV can be transmitted by intra partum route through genital tract secretions and via breast milk subsequently. Among CMV positive mothers, the virus is detectable in breast milk in 96%, with postnatal transmission occurring in approximately 38% of infants. 6-12% of CMV seropositive mothers transmit infection by contaminated cervical-vaginal secretions and 40% by breast milk to their infants. The risk of transmission to the fetus as a function of gestational age is uncertain but infection in early gestation carries a risk of severe fetal disease.

Almost all term infants who acquire infection perinatally from infected mothers remain asymptomatic. Many of these infections arise from mothers with reactivated viral excretion. In these cases, long-term developmental and neurologic abnormalities are infrequently seen. However, symptomatic perinatally acquired infections may occur at a higher frequency in preterm infants. Infection via breast milk rarely causes an illness or sequelae except in the very low birth weight or preterm. Occasionally, perinatally acquired CMV infection is associated with pneumonitis and sepsis-like syndrome. Premature and ill full-term infants may have neurologic sequelae and psychomotor retardation. Hearing abnormalities may also be detected in infants with perinatal CMV infection; therefore, hearing should be assessed in infants documented to have acquired CMV.

6. What are the common clinical features of CMV infection?

Infection with CMV is lifelong. Symptomatic congenital CMV infection was originally termed cytomegalic inclusion disease. Five percent of all congenitally infected infants have severe disease, 5% have mild involvement, and 90% are born with subclinical, but chronic CMV infection. Primary infection in a pregnant woman leads to the disease and 30–40% of the fetuses get infected. Fifteen percent of the infected fetuses get significant disease.

Congenital CMV is suspected in an infant having typical symptoms or having a maternal history of seroconversion or a mononucleosis like illness in pregnancy. One-third of the affected neonates are preterm and 1/3rd have intrauterine growth retardation. Congenital CMV is one of the leading causes of sensorineural hearing loss and developmental delay. The characteristic signs and symptoms of clinically manifested infections include intrauterine growth restriction, prematurity, hepatosplenomegaly and jaundice, blueberry muffin like rash, thrombocytopenia and purpura, microcephaly and intracranial calcifications. Other neurologic problems include chorioretinitis, sensorineural hearing loss, and mild increases in cerebrospinal fluid protein.

Symptomatic newborns are usually easy to identify. Congenital infections that are symptomatic, severe and those resulting in sequelae are more likely to be caused by primary infection in the mother. In a mother who is already infected prior to the pregnancy, rarely the fetus gets infected. This can happen only if the latent virus gets reactivated or the mother is infected by a different strain of the virus. Asymptomatic congenital CMV infection is likely a leading cause of sensorineural hearing loss, which occurs in approximately 7–10% of all infants, whether symptomatic at birth or not.

Symptomatic CMV infection of the fetus has the following presentations:
Early manifestation can be in the form of an acute fulminant infection involving multiple organ systems and carries a high risk of mortality (as much as 30%). Findings with this presentation include petechiae or purpura (79%), hepatosplenomegaly (74%), jaundice (63%), prematurity and "blueberry muffin spots" consistent with extramedullary hematopoiesis. Laboratory abnormalities include elevated hepatic transaminase and bilirubin levels (as much as half is conjugated), anemia and thrombocytopenia. Hyperbilirubinemia may be present at birth or develop over time. It usually persists beyond the period of physiologic jaundice. Approximately 1/3rd of these infants are preterm and 1/3rd have intrauterine growth restriction.

Infants who are symptomatic but without life-threatening complications —These neonates have IUGR or disproportionate microcephaly (48%) with or without intracranial calcifications which are classically periventricular but can be anywhere in the brain. Other central nervous system findings include ventricular dilatation, cortical atrophy, and migrational disorders like lissencephaly, pachygyria, demyelination and chorioretinitis seen in 10–15% of neonates. Developmental problems are in the form of motor abnormalities, intelligent quotient below 50, deafness, visual problems, mild language delay and learning disabilities. As sensorineural hearing loss is the most common sequelae of CMV infection, any infant failing the newborn hearing screen should be quickly assessed for the same.

Asymptomatic presentation—Those with asymptomatic CMV infection, 5% to 15% may have developmental abnormalities. These include hearing loss, mental retardation, motor spasticity and microcephaly. Other problems detected later in life include inguinal hernia and dental defects with abnormal enamel production.

CMV infection is more common with HIV-1 infected infants. These neonates have a rapid progression of HIV-1 disease. Hence, screening for CMV in HIV exposed infants is important.

7. What are the limitations of interpretation of serology report in congenital CMV infection?

The following are the tests for diagnosing congenital CMV infection and the limitations of these investigations:

CMV IgG and IgM

An IgG antibody test is of little diagnostic value because a positive result also reflects maternal antibodies, although a negative result excludes the diagnosis of congenital CMV infection. Demonstration of stable or rising titers in serial specimens during the first year of life does not help, because acquired infection in the first few months of life is common. Uninfected infants usually show a decline in IgG within 1 month and have no detectable titer by 4 to 9 months. Infected infants continue to produce IgG throughout the same time period.

IgM test is neither sensitive nor specific and is unreliable for diagnosis of CMV infection. CMV specific IgM is helpful in elucidating infant infection.

IgM antibody tests and the measurement of CMV IgG avidity can identify women at high risk for transmitting CMV in utero. Fetal infection can be confirmed by viral isolation from amniotic fluid. The sensitivity of this method is excellent after the 22nd week of gestation. The detection of viral genome by PCR in amniotic fluid is equally sensitive and specific.

The diagnosis of congenital CMV is, therefore, made if CMV is identified in urine, saliva, blood, or respiratory secretions within the first 2 weeks of life and as perinatal infection if detected after 4 weeks of life.

The other techniques for diagnosing CMV are:

Spin-enhanced culture or shell vial

CMV can be isolated from urine or saliva, but CMV is concentrated in high titers in urine. Urine should be maintained at 4°C for transport and storage. Virus can be detected with high sensitivity and specificity within 24 to 72 hours of inoculation. It is much more rapid than the standard tissue culture, which may take from 2 to 6 weeks for replication and identification.

CMV antigen

Peripheral blood can be centrifuged and the buffy coat spread on a slide. The neutrophils are then lysed and stained with an antibody to CMV pp65 antigen. Positive results confirm CMV infection and viremia; however, negative results do not rule out CMV infection. This test is usually used to follow efficacy of therapy.

CMV PCR

The sensitivity of using this test as a diagnostic modality is unknown in neonatal CMV disease. The demonstration of CMV DNA by PCR must be performed during the first 2 weeks of life because viral excretion afterwards may represent infection acquired at birth or shortly thereafter. Urine and saliva are the best specimens for culture and saliva, cord blood is best for PCR. Infants with CMV infection may excrete CMV in urine for several years.

8. What are the markers of favorable outcome in a neonate with congenital CMV infection?

The presence of microcephaly at birth, when carefully assessed by adjusting for gestational age and weight, was the most specific predictor of poor cognitive outcome in children with symptomatic congenital CMV infection.

Very low birthweight infants with transfusion-acquired or breast milk-acquired CMV infection have a much greater risk of morbidity.

Besides microcephaly, the presence of intracranial calcifications, or other CT scan abnormalities plus chorioretinitis correlates with a poor neurodevelopmental outcome; the absence of these factors predicts a normal or near-normal cognitive outcome.

The combination of normal findings on head CT scan and normal head circumference (HC) proportional to weight carried an almost universal prognosis for an IQ/DQ >70.

9. What are the risks and severity of congenital toxoplasmosis in different stages of gestation? How the mother should be managed in such condition?

When a mother acquires infection during gestation, organisms may disseminate hematogenously to the placenta. Infection may be transmitted to the fetus transplacentally or during vaginal delivery. The congenital infection risk increases when acute maternal infection occurs later in pregnancy. Untreated maternal infection acquired in the first-trimester leads to infection of 17% of the fetuses with a severe disease. Maternal infection in the third trimester leads to infection of 65% of the fetuses with a mild or inapparent disease and may approach 90% at term. Different rates of transmission and outcomes are most likely related to the placental blood flow, virulence, inoculum of *Toxoplasma gondii* and immunologic capacity of the mother to limit parasitemia.

The fetal disease severity, however, is inversely proportional to the gestational age. Without prenatal therapy, most fetuses infected in the first trimester die in utero or in the neonatal period, or have severe central nervous system and ophthalmologic disease. Conversely, most fetuses infected in the second trimester, and all infants infected in the third trimester, have mild or subclinical disease in the newborn period.

The immunocompetent pregnant woman who acquires *T. gondii* before conception does not need any treatment to prevent congenital infection of her fetus. Although data are not available to allow for a definitive time interval, if infection occurs during the 6 months prior to conception, it is reasonable to evaluate the fetus by amniotic fluid PCR and ultrasonography and treated to prevent congenital infection in the fetus in the same manner as described for the acutely infected pregnant patient.

Prompt treatment may prevent irreversible retinal and brain damage. The drug of choice for the treatment of the pregnant mother with toxoplasmosis is spiramycin. Spiramycin is recommended before 18 weeks gestation and until term if the fetus is uninfected by 18 week amniotic fluid PCR. This reduces or delays vertical transmission to the fetus through high placental levels. However, if transmission occurs, disease severity may be unaltered. Spiramycin is recommended in a dose of 1 g every 8 hours orally without food. It may cause paresthesias, rash, nausea, vomiting and diarrhea. Spiramycin is indicated when the mother develops acute toxoplasmosis during pregnancy and when there is uncertainty about the evidence of fetal infection.

Pyrimethamine, sulfadiazine, and folinic acid are recommended for confirmed fetal infections detected after 18 weeks gestation (or when unable to perform amniocentesis) and all acute maternal infections after 24 weeks. Fetal infections diagnosed before 17 weeks should be treated with sulfadiazine alone until after the first trimester as pyrimethamine is teratogenic. Treatment of infections acquired between 21 and 24 weeks with negative amniotic fluid PCR should be individualized. Recommended dose of pyrimethamine is 50 mg orally, sulfadiazine 1.5–2 g twice daily orally and leukovorin 10 mg once daily orally.

Prenatal diagnosis by amniotic fluid PCR should be performed, if possible, in every case of acute infection during pregnancy. After maternal treatment with pyrimethamine and sulfadiazine, diagnosis during infancy may be difficult as infants may lack typical clinical or serologic features. Ultrasonographic monitoring is also important as ventricular dilation is an indirect sign of fetal infection and may develop rapidly.

Therapeutic abortion is considered by some families. When infection occurs before 16 weeks gestation, prognosis can be dismal with necrosis of brain tissue despite lack of evidence of ventricular dilation by ultrasonography.

10. What are the common manifestations of Congenital toxoplasmosis?

Congenital toxoplasmosis presents as a mild to severe neonatal disease or with sequelae or relapse of a previously undiagnosed and untreated infection later in infancy or life.

There are four recognized patterns of presentation for congenital toxoplasmosis:
1. Neonatal symptomatic disease is usually severe and neurologic signs predominate.
2. Symptomatic disease in the first 3 months of age is most often seen with premature infants but can also be found in full-term neonates and can be severe.
3. Sequelae or relapse in infancy through adolescence of a previously undiagnosed infection with ocular or neurologic symptoms.
4. Subclinical infection—Most infants with congenital toxoplasmosis (80%-90%) do not have overt signs of infection at birth but may have retinal and CNS abnormalities when further testing is performed.

The classical triad of congenital toxoplasmosis is hydrocephalus, chorioretinitis, and intracranial calcifications.

The following is the clinical spectrum of the infected neonates:

Neurologic

Central nervous system findings include microcephaly or bulging fontanelle with increased head circumference, seizures, opisthotonos, paralysis, swallowing difficulties, respiratory distress, and deafness. Encephalitis may be present. There may be CSF abnormalities and intracranial calcifications. The neonate may have evidence of endocrine dysfunction or difficulties with temperature regulation depending on the areas of brain affected.

Ophthalmologic

Toxoplasmosis is one of the most common causes of chorioretinitis and can lead to visual impairment. Lesions not seen in the newborn period may develop during the first several years of life if congenital infection is not treated. Other findings include strabismus, nystagmus, cataracts, and microcornea. Focal necrotizing retinitis characterized by yellow-white cotton-like patches on the retina, is usually seen in both the eyes. Macular lesions are more common than peripheral. Inflammatory exudates may prevent visualization of the fundus. Retinal edema is common. Other manifestations include phthisis, retinal detachment, optic atrophy, iritis, scleritis, uveitis and vitreitis.

Other systemic findings include hepatosplenomegaly, persistent conjugated hyperbilirubinemia and thrombocytopenia. Some patients have lymphadenopathy, anemia, hypogammaglobulinemia or nephrotic syndrome.

Rare presentations include erythroblastosis and hydrops fetalis, myocarditis, vomiting, diarrhea, feeding problems, and respiratory distress (from interstitial pneumonitis, superinfection, or lesions affecting respiratory control centers).

11. What are confirmed case and presumptive cases for congenital syphilis?

Congenital syphilis results from transplacental passage of *Treponema pallidum*. The risk of transmission to the fetus correlates largely with the duration of maternal infection; the more recent the maternal infection, the more likely transmission to the fetus will occur. During the primary and secondary stages of syphilis, the likelihood of transmission from an untreated woman to her fetus is extremely high, approaching 100%. After the secondary stage, the likelihood of transmission to the fetus declines steadily until it reaches approximately 10% to 30% in late latency. Transplacental transmission of *T. pallidum* can occur throughout pregnancy.

Confirmed case

A laboratory confirmed case of syphilis is called a confirmed case. Demonstration of *T. pallidum* can be established by dark field microscopy, fluorescent antibody, or other specific stains in specimens from lesions, placenta, umbilical cord or autopsy material.

Presumptive case

The infection of an infant whose mother had untreated or inadequately treated syphilis at delivery, regardless of signs in the infant; or an infant or child who has a reactive treponemal test for syphilis and any one of the following:

> Any evidence of congenital syphilis on physical examination:
> - For children 0 to 2 years: Hepatosplenomegaly, rash, condyloma lata, snuffles, jaundice, pseudoparalysis, edema
> - For children >2 years: Interstitial keratitis, Sensorineural hearing loss, "Saber shins", frontal bossing, Hutchinson teeth, mulberry molars, saddle nose, rhagades and Clutton joints
> - Any evidence of congenital syphilis on long bone X-ray
> - A reactive cerebrospinal fluid (CSF) VDRL
> - An elevated CSF cell count or protein (without other cause)

For the purpose of the CDC case definition, inadequate treatment is defined by any non-penicillin therapy or any therapy (including penicillin) given less than 30 days before delivery. Other definitions of inadequate treatment may also include undocumented therapy, subtherapeutic or undocumented treatment response and inappropriate dose for maternal stage of disease.

12. What are the clinical manifestations of neonatal listeriosis?

Listeria monocytogenes is particularly virulent in pregnancy. The bacteria readily invades the placenta and can infect the developing fetus either by ascending infection, direct tissue invasion or hematogenous spread, causing spontaneous abortion or preterm labor and delivery and often fulminant early-onset disease or late onset neonatal infection. Over 90% of late-onset infections are complicated by meningitis.

Transplacental infection

It present as a nonspecific influenza like illness or gastroenteritis in pregnant women, during which the organism may infect the fetus either by spread across placenta or through amniotic fluid. First and second trimester infection may cause fetal death. Later in pregnancy, infection may precipitate preterm labor with fetal distress and meconium staining of the liquor. As meconium staining of the liquor is rare below 34 weeks, its presence should raise the suspicion of Listeriosis. A characteristic severe in utero infection, granulomatosis infantiseptica, may result from transplacental transmission. Infants with this disorder have disseminated abscesses and/or granulomas in multiple internal organs (liver, spleen, lungs, kidneys and brain). Skin lesions, papular or ulcerative, may develop. Most neonates with granulomatosis infantiseptica are stillborn or die soon after birth. Characteristically, small (2-3 mm) pinkish-grey cutaneous granulomas are present and, at autopsy, similar small granulomatous lesions are widespread in the internal organs.

Early-onset infection

60% of infants infected intrapartum are born before term and become ill within 24 hours of birth. Most have disseminated infection with pneumonia, meningitis, thrombocytopenia, anemia and sometimes conjunctivitis. Early onset sepsis is characterized by high neonatal mortality in association with maternal illness and premature delivery. Most cases are sporadic, but epidemics are described. The diagnosis of listerial bacteremia can only be established by obtaining blood cultures. There is no clinical way to distinguish this disorder from a number of other infectious diseases that manifest as fever and constitutional symptoms.

Late-onset infection

With late-onset disease, babies generally are full-term and have no history of perinatal complications. They may, however, present as meningitis, probably due to nosocomial infection. Median age of onset is about 2 weeks.

13. What are the available treatment options of various congenital infections ?

Cytomegalovirus

Ganciclovir in a dose of 6 mg/kg/dose every 12 hours for the first 6 weeks of life is the drug of choice. It prevents hearing deterioration and improves or maintains normal hearing function at 6 months of age and may prevent hearing deterioration that occurs after 1 year of age. Drug-related toxicity is common, with significant neutropenia developing in 63% of ganciclovir treated patients. The logistics of intravenous therapy for the first 6 weeks of life, can limit the benefits, and adverse effects may limit the use of this drug.

Valganciclovir administered orally to young infants at 16 mg/kg/dose every 12 hours, provides the same systemic exposure as does intravenous ganciclovir.

Antiviral therapy is not recommended routinely in neonates and young infants because of possible toxicity like neutropenia. Use of these drugs is limited to patients with symptomatic congenital CMV disease involving the central nervous system, who are able to start treatment within the first month of life.

Rubella

There is no specific treatment for congenital rubella syndrome (CRS). Management of neonates with CRS requires pediatric, cardiac, audiologic, ophthalmologic, and neurologic evaluation and follow-up to pick up late manifestations, if any. Hearing screening is of special importance.

Toxoplasmosis

All newborns infected with *T. gondii* should be treated whether or not they have clinical manifestations of the infection because treatment may be effective in interrupting acute disease that has the potential to damage vital organs. As current medications do not eradicate *T. gondii* and primarily act against the tachyzoite form and not tissue cysts (especially from neural tissue and the eye), extended therapy until 1 year of age is recommended.

Pyrimethamine in a dose of 2 mg/kg/day twice daily for 2 days, then 1 mg/kg/day for 2-6 months, and then 1 mg/kg/day every alternate day and sulfadiazine in a dose of 100 mg/kg/day twice daily given orally act synergistically and can result in symptom resolution within the first few weeks of therapy. Folinic acid (10 mg 3 times weekly until 1 week after pyrimethamine stopped) helps prevent bone marrow suppression, but temporary therapy cessation or dose modification may be required.

Side effects of sulfadiazine include crystalluria, hematuria, hypersensitivity and bone marrow suppression. Pyrimethamine can induce bone marrow suppression; patients should be monitored by a complete blood count, differential, and platelet count twice weekly. Neutropenia is more frequent than megaloblastic anemia or thrombocytopenia. Other less frequent side effects include gastrointestinal disturbances, convulsions, and tremor.

Prednisone (0.5 mg/kg every 12 hours) is recommended for active CNS disease (CSF protein exceeding 1 g/dL) or active chorioretinitis, which threatens vision. The dose can be tapered and discontinued when symptoms improve.

Herpes simplex virus

Treatment is indicated for all forms of neonatal HSV disease. Recommendations include treating infants with disease limited to the skin, eye, and mouth with 20 mg of acyclovir/kg/dose every 8 hours for 14 days, and those with CNS or disseminated disease for at least 21 days or longer if the CSF PCR remains positive. Infants with ocular involvement should have an ophthalmologic evaluation and consider topical ophthalmic agents (1% trifluridine, 0.1% iododeoxyruidine, or 3% vidarabine) in addition to parenteral therapy. Patients receiving high dose therapy should be monitored for neutropenia.

Approximately 50% of infants surviving neonatal HSV infection experience cutaneous recurrences. Use of oral acyclovir suppressive therapy for the 6 months following treatment of acute neonatal HSV disease has been shown to improve neurodevelopmental outcomes in infants with any classification of neonatal HSV. The dose is 300 mg/m^2/dose administered 3 times daily for 6 months. Absolute neutrophil counts should be assessed at 2–4 weeks after initiating therapy and then monthly during the treatment period.

Parvovirus

Treatment is generally supportive. Intravenous immunoglobulin (IVIG) has been used with reported success in a limited number of patients with severe hematologic disorders related to persistent parvovirus infection. In the carefully followed pregnancy in which hydrops fetalis is worsening, intrauterine blood transfusions may be considered, especially if the fetal hemoglobin is <8g/dL after assessing the risks and benefits of the procedure.

Hepatitis B

All infants born to mothers confirmed to be positive for HBsAg should receive HBIG in addition to recombinant Hepatitis B vaccine. The first immunization with Hepatitis B vaccine and HBIG are given within the first 12 hours of life. Hepatitis B vaccine is administered in a 3 dose schedule at 0, 1, and 6 months of age; 4 doses may be administered if a birth dose is given and a combination vaccine is used (at 2, 4, and 6 months) to complete the series.

Further Reading

1. Banatvala JE, Brown DW. Rubella. Lancet. 2004;363:1127.
2. Berrebi A, Bardou M, Bessieres MH, et al. Outcome for children infected with congenital toxoplasmosis in the first trimester and with normal ultrasound findings: a study of 36 cases. Eur J Obstet Gyn. 2007;135:53-7.
3. Boppana SB, Fowler KB, Britt WJ, et al. Symptomatic congenital cytomegalovirus infection in infants born to mothers with preexisting immunity to cytomegalovirus. Pediatrics. 1999;104:55.
4. Boyer K, Holfels E, Roizen N, et al. Risk factors for *Toxoplasma gondii* infection in mothers of infants with congenital toxoplasmosis: implications for prenatal management and screening. Am J Obstet Gynecol. 2005;192:564-71.

5. Britt W. Cytomegalovirus. Infectious Diseases of the Fetus and Newborn Infant, 7th ed. In: Remingtton JS, Klein JO, Wilson CB, et al (Eds). Elsevier Saunders, Philadelphia. 2011.p.706.
6. Bullens D, Koenraad S, Vanhaesebrouck P. Congenital rubella syndrome after maternal reinfection. Clin Pediatr. 2000;39:113-6.
7. Burchett SK, Dalgic N. Viral Infections. Manual of Neonatal Care, 6th Ed. Lippincott Williams & Wilkins Publishers; 2008;23A:244.
8. Burchett SK, Dalgic N. Viral Infections. Manual of Neonatal Care, 6th Ed. Lippincott Williams & Wilkins Publishers. 2008;23A:271.
9. Burchett SK, Dalgic N. Viral Infections. Manual of Neonatal Care, 6th Ed. Lippincott Williams & Wilkins Publishers. 2008;23A:270-2.
10. Burchett SK, Dalgic N. Viral Infections. Manual of Neonatal Care, 6th Ed. Lippincott Williams & Wilkins Publishers. 2008;23A:244-6.
11. Burchett SK, Dalgic N. Viral Infections. Manual of Neonatal Care, 6th Ed. Lippincott Williams & Wilkins Publishers. 2008;23A:246.
12. Burchett SK, Dalgic N. Viral Infections. Manual of Neonatal Care, 6th Ed. Lippincott Williams & Wilkins Publishers. 2008;23A:251.
13. Burchett SK, Dalgic N. Viral Infections. Manual of Neonatal Care, 6th Ed. Lippincott Williams & Wilkins Publishers. 2008;23A:254.
14. Burchett SK, Dalgic N. Viral Infections. Manual of Neonatal Care, 6th Ed. Lippincott Williams & Wilkins Publishers. 2008;23A:264-5.
15. Burchett SK, Dalgic N. Viral Infections. Manual of Neonatal Care, 6th Ed. Lippincott Williams & Wilkins Publishers. 2008;23A:247-8.
16. Centers for Disease Control and Prevention. Congenital syphilis (*Treponema pallidum*) case definition. Available at: http://www.cdc.gov/ncphi/od/ai/casedef/syphilisccurrent.htm. (Accessed September, 2010).
17. Centers for Disease Control and Prevention: Achievements in public health: elimination of rubella and congenital rubella syndrome—United States, 1969-2004. MMWR Morb Mortal Wkly Rep. 2005;54:279-82.
18. Centers for Disease Control and Prevention: Progress toward control of rubella and prevention of congenital rubella syndrome—worldwide, 2009. MMWR 2010; 59(40):1307-10.
19. Centers for Disease Control and Prevention; Progress toward elimination of rubella and congenital rubella syndrome—the Americas, 2003-2008. MMWR Morb Mortal Wkly Rep. 2008;57:1176-9.
20. Coles FS. Viral Infections of the Fetus and Newborn. Avery's Diseases of the Newborn, 7th ed. In: Taeusch WH, Ballard RA (Eds). Saunders, Philadelphia. 1998. p.471.
21. Contopoulos-Ioannidis D, Montoya JG. *Toxoplasma gondii* (toxoplasmosis). Principles and Practice of Pediatric Infectious Diseases, 4th. Long SS, Pickering LK, Prober CG (Eds). Elsevier Saunders, Edinburgh. 2012.p.1308.
22. Cooper LZ, Ziring PR, Ockerse AB, et al. Rubella: clinical manifestations and management. Am J Dis Child. 1969;118:18-29.
23. Cullen A, Brown S, Cafferkey M, et al. Current use of the TORCH screen in the diagnosis of congenital infection. J Infect. 1998;36:185.
24. Daffos F, Forestier F, Capella-Pavlovsky M, et al. Prenatal management of 746 pregnancies at risk for congenital toxoplasmosis. N Engl J Med. 1988;318:271-5.
25. de Jong EP, Vossen AC, Walther FJ, Lopriore E. How to use. neonatal TORCH testing. Arch Dis Child Educ Pract Ed. 2013;98:3.

26. Desmonts G, Couvreur J. Natural history of congenital toxoplasmosis. Ann Pediatr 1984;31:799-802.
27. Dwyer DE, Robertson PW, Field PR. Clinical and laboratory features of rubella. Pathology. 2001;33:322-8.
28. Fortunov RM. Congenital Toxoplasmosis. Manual of Neonatal Care, 6th Ed. Lippincott Williams & Wilkins Publishers. 2008;23F:317-22.
29. Fortunov RM. Congenital Toxoplasmosis. Manual of Neonatal Care, 6th Ed. Lippincott Williams & Wilkins Publishers. 2008;23F:317-8.
30. Fortunov RM. Congenital Toxoplasmosis. Manual of Neonatal Care, 6th Ed. Lippincott Williams & Wilkins Publishers. 2008;23F:321-2.
31. Fowler KB, Stagno S, Pass RF. Maternal immunity and prevention of congenital cytomegalovirus infection. JAMA. 2003;289:1008-11.
32. Kessler SL, Dajani AS. Listeria meningitis in infants and children. Pediatr Infect Dis J. 1990;9:61.
33. Kimberlin DW, Lin CY, Jacobs RF, et al. Safety and efficacy of high-dose intravenous acyclovir in the management of neonatal herpes simplex virus infections. Pediatrics. 2001;108:230.
34. Kimberlin DW. Neonatal herpes simplex infection. Clin Microbiol Rev. 2004;17:1.
35. Kinney JS, Kumar ML. Should we expand the TORCH complex? A description of clinical and diagnostic aspects of selected old and new agents. Clin Perinatol. 1988;15:727.
36. Koch WC. Parvovirus B19. Nelson Textbook of Pediatrics, 19th Ed. Elsevier Saunders Publishers. 2011;243:1095-7.
37. Kodjikian L, Wallon M, Fleury J, et al. Ocular manifestations in congenital toxoplasmosis. Graefes Arch Clin Exp Ophthalmol. 2006;244:14-21.
38. Lamont RF, Sobel J, Mazaki-Tovi S, et al. Listeriosis in human pregnancy: a systematic review. J Perinat Med. 2011;39:227.
39. Lazzarotto T, Guerra B, Lanari M, et al. New advances in the diagnosis of congenital cytomegalovirus infection. J Clin Virol. 2008;41:192-7.
40. Lee C, Gong Y, Brok J, et al. Hepatitis B immunisation for newborn infants of hepatitis B surface antigen-positive mothers. Cochrane Database Syst Rev. 2006; CD004790.
41. Leland D, French ML, Kleiman MB, Schreiner RL. The use of TORCH titers. Pediatrics. 1983;72:41.
42. Lombardi G, Garofoli F, Villani P, et al. Oral valganciclovir treatment in newborns with symptomatic congenital cytomegalovirus infection. Eur J Clin Microbiol Infect Dis. 2009;28:1465.
43. Lorber B. *Listeria monocytogenes*. Principles and Practice of Infectious Diseases, 7th ed. In: Mandell GL, Bennett JE, Dolin R (Eds). Churchill Livingstone, Philadelphia. 2010.p.2707.
44. Maldonado YA, Nizet V, Klein JO, et al. Current concepts of infections of the fetus and newborn infant. Infectious Diseases of the Fetus and Newborn Infant, 7th ed, Remington JS, Klein JO, Wilson CB, et al (Eds). Elsevier Saunders, Philadelphia. 2011.p.2.
45. Maldonado YA, Nizet V, Klein JO, et al. Current concepts of infections of the fetus and newborn infant. Infectious Diseases of the Fetus and Newborn Infant, 7th ed. In: Remington JS, Klein JO, Wilson CB, et al (Eds). Elsevier Saunders, Philadelphia. 2011.p.2.
46. Mason WH. Rubella. Nelson Textbook of Pediatrics, 19th Ed. Elsevier Saunders Publishers. 2011;239:1075-6.

47. Mason WH. Rubella. Nelson Textbook of Pediatrics, 19th Ed. Elsevier Saunders Publishers. 2011;239:1075-8.
48. McAuley JB, Boyer KM, Remington JS, McLeod RL. Toxoplasmosis. Textbook of Pediatric Infectious Diseases, 6th ed. Feigin RD, Cherry JD, Demmler-Harrison GJ, Kaplan SL (Eds). Saunders, Philadelphia. 2009.p.2954.
49. McLeod R, Boyer K, Roizen N, et al. The child with congenital toxoplasmosis. Curr Clin Top Infect Dis. 2000;20:189-208.
50. McLeod R. Toxoplasmosis (*Toxoplasma gondii*). Nelson Textbook of Pediatrics, 19th Ed. Elsevier Saunders Publishers. 2011;282:1208-16.
51. Mets MB, Holfels E, Boyer KM, et al. Eye manifestations of congenital toxoplasmosis. Am J Ophthalmol. 1997;123:1-16.
52. Miller E, Cradock-Watson JE, Pollock TM. Consequences of confirmed maternal rubella at successive stages of pregnancy. Lancet. 1982;2:781-4.
53. Montoya JG, Liesenfeld O. Toxoplasmosis. Lancet. 2004;363:1965-76.
54. Mylonakis E, Paliou M, Hohmann EL, et al. Listeriosis during pregnancy: a case series and review of 222 cases. Medicine (Baltimore). 2002;81:260.
55. Nassetta L, Kimberlin D, Whitley R. Treatment of congenital cytomegalovirus infection: implications for future therapeutic strategies. J Antimicrob Chemother. 2009;63:862-7.
56. Noyola DE, Demmier GJ, Nelson CT, et al. Early predictors of neurodevelopmental outcome in symptomatic congenital cytomegalovirus infection. The journal of Pediatrics. 2001;325-31.
57. Noyola DE, Demmler GJ, Nelson CT, et al. Early predictors of neurodevelopmental outcome in symptomatic congenital cytomegalovirus infection. J Pediatr. 2001;138:325.
58. Pass RF. Congenital cytomegalovirus infection: screening and treatment. J Pediatr. 2010;157(2):179-80.
59. Plotkin SA, Reef SE, Cooper LZ, Alford CA. Rubella. Infectious Diseases of the Fetus and Newborn Infant, 7th ed. Remington JS, Klein JO, Wilson CB, et al. (Eds). Elsevier Saunders, Philadelphia. 2011.p.861.
60. Plotkin SA, Reef SE, Cooper LZ, Alford CA. Rubella. Infectious Diseases of the Fetus and Newborn Infant, 7th Edn: Remington JS, Klein JO, Wilson CB, et al. (Eds). Elsevier Saunders, Philadelphia. 2011. p. 861.
61. Ramirez MM, Mastrobattista JM. Diagnosis and management of human parvovirus B19 infection. Clin Perinatol. 2005;32:697-704.
62. Remington JS, McLeod R, Thulliez P, Desmonts G. Toxoplasmosis. Infectious Disease of the Fetus adn Newborn Infant, 6th ed. In: Remington JS, Klein J, Wilson CB, Baker CJ (Eds). Elsevier Saunders, Philadelphia. 2006.p.947.
63. Remington JS, McLeod R, Wilson CB, Desmonts G. Toxoplasmosis. Infectious Diseases of the Fetus and Newborn Infant, 7th ed. In: Remington JS, Klein JO, Wilson CB, et al (Eds). Elsevier Saunders, Philadelphia. 2011.p.918.
64. Report of the committee on Infectious diseases. Cytomegalovirus. Red book, 29th Ed. American Academy of Pediatrics. 2012;300-4.
65. Report of the committee on Infectious diseases. Hepatitis B. Red book, 29th Ed. American Academy of Pediatrics. 2012:374-8.
66. Report of the committee on Infectious diseases. Herpes Simplex Virus. Red book, 29th Ed. American Academy of Pediatrics. 2012:402.
67. Report of the committee on Infectious diseases. Rubella. Red book, 29th Ed. American Academy Of Pediatrics. 2012:629-30.
68. Report of the committee on Infectious diseases. Rubella. Red book, 29th Ed. American Academy of Pediatrics. 2012;631.

69. Report of the committee on Infectious diseases. Toxoplasmosis. Red book, 29th Ed. American Academy of Pediatrics. 2012.p.727-8.
70. Report of the committee on Infectious diseases. Toxoplasmosis. Red book, 29th Ed. American Academy of Pediatrics. 2012:720-1.
71. Report of the committee on Infectious diseases. Toxoplasmosis. Red book, 29th Ed. American Academy of Pediatrics. 2012;725-8.
72. Revello MG, Gerna G. Diagnosis and management of human cytomegalovirus infection in the mother, fetus, and newborn infant. Clin Microbiol Rev. 2002; 15:680-715.
73. Rima McLeod. Toxoplasmosis (*Toxoplasma gondii*). Nelson Textbook of Pediatrics, 19th Ed. Elsevier Saunders Publishers. 2011;282:1208-16.
74. Sanchez PJ, Demmler-Harrison GJ. Viral infections of the fetus and newborn. In: Feigin and Cherry's Textbook of Pediatric Infectious Diseases, 6th ed. In: Feigin RD, Cherry JD, Demmler-Harrison GJ, Kaplan SL (Eds). Saunders, Philadelphia. 2009.p.895.
75. Selbing A, Josefsson A, Dahle LO, Lindgren R. Parvovirus B19 infection during pregnancy treated with high-dose intravenous gammaglobulin. Lancet. 1995; 345:660.
76. Stagno S. Cytomegalovirus. Nelson Textbook of Pediatrics, 19th Ed. Elsevier Saunders Publishers. 2011;247:1115-7.
77. Stamos JK, Rowley AH. Timely diagnosis of congenital infections. Pediatr Clin North Am 1994;41:1017.
78. Stanberry LR. Herpes Simplex Virus. Nelson Textbook of Pediatrics, 19th Ed. Elsevier Saunders Publishers. 2011;244:1097-104.
79. Stoll BJ. Infections of the Neonatal Infant. Nelson Textbook of Pediatrics, 19th Ed. Elsevier Saunders Publishers. 2011;103:629-44.
80. SYROCOT (Systematic Review on Congenital Toxoplasmosis) study group, Thiébaut R, Leproust S, et al. Effectiveness of prenatal treatment for congenital toxoplasmosis: a meta-analysis of individual patients' data. Lancet. 2007;369:115.
81. The SYROCOT (Systematic Review on Congenital Toxoplasmosis) study group: Effectiveness of prenatal treatment for congenital toxoplasmosis: a meta-analysis of individual patient's data. Lancet. 2007;369:115-22.
82. Van der Weiden S, de Jong EP, Te Pas AB, et al. Is routine TORCH screening and urine CMV culture warranted in small for gestational age neonates? Early Hum Dev. 2011;87:103.
83. Vaudry W, Ettenger R, Jara P, et al. Valganciclovir dosing according to body surface area and renal function in pediatric solid organ transplant recipients. Am J Transplant. 2009;9:636-43.
84. Vergnano S, Sharland M, Kasembe P, et al. Neonatal sepsis: an international perspective. Arch Dis Child Fetal Neonatal Ed. 2005;90:220-4.
85. Whitley RJ, Cloud G, Gruber W, et al. Ganciclovir treatment of symptomatic congenital cytomegalovirus infection: results of a phase II study. National Institute of Allergy and Infectious Diseases Collaborative Antiviral Study Group. J Infect Dis. 1997;175:1080.
86. World Health Organization. Immunization, Vaccines and Biologicals. Hepatitis B vaccine. Available at: www.who.int/vaccines/en/hepatitisb.shtml (Accessed May, 2006).
87. Young NS, Brown KE. Parvovirus B19. N Engl J Med. 2004;350:586-97.
88. Zaidi AKM, Thaver D, Asas S, Khan TA. Pathogens associated with sepsis in newborns and young infants in developing countries. Pediatr Infect Dis J. 2009; 28:S10-8.

41. Primary Immunodeficiency

Subhasish Bhattacharyya

1. When to suspect Primary Immunodeficiency (PID)?

i. Six or more new ear infections within 1 year.
ii. Two or more serious sinus infections within 1 year.
iii. Two or more severe pneumonias within 1 year.
iv. Two or more months on antibiotics with little effect.
v. Failure of an infant to thrive.
vi. Persistent oral thrush or cutaneous candidiasis after 1 year of age.
vii. Two or more deep-seated infections like sepsis, meningitis, cellulitis and osteomyelitis.
viii. Absolute lymphocyte count <2000/mm^3.
ix. Serious infections occurring at unusual sites (liver and brain abscess)
x. Infections with unusual pathogens (PCP, Aspergillus, Serratia marcescens and Nocardia).
xi. Infections with common childhood pathogens but of unusual severity.
xii. A family history of primary immunodeficiency.

2. What is the classification of PID?

i. Predominantly antibody deficiencies.
ii. Severe combined immunodeficiencies.
iii. Other cellular deficiencies (DiGeorge, WishKott-Aldrich and Ataxia-telangiectasia).
iv. Defects of phagocytic functions (i.e. chronic granulomatous disease and leucocyte adhesion defect).
v. Complement deficiencies.
vi. Immunodeficiencies associated with other diseases (i.e. Fanconi anemia, down syndrome, anhidrotic ectodermal dysplasia).

3. How common are PID?

Incidence is 1:10,000
i. B-cell defect—50%.
ii. Combined cellular and antibody deficiency—20%.
iii. T-cell defect—10%.
iv. Phagocytic disorder—18%.
v. Complement component disorder—2%.

4. What are the common organisms associated with different PIDs?

i. Predominat B-cell: Gram positive or gram negative (encapsulated) bacteria, i.e. Streptococcus pneumonia, staphylococcus aureus, Hemophilus influenzae and Neisseria meningitidis, Pseudomonas and Campylobacter species, enterovirus, rotavirus, Mycoplasma, Giardia, Cryptosoradium, Pneomocystis Jiroveci.

ii. Predominant T-cell deficiency: Encapsulated bacteria (i.e. *S. pnemoniae, H. influenzae,* Mycobacterium tuberculosis and other Mycobacteria infection, Intracellular bacteria (i.e. *L. monocytogenes*), *E. coli, P. aeruginosa,* Klebsiella, serratia and Salmonella, Nocardia. Viruses: CMV, Herpes Simplex, Varicella-Zoster virus, EBV, Rotavirus, Measles and RSV. Protozoa: *T. gondi,* Cryptosporidium. Fungi, i.e. Candida, Cryptococcus neoformans, Histoplasma capsulatun and Pneumocystis jiroveci).

iii. Phagocytic defects: Gram positive or gram negative bacteria catalase positive organisms including fungus, i.e. Aspergillus.

iv. Complement defects: Streptococcus and Neisseria.

5. What are the lab investigations in a suspected case of PID?

Most immunologic defects can be excluded at minimal cost by proper choice of screening test.

i. Complete blood count (CBC)

ii. Manual differential count—High neutrophil count in the absence of any signs of infection, a leukocyte adhesion deficiency should be suspected. If absolute lymphocyte count is normal, the patient is not likely to have a severe T-cell defect. Normal platelet size or count excludes Wishkott-Aldrich Syndrome.

iii. ESR (Normal ESR excludes chronic bacterial and fungal infection.)

iv. Quantification of Immunoglobulin levels. (IgM, IgG, IgE and IgA)

v. Tests for the specific evaluation of T-cell function-
   a. Total lymphocyte count
   b. T-cell subpopulations
   c. Delayed type hypersensitivity
   d. Cytotoxic assay.

vi. Proliferative responses to mitogens

vii. Tests for complement cascade:
   a. CH_{50} screening (quality of complement necessary for 50% lysis of sheep red blood cells)
   b. C_3 and C_4 level assay.

6. What is chronic granulomatous disease (CGD), and how to recognize and manage it?

In CGD, there is profound defect in the oxygen metabolic burst in myeloid cells following the phagocytosis of microbes. There is defect in NADPH and oxidase, leads to defects in the production of superoxide, peroxide and free oxygen radicals. Patients with CGD cannot kill Catalase positive pathogenic bacteria and fungus (i.e. *Staphylococcus, Nocardia, Serratia* and *Aspergillus*). Usual presentations are with superficial staph infections around nose, eyes and anus, adenitis, osteomyelitis and recurrent pneumonia. A male child with a pyogenic liver abscess should be considered to have CGD. The screening tests for the production of superoxide are the slide nitroblue tetrazolium reduction test and the flow cytometry using dihydrorhodamine 123 (DHR) to measure oxidant production. Few patients of CGD may have severe G6PD deficiency. Hematopietic stem cell transplantation is the only cure for CGD. Daily oral co-trimoxazole, itraconazole reduces the frequency of bacterial and fungal infections. Interferon-γ 50 µg/m^2 three times a week reduces the number of hospitalizations and serious infections.

7. What is X-linked agammaglobunemia (XLA)? What is the management of XLA?

XLA patients have a profound defect in B-lymphocyte development resulting in severe hypogammaglobunemia. Serum immunoglobulin values for IgG, IgM and IgA are below two standard deviations of the normal for age with less than 2% peripheral B-cell. There are no tonsillar tissue and palpable lymph nodes. After neonatal period symptoms begin at the age of 4-12 months, there is poor to absent response to vaccines. Infections are the most common clinical manifestation and mostly due to *Staphylococcus*, *Salmonella, Campylobacter*, capsulated bacteria, *Mycoplasma* and *Giardia*. Infections may be localized to the respiratory tract, skin, gastrointestinal tract and may be hematogenous. XLA patients are most susceptible to enterovirus (polio, coxsackie and ECHO) infections. Vaccine-associated poliomyelitis is increased. Major causes of death in these patients are enteroviral infections. IVIg and antimicrobials are the treatment of choice for these patients.

8. What are the common infections in common variable immune deficiencies (CVID), how are they diagnosed and what problem do they face?

CVID is characterized by hypogammaglobulinemia with phenotypically normal B-cells. The symptom of CVID may first occur during childhood, but they more often occur after puberty. Most cases of CVID are sporadic or follow an autosomal dominant pattern of inheritance. The serum immunoglobulin and antibody deficiency in CVID is profound with often development of autoantibody. Recurrent infections include pneumonia, sinusitis, diarrhea due to bacteria and giardia, may occur and lead to bronchiectasis, chronic malabsorption, nodular lymphoid hyperplasia and gastric atrophy. Sepsis and meningitis with encapsulated bacteria may occur more frequently and live polio vaccine may produce paralysis.

Lab evaluation in CVID patients demonstrates low IgG levels and low and absent IgA and IgM serum concentration. Patients with CVID exhibit a depressed switch from IgM to IgG.

Treatment of CVID includes IgG substitution antibiotic and physiotherapy for chest diseases.

9. What are the common infections in T-cell deficiencies, and what are the consequences of T-cell deficiency?

Patients with defects in T-cell function have infections or other clinical problems that are more severe than in patients with antibody deficiency disorders. Usually have an early onset, by 2-6 months of age. They are susceptible to low-grade opportunistic pathogens, including fungi, viruses, candida and *Pneumocystis jiroveci*. Among the viruses are CMV, EBV, adenovirus, varicella and enteroviruses. Among the bacterial infections are gram positive and negative bacteria and mycobacteria. There may be extensive mucocutaneous candidiasis and protracted diarrhea; increased incidence of GVHD following blood transfusion and postvaccination dissemination of BCG and varicella.

10. What is leukocyte adhesion defect (LAD)?

LAD (1, 2, 3) are rare autosomal recessive disorders of leukocyte function, characterized by recurrent bacterial and fungal infections. There may be delayed separation of umbilical cord with omphalitis. Pathogens are similar to those affecting patients with severe neutropenia (i.e. *Staphylococcus* and *E. coli*). Typical sign of inflammation may be absent, usually pus does not form but circulating neutrophil count during infection may exceed 30,000/μL to 1 lakh/μL. Early allogenic hematopoietic stem cell transplantation is the treatment of choice for severe LAD.

11. What are the hyper IgE syndrome and hyper IgM syndrome?

Hyper IgE syndrome is rare autosomal dominant disorder characterized by recurrent severe staphylococcal abscess of the skin, lungs, sinuses and other visceral organs. There may be osteopenia with unusual facial features (prominent forehead, deep set wide-spaced eyes and broad nasal bridge).

Hyper IgM presents with recurrent pyogenic infections, sinusitis and tonsilitis. There may be increased incidence of *P. jiroveci* pneumonia, extensive verruca vulgaris lesions and cryptosporidium enteritis.

12. What are the common complement deficiencies and their clinical presentations?

Deficiencies of early complements (C1, C2, C3 and C4) are associated with diseases like acute glomerulonephritis, systemic lupus erythematosis and vasculitis, terminal (C5, C6, C7, C8 and C9) complement deficiency possibly associated with recurrent neisserial infections.

13. Which primary immune defects are associated with albinism? How to diagnose this?

Chediak-Higashi syndrome (CHS) is associated with partial oculocutaneous albinism. Patients of CHS have light skin, silvery hair and solar sensitivity and sensory motor neuropathy. CHS is diagnosed by finding large inclusions in all the nucleated blood cells.

Further Reading

1. Buckley Rebecca H. Evaluation of Immunology. In: Cliegman, Stanton, St. Jame, et al. Nelson Textbook of Pediatrics, 19th ed. Philadelphia: Elsevier; 2011. p. 7150-738.
2. Immune Deficiency Foundation: www.primaryimmune.org.
3. Polin Richard A and Ditmark Mark F. Pediatric Secrets. 4th ed. Philadelphia: MOSBY;2005.p.295-309.

42 Sepsis Syndrome

Tanu Singhal

1. What are the different nomenclature for disorders related to sepsis and how they are helpful?

The various terms used in this context are Systemic Inflammatory Response Syndrome (SIRS), infection, sepsis, severe sepsis, septic shock and Multiple Organ Dysfunction Syndrome (MODS).

- SIRS is used in the presence of at least two of the following four criteria, one of which must be abnormal temperature or leukocyte count. These criteria include core (oral or rectal) temperature of > 38.5° C or < 36° C, tachycardia/bradycardia, tachypnea for an acute process not related to underlying neuromuscular disease and leukocyte count elevated or depressed for age (not secondary to chemotherapy induced leucopenia) or > 10% immature neutrophils. SIRS can be caused by infectious or non infectious causes (such as trauma, injury, surgery)
- The term sepsis is used when SIRS results from a suspected/proven infection
- Severe sepsis is sepsis plus one of the following: cardiovascular dysfunction or acute respiratory distress syndrome or two or more other organ dysfunctions
- The term septic shock is employed if there is circulatory impairment in the form of hypotension or need for vasoactive drug to maintain BP above 5th centile or signs of hypoperfusion such as decreased pulse volume/tachycardia/poor capillary refill/increased core and peripheral temperature gap
- Multiorgan dysfunction syndrome is used when two or more organs are dysfunctional.

These terms indicate the severity of the sepsis process, assist in prognostication and insure uniformity in clinical trials related to sepsis.

2. What are the common organisms causing sepsis in immunocompetent child?

Neonates and young infants (0–3 months)

The common organisms in India are predominantly gram negative bacteria such as *Klebsiella, E. coli, pseudomonas, Enterobacter* and *Citrobacter*. Other pathogens include *S. aureus*, *Enterococcus*, *Candida* and less commonly *Hib* and *pneumococcus*. *Listeria monocytogenes* and Group B Streptococcus are infrequently encountered in the Indian setting.

Bacteremia/viremia/parasitemia/toxemia in children

The common pathogens include bacteremia due to *S. pneumoniae*, *H. influenzae* and meningococcus, particularly in children below 36 months of age. *Salmonella typhi* and *paratyphi* bacteremia is also very common but uncommonly causes severe sepsis/septic shock owing to low virulence. Dengue and falciparum malaria occur at all ages, particularly in the monsoon season. Leptospirosis, rickettsial infections such as scrub typhus and spotted fever are important in particular epidemiologic settings. Finally toxic shock syndromes due to infection with toxigenic strains of staphylococci and streptococci should not be forgotten.

Site specific infections

These include acute bacterial meningitis (due to *S. pneumoniae*, *H. influenzae* and meningococcus), lower respiratory infections and pneumonia (due to viruses such as influenza, parainfluenza, RSV, adenovirus, coronavirus, bacteria including *S. pneumoniae*, *H. influenzae* and *Staphylococcus aureus* and atypical organisms such as *Mycoplasma*), urinary tract infections (most commonly due to *E. coli* and less often due to *Klebsiella pneumoniae*, Proteus), complicated gastrointestinal and intrabdominal infections (due to *Shigella*, *E. coli*, anaerobes and enterococci), complicated skin and soft tissue infections such as cellulitis, pyomyositis and necrotizing fascitis (due to *S. aureus* or *S. pyogenes* and rarely anaerobes and Gram negative infections; rising incidence of CA (community associated) MRSA is now being reported) and finally bone and joint infections (most commonly due to *S. aureus*).

Nosocomial infection

The commonest etiologic agents in the Indian setting are Gram negative pathogens such as *E. coli*, *Klebsiella*, *Pseudomonas* and *Acinetobacter*. Most of these are multidrug resistant due to production of extended spectrum beta- lactamases (ESBL), Amp C or now even carbapenem destroying enzymes. Next in the list are Gram positive pathogens such as enterococcus, methicillin sensitive and resistant *S. aureus*. *Candida* predominantly non albicans species such as *C. tropicalis* have also become increasingly common causes of nosocomial infections.

3. **What are the laboratory investigations to determine the cause, progress and severity of the disease?**

The laboratory investigations are shown in Table 1.

Table 1: Laboratory investigations
Essential investigations
CBC with platelet count
Smear for Malarial parasite or rapid malaria antigen test
At least 1 set of blood cultures
Urine routine and urine culture
CXR (Chest X-ray)
US abdomen
CRP and if available PCT
Other investigations (depending on clinical suspicion/ preliminary investigations)
LP and CSF analysis
Dengue NS1 antigen
Leptospira IgM, Weil Felix, IgM for scrub typhus/ spotted fever
CT chest and abdomen
Pus or tissue cultures
Investigations that help in supportive care
Liver and renal functions
Arterial blood gas
Serum lactate
Coagulation profile

4. Comparison of various inflammatory markers of sepsis?

The acute phase reactants are commonly estimated in patients with suspected sepsis to help differentiate between non infectious SIRS and sepsis, viral and bacterial causes of sepsis and also to assess severity and follow response to therapy.

The *ESR or erythrocyte sedimentation rate* is cheap and widely available, but unfortunately of limited sensitivity and specificity. A high ESR may be seen in anemia and other non infectious conditions while the ESR may be normal in full blown sepsis. The micro ESR, a component of neonatal septic screen in the past has been largely supplanted by CRP.

The *C reactive protein (CRP)* is an acute phase reactant produced by the liver in response to IL-6, TNF-α and other cytokines. It rises in 6 hours, peaks within 48 hours and has a half life of 8 hours. A level of more than 6 mg/L is considered positive. It rises and falls more quickly than ESR. A rise of C reactive protein may be seen in any SIRS including infections, trauma, necrosis and inflammation. Hence, it does not distinguish infectious from non infectious causes of SIRS. It rises in both viral and bacterial infections, though the rise is more in bacterial than viral. There is no accurate cut off that distinguishes viral from bacterial infections; however, if the CRP is very high (> 100 mg/liter), bacterial etiology is more likely. The CRP is an important component of neonatal septic screen and in evaluation of fever without focus. Serial CRP's help in tracking the progress of infections, especially in patients with bone and joint infections.

Procalcitonin is a newly evaluated acute phase reactant, and is produced by most cells of the body in response to injury and infection. It rises and falls earlier than CRP and does not rise in many inflammatory and neoplastic conditions. Studies have shown that it is more reliable than CRP in distinguishing infectious from non infectious causes of SIRS and in differentiating viral from bacterial infections. A level of more than 2 mg/mL is highly specific for serious bacterial infection. Moreover, its levels correlate with severity of infection and prognosis. Very high Procalcitonin (PCT) levels at onset and failure of PCT to decline with treatment have been associated with poor outcome. PCT estimation is however more expensive than CRP. Some studies have shown that procalcitonin is not significantly better than CRP in evaluation of neonatal sepsis or fever without focus.

IL-18 and *CD64* are other biomarkers being evaluated. At present, serum PCT is the best biomarker for diagnosis and prognosis of pediatric sepsis.

5. How should we select empiric antibiotic in a child with community acquired septic shock in a normal child?

Appropriate antibiotics must be initiated at the earliest in suspected pediatric sepsis, since delaying antibiotics or inappropriate choice of antibiotics increase mortality. The choice of initial antibiotic depends on various factors such as likely pathogen and its antimicrobial susceptibility, prior antibiotic exposure, severity of illness, host comorbidities and site of infection.

Neonates

In antibiotic naïve community acquired neonatal sepsis, initial antibiotic therapy with a third generation cephalosporin such as cefotaxime/ceftriaxone and an aminoglycoside should be initiated.

Infants and children

In children beyond the neonatal period who have severe sepsis with no localizable focus, a combination of ceftriaxone with aminoglycoside is recommended as it adequately covers common bacterial pathogens such as *pneumococcus*, *Hib*, *Salmonella* and Gram negative pathogens causing urinary tract infections and intrabdominal infections. If malaria is suspected, IV artesunate should be initiated till smear reports are available. Empirical monotherapy with ceftriaxone is adequate for children with suspected bacterial meningitis and most children with community acquired pneumonia (CAP). In children with CAP due to suspected atypical pathogens, addition of macrolide to ceftriaxone is recommended. With increasing incidence of community acquired urinary tract infections due to ESBL producing Gram negative pathogens, addition of an aminoglycoside to ceftriaxone in children with suspected UTI who have received prior antibiotics is advisable. Children with suspected intrabdominal sepsis should receive a combination of metronidazole and ceftriaxone or a monotherapy with a β-lactam/ β-lactam inhibitor (BLBLI) combination such as piperacillin tazobactam/ cefoperazone sublactam or cefepime tazobactam. Children with skin, soft tissue and musculoskeletal infections below the age of 5 years should be treated with a combination of ceftriaxone and cloxacillin and those above 5 years can be treated with cloxacillin monotherapy. An increasing incidence of community acquired MRSA has been noted; infection due to CA MRSA are characterized by severe toxicity, necrosis and leukopenia. If CA MRSA is suspected then addition of an antiMRSA agent such as vancomycin/ teicoplanin/linezolid to cloxacillin is recommended. For children with severe gram positive infections and necrotizing fasciitis, a toxin inhibiting drug such as clindamycin or linezolid should be added to the antibiotic regime.

6. How should we select empiric antibiotics for sepsis in an immunocompromised child?

Empirical antimicrobial therapy is complex and depends on the type and severity of the immunocompromised state, and hence, the likely etiologic agents. Broadly speaking, treatment should be initiated with a potent Gram negative cover such as BL-BLI combination or carbapenems with or without aminoglycoside. Additional antiMRSA, broad spectrum antifungal therapy (echinocandins/voriconazole/amphotericin B), antiviral therapy and therapy for pneumocystis carinii may be considered on a case by case basis.

7. When should we use antifungal and for how long?

Candida is emerging as an important cause of nosocomial blood stream infections in both the neonatal and pediatric intensive care unit. Risk factors for candidemia include low birth weight and prematurity, prolonged ICU stay, receipt of broad spectrum antibiotics, presence of central line, use of intralipids, dialysis, renal failure, use of corticosteroids, abdominal surgery and multisite colonization with *Candida* (in urine, stool, respiratory secretions). Children with nosocomial sepsis and a combination of these risk factors merit empirical antifungal therapy after sending blood cultures. Instituting antifungals only after receipt of a positive culture report is associated with increased mortality due to delay in therapy and missing 50% of cases of invasive candidiasis which are culture negative. Choice of empirical therapy depends on severity of illness, history of azole exposure and local epidemiology. In children with severe illness or history of azole exposure or where there is high prevalence of azole resistant *Candida* amphotericin B/echinocandins should be used. In other cases, fluconazole usually suffices in doses of 12 mg/kg/day. If the cultures are positive, therapy should be modified as per susceptibility and continued for 2 weeks (3 weeks in neonates) after the last negative cultures. Central lines should be removed. Neonates should undergo ophthalmic and CSF examination to rule out end-ophthalmitis and meningitis.

Antifungal therapy should not be initiated in children who grow *Candida* in fecal/respiratory or urinary samples in the absence of features of sepsis, since this just indicates colonization. Certain NICU's may initiate prophylactic intravenous fluconazole at 3-6 mg/kg twice weekly in very low birth weight babies till they are on intravenous therapy. Prophylactic use of antifungals in pediatric intensive care units is not normally recommended.

8. What is the role of immunoglobulins and steroids in sepsis?

A very recent Cochrane review published in 2013 concluded that though there was significant reduction in mortality in adults with sepsis with use of polyclonal intravenous immunoglobulin (IVIG) compared to placebo or no intervention (relative risk 0.81 and 0.66, respectively) this effect disappeared when only studies with low risk of bias were included. Conversely in neonates, there is now sufficient and robust evidence to show that adjunctive therapy with IVIG is not beneficial. The use of IVIG may however be considered in children with toxic shock syndrome, not responding to standard antibacterial therapy.

Several trials and systematic reviews have examined the efficacy and safety of corticosteroids in patients with sepsis and septic shock with conflicting results. Some trials and systematic reviews have demonstrated significant reduction in 28 days mortality, while others have demonstrated only significant benefits in time to reversal of shock. Large trials are ongoing. The consensus guidelines for pediatric sepsis management in resource limited countries recommend corticosteroid therapy only in children with vasopressor refractory shock or those with documented adrenocortical insufficiency.

Further Reading

1. Alejandria MM, Lansang MA, Dans LF, Mantaring Iii JB. Intravenous immunoglobulin for treating sepsis, severe sepsis and septic shock. Cochrane Database Syst Rev. 2013 Sep 16; 9: CD001090. doi: 10.1002/14651858.CD001090. pub2.
2. Goldstein B, Giroir B, Randolph A; International Consensus Conference on Pediatric Sepsis. International pediatric sepsis consensus conference: Definitions for sepsis and organ dysfunction in pediatrics. Pediatr Crit Care Med. 2005; 6:2-8.
3. Gupta A, Kapil A, Lodha R, Kabra SK, Sood S, Dhawan B, Das BK, Sreenivas V. Burden of healthcare-associated infections in a pediatric intensive care unit of a developing country: A single center experience using active surveillance. J Hosp Infect. 2011; 78: 323-6.
4. Khilnani P, Singhi S, Lodha R, Santhanam I, Sachdev A, Chugh K, et al. Pediatric Sepsis Guidelines: Summary for resource-limited countries. Indian J Crit Care Med. 2010;14:41-52.
5. Pappas PG, Kauffman CA, Andes D, Benjamin DK, Calandra TF, Edwards JE, et al. Clinical Practice Guidelines for the Management of Candidiasis: 2009 Update by the Infectious Diseases Society of America. Clinical Infectious Diseases 2009; 48:503-35.

6. Sligl WI, Milner DA, Sundar S, Mphatswe W, Majumdar SR. Safety and efficacy of corticosteroids for the treatment of septic shock: A systematic review and meta-analysis. Clin Infect Dis. 2009 Jul 1; 49(1):93-101.
7. Standage SW and Wong HR. Biomarkers for pediatric sepsis and septic shock Expert Rev Anti Infect Ther. 2011;9(1):71-9. doi:10.1586/eri.10.154.
8. Viswanathan R, Singh AK, Basu S, Chatterjee S, Sardar S, Isaacs D. Multi-drug resistant Gram negative bacilli causing early neonatal sepsis in India. Arch Dis Child Fetal Neonatal Ed. 2012; 97: F182-7.

43 Febrile Neutropenia

Kheya Ghosh Uttam

1. How do you classify Neutropenia?

Normal Absolute Neutrophil Count (ANC) is 1500 to 8000 cells/mm^3. Neutropenia is defined as ANC less than two standard deviation of the normal mean. In other words, it can be defined as ANC < 1500 cells/mm^3.

Depending upon the ANC, neutropenia is further classified as:
- Mild Neutropenia: 1000–1500 cells/mm^3
- Moderate Neutropenia: 500–999 cells/mm^3
- Severe Neutropenia: < 500 cells/mm^3
- Profound Neutropenia: <100 cells/mm^3.

Neutropenia may be classified according to the etiology into three groups:
- Extrinsic to marrow myeloid cells (Infections, drugs, immunological, radiation)
- Acquired disorder of myeloid cells (Aplastic anemia, leukemia, myelodysplasis, Vit B12 or folate deficiency)
- Intrinsic disorders of myeloid precursor cells (Genetic disorders like cyclic neutropenia, Shwachman Diamond's syndrome, Kostmann's syndrome)

2. What is febrile neutropenia?

Febrile neutropenia is defined as an axillary temperature >38.5°C lasting >1 hour in the context of an absolute neutrophil count (ANC) < 500 cells/mm^3. Fever has also been defined as a single oral temperature of 38.3°C (101°F) or a temperature of 38°C (100.4°F) for >1 hour.

3. Which infections affect neutropenic patients?

Children with chronic isolated neutropenia may not suffer from serious infections as the rest of the immune system remains intact. Whereas children with acquired neutropenia due to cytotoxic drugs, radiation develop serious infections.

The most common pathogen causing infections in neutropenic patients are *Staphylococcus aureus* and Gram negative bacteria.

In case of acquired neutropenia due to malignancy or cytotoxic drugs, organisms causing infection depend upon the associated underlying malig-nancies and resultant disruption of normal barrier function. Like in leukemia and lymphoma where there is lack of T cells, there will be infection with intracellular organisms. Thus in these children, infection with *Mycobacterium tuberculosis*, herpes virus, fungi and other intracellular parasites are common. As lymph nodes and splenic reticuloendothelial cells are also involved in these diseases, Staphylococci, *Streptococcus pneumoniae*, *Hemophilus influenzae*, *Neisseria meningitidis* may also occur. Irrespective of underlying malignancies, the organism causing infections are Gram negative bacteria like *Pseudomonas species*, *E. coli*, *Klebsiella sp*, *Acinetobacter* and Gram positive bacteria like Coagulase negative *Staphyloccus*, *S. aureus*, *Streptococcus sp*. If there is associated pulmonary compromise infection with *Legionella*, *pneumocystis*, and fungal (*Candida* and *Aspergillus*) are common. Fungal infection is also common in patients with prolonged neutropenia. Viral infections like adeno, cytomegalo, Herpes simplex and Varicella zoster may also occur specially after bone marrow transplant.

4. How to investigate a child with febrile neutropenia?

Always search for focus of infection in different systems including skin and mucosa. Indwelling intravenous cannula, indwelling catheter are often potential source of infection. Initial investigation includes the following:
  i. Complete hemogram to assess bone marrow function
  ii. Renal and liver function test
  iii. Coagulation screen
  iv. C-reactive protein
  v. Blood cultures (minimum two sets) including cultures from intravenous catheter. Most centers limit blood draws to not more than 1% of patients total blood volume. Blood culture sent from all central venous catheter lumens, as well as one from a peripheral vein is advocated
  vi. Urine and sputum (If available) analysis and culture
  vii. Other investigations depending upon the systems involved—
    a. Stool microscopy and culture (if diarrhea present)
    b. Skin lesions (aspirate/biopsy/swab)
    c. Chest radiograph (if respiratory symptoms present or outpatient therapy considered).

5. What is the empirical antibiotic used in febrile neutropenia?

Empiric antibiotic will depend upon presence or absence of risk factors. High risk patients are children with any of the following criteria:
  i. Profound neutropenia (ANC< 100/cmm) anticipated to last > 7 days.
  ii. Presence of any associated co-morbid medical problems:
    - Hemodynamic instability
    - Oral or gastrointestinal mucositis
    - Abdominal symptoms like pain, nausea, vomiting or diarrhea
    - Neurological or mental status changes of new onset
    - IV catheter infection especially catheter tunnel infection
    - New pulmonary infiltrate or hypoxemia, or underlying chronic lung disease.

Table 1: MASCC scoring index

Characteristic	Score
Burden of illness: no or mild symptoms	5
No hypotension	5
No chronic obstructive pulmonary disease	4
Solid tumor or no previous fungal infection	4
No dehydration	3
Burden of illness: moderate symptoms	3
Outpatient status (at onset of fever)	3
Age <20 years	2

iii. Hepatic insuffiency (SGPT > 5X normal values) or renal insufficiency (creatinine clearance < 30 mL/ minute).

vi. MASCC index (Multinational Association for Supportive Care in Cancer (MASCC) index) < 21 (Table 1).

High risk patients should be admitted for IV empirical antibiotic therapy. Monotherapy with an anti-pseudomonal agent like ceftazidime, a carbapenem (meropenem or imipenem-cilastatin) or piperacillin-tazobactam is recommended. Other antibiotics (aminoglycosides or fluroquinolones and/or vancomycin) maybe added to counteract complications or if antibiotic resistance is suspected or proven.

Indications of vancomycin therapy

i. Severe mucositis.
ii. Obvious catheter related infection.
iii. Colonization with methicillin resistant *Staphylococcus aureus* (MRSA).
iv Hypotension.
v. Patient on quinolone prophylaxis.
vi. Skin or soft tissue infection/pneumonia.

If the patient has associated diarrhea, *Clostridium difficile* should be suspected and metronidazole should be added.

Those without high risk criteria may initially receive oral antibiotics instead of IV medications, or may be initiated with IV and converted to outpatient oral treatment at the earliest.

Ciprofloxacin plus coamoxyclav is commonly recommended for oral treatment. Others like levofloxacin or ciprofloxacin alone or ciprofloxacin plus clindamycin are also commonly used. Patients on fluroquinolone prophylaxis should not receive empirical oral therapy with fluroquinolone. Hospital admission is required for persistent fever or signs of worsening infection.

6. How long empiric antibiotic therapy should be continued?

Duration of therapy will depend on particular organism and site of infection, and should continue till marrow recovery (ANC > 500/cmm). Alternatively, if therapy has been completed and patient is afebrile and stable, but remains neutropenic, oral fluroquinolone prophylaxis may be initiated till marrow recovery.

7. Whom should we give prophylactic antibiotics following recovery from fever?

Fluoroquinolone (levofloxacin or ciprofloxacin) prophylaxis should be given to patients with expected prolonged (> 7 days) and severe neutropenia (ANC < 100/cmm).

Addition of an antigram-positive agent is generally not required.

Low risk patients with expected short (< 7 days) duration of neutropenia are generally not put on antibiotic prophylaxis.

Prophylaxis against *Candida* infections is recommended in high risk groups like allogeneic Hematopoietic stem cell transplantation (HSCT) receipients or those undergoing intensive remission induction chemotherapy for acute leukemia. Fluconazole, itraconazole, voricanazole, posaconazole and caspofungin are all acceptable alternatives.

Prophylaxis against invasive *Aspergillus* with posaconazole should be considered for selected patients > 13 years, undergoing intensive chemotherapy for acute myeloid leukemia or myeloid dysplasia.

8. When to give antivirals?

HSV-seropositive patients undergoing allogeneic HSCT or leukemia induction should receive acyclovir. Treatment for HSV or VZV is indicated only if there is evidence of active viral disease. Influenza infection should be treated if the infecting strain is susceptible, and during influenza outbreaks, all symptomatic neutropenic patients should receive empirical treatment. Respiratory syncytial virus (RSV) treatment should not be given to patients who present with upper respiratory tract symptoms.

Further Reading

1. Edward A S, Dan L L. Principles of Cancer Treatment. In: Fauci, Braunwald, kasper, Hauser, longo, Jameson, Loscalzo, editors. Harrison's Principles of Internal Medicine, 17th edition. Mc Graw Hill, 2008;1.
2. Laurence AB. Leukopenia. In Kliegman, Behrman, Jenson, Stanton, editors. Nelson Textbook of Pediatrics, 18th edition. Elsevier, 2007.

44 Lymphadenitis

Ritabrata Kundu

1. What are the different types of lymphadenopathy according to the pattern of lymph node involvement?

Lymph nodes are enlarged either by proliferation of normal lymphoid tissues or when they are infiltrated by other cells like malignant or phagocytic cells. Normal nodes in cervical and axillary regions are less than 1 cm diameter whereas inguinal nodes may be up to 1.5 cm in diameter.

Lymph node enlargement can be generalized or localized as shown in Flow chart 1. Enlargement of more than two non contiguous lymph node group are generalized lymphadenopathy. Localized lymphadenopathy may be cervical or others. Cervical lymphadenopathy may be further divided into three groups acute unilateral cervical, acute bilateral cervical or chronic/sub acute lymphadenopathy.

Flow chart 1: Different types of lymphadenopathy

```
                    ┌─→ Generalized          ┌─→ Acute unilateral
Lymphadenopathy ────┼─→ Cervical      ───────┼─→ Acute bilateral
                    └─→ Localized            └─→ Chronic/Subacute
                         │
                         └─→ Others, e.g.
                             abdominal
```

2. What are the causes of generalized lymphadenopathy in infants and children?

Generalized lymphadenopathy is often associated with systemic viral illnesses but it may be a manifestation of other systemic diseases with abnormal findings in other systems :

Causes of generalized lymphadenopathy
1. Viral infections
   i. EBV, CMV, HHV-6

    ii. HIV
    iii. Parvovirus B19
    iv. Rubella, Measles, Adenovirus
    v. Hepatitis A and B, Enterovirus
    vi. Dengue, Chikungunya
2. Bacterial infection
    i. Tubeculosis
    ii. *Salmonella typhi*
    iii. Scarlet fever
    iv. Rickettsia
    v. Brucella
    vi. Cat scratch disease
3. Fungal infections
    i. Histoplasmosis
    ii. Coccidiomycosis
4. Parasitic infections
    i. Toxoplasmosis
    ii. Filaviasis
5. Non infection causes
    i. Malignancy (lymphomas)
    ii. Hemophagocytic lymphohistiocytosis
    iii. Primary immuno deficiency (Chronic granulomatous disease, Wiskott-Aldrich syndrome, Chediak Higashi disease, hyper IgE syndrome)
    iv. Rheumatological disorders (Systemic onset JIA, SLE)
    v. Sarcoidosis
    vi. Drug reaction (e.g. phenytoin)
6. Syndromal causes
    i. Kikuchi Fujimoto disease
    ii. Rosai Dorfman disease
    iii. Castleman's disease

3. What are the causes of acute unilateral cervical, acute bilateral cervical and chronic cervical lymphadenitis?

Acute cervical lymphadenopathy:

These are mostly due to pyogenic infection. *S aureus* and *S pyogenes* account for majority of the cases. GBS may be an important cause in neonates associated with features of sepsis. In children with caries teeth and periodical disease anaerobes may be responsible.

Kawasaki disease constitute an important cause of unilateral acute cervical lymphadenpathy but may be bilateral.

Acute unilateral cervical lymphadenopathy
    i. *Staphylococcus aureus*
    ii. *Streptococcus pyogenes*
    iii. Group B *streptococcus*
    iv. Anerobes
    v. Kawasaki disease

Acute bilateral cervical lymphadenopathy
  i. Systemic viral infection
  ii. Acute viral pharyngitis
  iii. Acute bacterial tonsillitis
  iv. Pharyngeal diphtheria
  v. *Mycoplasma pneumoniae* infection
  vi. Malignancy
  vii. Periodic fever (PFAPA)

Chronic cervical lymphadenopathy
  i. Tuberculosis
  ii. NTM (Nontuberculous mycobacteria)
  iii. Toxoplasmosis
  iv. Cat scratch disease.

4. When should you consider malignancy in patients with lymphadenopathy?

A detailed history and meticulous clinical examinations is essential to diagnose the condition. Lymphadenpathy due to neoplasia is more common in adolescent age group often, with a history of weight loss and night sweats.

The nodes are usually non-tender, firm to hard in feel with no erythema or warmth of the overlying skin unless they are secondarily infected. They at times grow rapidly and may become fixed to underlying structure.

Supraclavicular lymph node enlargement are uncommon following infection, and malignancy should be considered in such cases. Particularly, left supraclavicular lymph node, virchow's node, drains lymphatics from thorax and abdomen. Other palpable nodes at unusual site like epitrochlear and popliteal should always be considered abnormal and investigated.

5. How to approach a case of lymphadenopathy?

A thorough history may provide many important clues to diagnose the etiology. A history of contact with animals or visit to forest areas may suggest brucella or tick borne rickettsia. Risk factors for TB, hepatitis B and HIV should be sought. Immunization history against MMR, hepatitis A and B is important.

Standard lymph node examination should include following points:
  i. Sites
  ii. Single or multiple
  iii. Consistency (Soft, fluctuant, firm, rubbery or hand)
  iv. Attachment (Superficial or deep)
  v. Skin changes
  vi. Tenderness

Full systemic examination should include examination of all other lymph node groups along with assessment of splenomegaly and hepatomegaly. Look for infection in the area drained by affected nodes. Skin should be examined for viral exanthems or rashes and document fever and weight loss.

6. How to diagnose tuberculous lymphadenitis?

This is most common from of extrapulmonary tuberculosis. Persistent lymphadenopathy more than 2 cm in size should be investigated. Though tuberculin test may be positive in a significant proportion of cases but isolated positivity doesn't prove the diagnosis. A course of antibiotics other than quinolones for 7 days are usually prescribed. In case of non response after 2 weeks or if the nodes are matted, fluctuant with minimal tenderness or non-tender or with discharging sinus to start with should be investigated. Smear examination for AFB of pus from discharging sinus or aspirate from lymph node should be done. If facilities exist then fine needle aspiration for cytology (FNAC) may be done as it correlates with biopsy in more than 90% cases. Diagnosis is confirmed if AFB is positive in FNAC aspirate or histopathology shows necrosis and epitheloid grannuloma. If FNAC is inconclusive then lymph node biopsy is necessary for confirmation of diagnosis. According to the National Consultation on Diagnosis and Treatment of Pediatric Tuberculosis, isolated tuberculin test positively without suggestive findings in either FNAC or lymph node biopsy should not be treated with anti tuberculous drugs.

Further Reading

1. Ishimine P. Fever without source in children 0-36 months of age. Pediatr Clin N Am. 2006;53:167-94.
2. Nark JW. Fever without source in children: recommendations for outpatient care in those up to 3. Postgrad Med. 2000;107(2):259-66.
3. National Neonatal Perinatal Database: Report 2002-2003 ICMR, New Delhi Publications. 2005.p.45-57.
4. Powell RK. Fever without a focus. In : Behrman ER, Kliegman MR, Jenson BH (Eds). Nelson Textbook of Pediatrics USA: Saunders 2004.p.841-6.

45 HIV Infection

Ira Shah

1. What is the epidemiology of HIV of children in India?

An estimated 25,000 HIV infections occur annually among Indian children. Most of these children are infected during pregnancy, delivery or soon after birth through mother-to-child transmission. Approximately, 5,000 HIV-infected Indian children progress to AIDS, annually. Although, an unknown number of HIV-infected Indian children die each year. About 70,000 children are estimated to be living with HIV infection in India. One out of every 25 HIV-infected children worldwide lives in India.

2. How HIV is transmitted in children?

Transmission of HIV in children is predominantly vertical. Rarely transmission occurs due to blood product transfusions or through sexual route. HIV can be transmitted vertically through the placenta (intrauterine transmission), exposure to vaginal fluids at the time of labor (intrapartum transmission) and through breast milk (breastfeeding—postpartum transmission). Pooled data from various cohort studies conducted prior to preventive interventions estimated the risk of in-utero transmission to be approximately 10%, the risk of intrapartum transmission, i.e. during labor and delivery, to be approximately 15%, and the risk of postpartum transmission to be between 10 and 15%, depending on the duration of breastfeeding.

3. What is the clinical staging of HIV in children?

For the simplification of management of HIV infected children, Center for Diseases Control and Prevention in 1994 categorized HIV in children below 13 years of age into 4 groups: N, A, B and C based on signs, symptoms, or diagnoses related to HIV infection as shown in Table 1. Category N, not symptomatic, includes children with no signs or symptoms considered to be the result of HIV infection or with only one of the conditions listed in Category A, mildly symptomatic. Category N was separated from Category A partly because of the substantial amount of time that can elapse before a child manifests the signs or symptoms defined in Category B, moderately symptomatic. Category B includes all children with signs and symptoms thought to be caused by HIV infection but not specifically outlined under Category A or Category C, severely symptomatic. Category C includes all AIDS-defining conditions except lymphoid interstitial pneumonitis (LIP).

Table 1: 1994 Revised CDC clinical categories of HIV in children <13 years

CATEGORY N: NOT SYMPTOMATIC
Children who have no signs or symptoms considered to be the result of HIV infection or who have only one of the conditions listed in Category A

CATEGORY A: MILDLY SYMPTOMATIC
Children with two or more of the conditions listed below but none of the conditions listed in categories B and C:
- Lymphadenopathy ($\geq$ 0.5 cm at more than two sites; bilateral = one site)
- Hepatomegaly
- Splenomegaly
- Dermatitis
- Parotitis
- Recurrent or persistent upper respiratory infection, sinusitis, or otitis media

CATEGORY B: MODERATELY SYMPTOMATIC
Children who have symptomatic conditions other than those listed for category A or C that are attributed to HIV infection. Examples of conditions in clinical category B include but are not limited to:
- Anemia (<8 g/dL), neutropenia (<1,000/mm^3), or thrombocytopenia (<100,000/mm^3) persisting $\geq$ 30 days
- Bacterial meningitis, pneumonia, or sepsis (single episode)
- Candidiasis, oropharyngeal (thrush), persisting (>2 months) in children > 6 months of age
- Cardiomyopathy
- Cytomegalovirus infection, with onset before 1 month of age
- Diarrhea, recurrent or chronic
- Hepatitis
- Herpes simplex virus (HSV) stomatitis, recurrent (more than two episodes within 1 year)
- HSV bronchitis, pneumonitis, or esophagitis with onset before 1 month of age
- Herpes zoster (shingles) involving at least 2 distinct episodes or more than one dermatome
- Leiomyosarcoma
- Lymphoid interstitial pneumonia (LIP) or pulmonary lymphoid hyperplasia complex
- Nephropathy
- Nocardiosis
- Persistent fever (lasting >1 month)
- Toxoplasmosis, onset before 1 month of age
- Varicella, disseminated (complicated chickenpox)

CATEGORY C: SEVERELY SYMPTOMATIC
- Serious bacterial infections, multiple or recurrent (i.e. any combination of at least two culture-confirmed infections within a 2-year period), of the following types: septicemia, pneumonia, meningitis, bone or joint infection, or abscess of an internal organ or body cavity (excluding otitis media, superficial skin or mucosal abscesses, and indwelling catheter-related infections)
- Candidiasis, esophageal or pulmonary (bronchi, trachea, lungs)
- Coccidioidomycosis, disseminated (at site other than or in addition to lungs or cervical or hilar lymph nodes)
- Cryptococcosis, extrapulmonary
- Cryptosporidiosis or isosporiasis with diarrhea persisting >1 month
- Cytomegalovirus disease with onset of symptoms at age >1 month (at a site other than liver, spleen, or lymph nodes)
- Encephalopathy (at least one of the following progressive findings present for at least 2 months in the absence of a concurrent illness other than HIV infection that could explain the findings): a) failure to attain or loss of developmental milestones or loss

Contd...

Contd...

> of intellectual ability, verified by standard developmental scale or neuropsychological tests; b) impaired brain growth or acquired microcephaly demonstrated by head circumference measurements or brain atrophy demonstrated by computerized tomography or magnetic resonance imaging (serial imaging is required for children <2 years of age); c) acquired symmetric motor deficit manifested by two or more of the following: paresis, pathologic reflexes, ataxia, or gait disturbance
> - Herpes simplex virus infection causing a mucocutaneous ulcer that persists for >1 month; or bronchitis, pneumonitis, or esophagitis for any duration affecting a child >1 month of age
> - Histoplasmosis, disseminated (at a site other than or in addition to lungs or cervical or hilar lymph nodes)
> - Kaposi's sarcoma
> - Lymphoma, primary, in brain
> - Lymphoma, small, noncleaved cell (Burkitt's), or immunoblastic or large cell lymphoma of B-cell or unknown immunologic phenotype
> - Mycobacterium tuberculosis, disseminated or extrapulmonary
> - Mycobacterium, other species or unidentified species, disseminated (at a site other than or in addition to lungs, skin, or cervical or hilar lymph nodes)
> - *Mycobacterium avium* complex or *Mycobacterium kansasii*, disseminated (at site other than or in addition to lungs, skin, or cervical or hilar lymph nodes)
> - *Pneumocystis carinii* pneumonia
> - Progressive multifocal leukoencephalopathy
> - *Salmonella* (nontyphoid) septicemia, recurrent
> - Toxoplasmosis of the brain with onset at >1 month of age
> - Wasting syndrome in the absence of a concurrent illness other than HIV infection that could explain the following findings: a) persistent weight loss >10% of baseline OR b) downward crossing of at least two of the following percentile lines on the weight-for-age chart (e.g. 95th, 75th, 50th, 25th, 5th) in a child ≥ 1 year of age or c) <5th percentile on weight-for-height chart on two consecutive measurements, ≥ 30 days apart PLUS a) chronic diarrhea (i.e. at least two loose stools per day for > 30 days) OR b) documented fever (for ≥ 30 days, intermittent or constant)

In 1986, World Health Organization (WHO) developed a provisional clinical AIDS case definition for adults and children to report AIDS cases in resource-constrained settings. It was modified in 1994 to accommodate 1993 revisions to European and United States Centers for Disease Control and Prevention definitions as shown in Table 2. Studies in African settings suggested that the original WHO clinical case definitions for AIDS in children were not very sensitive or specific. Thus, in 2006, WHO revised the clinical staging in children below 15 years of age. The clinical stage is useful for assessment at baseline (first diagnosis of HIV infection) or entry into long-term HIV care and in the follow-up of patients along with decision when to start cotrimoxazole prophylaxis and when to start antiretroviral therapy.

Table 2: WHO clinical staging of HIV/AIDS for children with confirmed HIV

CLINICAL STAGE 1
- Asymptomatic
- Persistent generalized lymphadenopathy

Contd...

Contd...

CLINICAL STAGE 2
- Unexplained persistent hepatosplenomegaly
- Papular pruritic eruptions
- Fungal nail infection
- Angular cheilitis
- Lineal gingival erythema
- Extensive wart virus infection
- Extensive molluscum contagiosum
- Recurrent oral ulcerations
- Unexplained persistent parotid enlargement
- Herpes zoster
- Recurrent or chronic upper respiratory tract infections (otitis media, otorrhea, sinusitis or tonsillitis)

CLINICAL STAGE 3
- Unexplained moderate malnutrition or wasting not adequately responding to standard therapy
- Unexplained persistent diarrhea (14 days or more)
- Unexplained persistent fever (above 37.5°C intermittent or constant, for longer than one month)
- Persistent oral candidiasis (after first 6–8 weeks of life)
- Oral hairy leukoplakia
- Acute necrotizing ulcerative gingivitis or periodontitis
- Lymph node tuberculosis
- Pulmonary tuberculosis
- Severe recurrent bacterial pneumonia
- Symptomatic lymphoid interstitial pneumonitis
- Chronic HIV-associated lung disease including bronchiectasis
- Unexplained anemia (< 8 g/dL), neutropenia (< 0.5×10^9 per liter) and or chronic thrombocytopenia (< 50×10^9 per liter)

CLINICAL STAGE 4
- Unexplained severe wasting, stunting or severe malnutrition not responding to standard therapy
- Pneumocystis pneumonia
- Recurrent severe presumed bacterial infections (e.g. empyema, pyomyositis, bone or joint infection, meningitis, but excluding pneumonia)
- Chronic herpes simplex infection; (orolabial or cutaneous of more than one month's duration or visceral at any site)
- Extrapulmonary tuberculosis
- Kaposi sarcoma
- Esophageal candidiasis (or candida of trachea, bronchi or lungs)
- Central nervous system toxoplasmosis (outside the neonatal period)
- HIV encephalopathy
- Cytomegalovirus (CMV) infection; retinitis or CMV infection affecting another organ, with onset at age over 1 month
- Extrapulmonary cryptococcosis including meningitis
- Disseminated endemic mycosis (extrapulmonary histoplasmosis, coccidiomycosis, penicilliosis)
- Chronic cryptosporidiosis
- Chronic isosporiasis
- Disseminated non-tuberculous mycobacteria infection
- Acquired HIV-associated rectal fistula
- Cerebral or B cell non-Hodgkin lymphoma
- Progressive multifocal leukoencephalopathy
- Symptomatic HIV-associated nephropathy or HIV-associated cardiomyopathy

HIV Infection

4. What are the diagnostic modalities of HIV in children in various age groups?

Diagnosis of HIV in infants

All infants born to HIV-infected mothers carry maternal IgG antibodies which cross the placenta freely. These maternal antibodies may remain detectable in the infant's serum for up to 12–15 months after birth. As a result, serological diagnosis of HIV infection is only reliable after 15–18 months of age. Tests that can be done for diagnosis of HIV infection in children below 18 months of age are HIV culture, detection of HIV proviral DNA by polymerase chain reaction (PCR) or HIV antigen (p24). Detection of p24 antigen is cheaper, highly specific and easy-to-perform but it is less sensitive than other virologic tests. Also false negativity is high in younger children as most of the p24 antigen is bound to maternal antibodies. PCR is now the preferred tool for diagnosis of HIV in infants. It should be done at 4–6 weeks after birth in non-breast fed infants and 6–8 weeks after cessation of breast milk in breastfed infants. HIV culture is done from peripheral blood mononuclear cells (PBMCs) but is technically difficult and time consuming. It is expensive and done in research institutes.

Diagnosis of HIV in children above 18 months of age

ELISA is the time-tested reliable method for detection of anti-HIV antibodies with a sensitivity of >99.5% and specificity of 99%. Confirmation of positive HIV status can be done by 2 or 3 ELISA tests using different kits on the same sample (one of which is a Rapid ELISA).

5. What are the various opportunistic infections (OI) and what is the management?

Children with HIV/AIDS show a gradual decline in both humoral and cell mediated immunity placing them at higher risk for infections from bacterial, viral, fungal and protozoal agents. The manifestations may be due to an unusual organism or due to unusual manifestation of a known organism.

Bacterial infections

Recurrent bacterial infections are the commonest opportunistic infections (OI) in HIV infected children. Whenever, a child presents with a longer duration of bacterial infection than expected for that infection or infection at a site unusual for a particular pathogen or takes a longer than normal time for recovery, an underlying immunodeficiency (be it acquired or infected) should be suspected. Treatment of these infections is essentially the same as per standard guidelines for similar infections in HIV naïve patients. However, the duration of treatment may be prolonged as the already weak immune system of the HIV infected child will take time to clear the infection. Prophylaxis with trimethoprim-sulfamethoxazole (TMP-SMX), routine vaccination, pneumococcal and Hib vaccine along with an effective screening of children for opportunistic infections will help to keep the rate of bacterial infection at a low level.

Viral infections

The common viruses that infect children with HIV include herpes simplex, varicella zoster, hepatitis B, C and cytomegalovirus (CMV). The lesser common viruses include John Cunnigham (JC) virus, which is the agent responsible for progressive multifocal leukoencephalopathy (PML) and human herpes virus 8 (responsible for Kaposi's sarcoma). Herpes simplex virus 1 (HSV 1) can cause recurrent gingivostomatitis while HSV 2 can cause perirectal disease. HSV 1 infection can be complicated by local and distant cutaneous spread as well herpes encephalitis. Disseminated and severe chickenpox is common in HIV infected children. Herpes zoster is the latent form of varicella zoster virus. With a dip in immunity, there is a reactivation of the virus dormant in the dorsal sensory root ganglion. In immunocompetent individual, it occurs in adults with a past history of chicken pox. The appearance of herpes zoster in children itself announces the presence of underlying immunodeficiency. It may be limited to one dermatome or may be extensive affecting large areas of skin. Treatment is with oral acyclovir (10 mg/kg/dose 3-4 times a day) for 14-21 days. Varicella vaccine may be protective against both chicken pox and shingles.

With the steady decline in the incidence of PCP due to effective prophylaxis, CMV infection has become one of the most common opportunistic infection in children. CMV infection is an AIDS defining illness. Low CD4 counts (< 50/mm^3) predisposes the child to disseminated CMV infection with a variety of clinical presentations like chorioretinitis, hepatitis, pneumonia, anemia due to bone marrow suppression and rarely colitis and encephalitis. High degree of clinical suspicion, regular fundus examination can pick up the diagnosis which can be confirmed by virus isolation and/or IgG and IgM antibody titers. Ganciclovir (5 mg/kg/dose twice daily IV) administered over 1-2 hours for 14-21 days or valganciclovir in dose of 16 mg/kg/day or foscarnet (60 mg/kg thrice daily IV) for 14-21 days are the drugs of choice.

Molluscum contagiosum

Molluscum contagiosum is a superficial cutaneous viral infection manifested as 2 to 3-mm flesh-colored hemispheric papules. Characteristically, a faint whitish core is at the center of each papule, some of which may be slightly umbilicated. Early in the infection, the lesions are usually mild and localized to the groin or face. Extensive molluscum contagiosum is a cutaneous marker of advanced HIV disease. Treatment consists of light cryotherapy using liquid nitrogen or pricking the lesion with a large-gauge needle and removing the white core (molluscum body) may also be effective. For refractory lesions, curettage without cautery can be done.

Fungal infections

Oral thrush in an infant more than 6 months of age can be one of the first signs of an underlying immunodeficiency. About 20% of children with oral thrush progress to acquire esophageal candidiasis which presents as substernal or abdominal pain, dysphagia, fever and weight loss. Systemic spread with pulmonary and urinary candidiasis is associated with severe immune destruction. Diagnosis of oral thrush can be made by clinical examination and KOH mount examination of scrapings. Esophageal candidiasis can be diagnosed by esophageoscopy with scrapping of white fluffy patches. A barium swallow in older children can also pick up the diagnosis. Oral thrush can be treated by local application of nystatin or clotrimazole. In non-responders or those with esophageal extension, oral/intravenous fluconazole (12 mg/kg/day) can be given. Pulmonary, urinary or systemic disease warrants the use of intravenous amphotericin B.

Other fungal infections

Apart from candidiasis, other fungal infections that can occur in children include cyptococcosis. Cryptococcus causes meningitis in children which can be diagnosed by India ink preparation of CSF or by cryptococcal antigen detection in CSF. Amphotericin B is used to treat it.

Parasitic infestations

Toxoplasmosis: *Toxoplasma gondii*, the causative agent of toxoplasmosis infects children with HIV and causes severe CNS disease characterized by meningitis and/or chorioretinitis. Ring enhancing lesions on CT brain is a diagnostic feature of toxoplasmosis supported by positive anti-toxoplasma IgM antibodies or CSF Toxoplasma IgG > Toxoplasma IgG levels in blood. It is treated by pyrimethamine (1mg/kg/day) and sulfadiazine (100mg/kg/day) for 6 weeks after the resolution of lesions. Prophylaxis with TMP-SMX is effective in prevention.

Other parasitic infections

Cryptospora, microspora, i*sospora* and *giardia* can cause opportunistic infection in HIV infected children living in endemic regions. It presents with severe chronic diarrhea and HIV related enteropathy often leading to malnutrition. Thus in any HIV infected child with chronic diarrhea, screening for these opportunistic organisms should be done. Treatment of *isospora* consists of TMP-SMX and that of *cryptosporidia* is nitazoxanide. Few cases of *microsporidia* are reported to be treated successfully with albendazole.

Scabies: In HIV-infected persons, it is usually presents with the typical pattern of pruritic papules with accentuation in the intertriginous areas, genitalia, and finger webs. Gamma-benzene hexachloride (lindane) applied from the neck down for 8 to 24 hours is usually curative. Other treatment option is 5% permethrin cream. In rare cases, true crusted (Norwegian) scabies may occur in patients with advanced HIV disease. Norwegian scabies is non-pruritic and appears as thick crusts over some areas of the body. These crusts teem with mites and are highly contagious. Treatment is difficult. Permethrin

5% cream repeated at least weekly until cutaneous manifestations clear is recommended. Additionally, ivermectin (200 μg/kg/day) may be added.

Tuberculosis (TB): It is the leading cause of death among HIV infected people and WHO estimates that TB accounts for up to a third of AIDS deaths worldwide. TB is harder to diagnose in HIV positive people, progresses faster and is more fatal. TB occurs earlier in the course of HIV infection than other opportunistic infections. All forms of tuberculosis may be seen in HIV infected children. Children are also more susceptible to atypical mycobacteria *Mycobacterium Avium Complex* (MAC) with incidence of disseminated MAC TB in HAART naïve patients being up to 10%. Treatment is with standard anti-tuberculous therapy (ATT). In patients with HIV-TB coinfection, it is necessary to treat TB completely before starting antiretroviral therapy (ART) ideally because of the risk of IRIS and the potential for additive drug toxicities, drug interactions and excessive pill burden. However, in situations where ART is needed then at least intensification phase of antituberculous therapy (ATT) should be completed before starting ART. In very rare situations, only ART and ATT should be given together. One caution to be exercised is that, rifampicin should not be given along with protease inhibitors (PI) and non-nucleotide reverse transcriptase inhibitors (NNRTI) dose adjustment may be needed as it reduces the level of these anti-retroviral drugs by enzymatic induction.

Pneumocystis jirovecii: PCP infection in HIV infected children is common in the first year of life and is associated with mortality more than 35%. Pneumocystis is an organism with biological characteristics similar to that of fungi and protozoa. It is now renamed as *Pneumocystis jiroveci* (for the human strain). *P. carinii* is now referred to the organism found in rats. In immunocompetent infants, it may lead to mild respiratory symptoms or children are usually asymptomatic. In immunodeficient individuals it infects the alveoli leads to interstitial edema and results in progressive hypoxemia and respiratory failure. It is not clinically or radiologically possible to distinguish PCP from other severe pulmonary interstitial infections in infants, and the diagnosis should be confirmed by bronchoalveolar lavage (BAL). Gomori's methenamine silver stain, toluidine stain or Giemsa stain are used to depict the cysts. Immunoflorescent antibodies stain the cyst wall and is most sensitive. PCP should be treated on suspicion with high-dose cotrimoxazole [15-20 mg/kg/day of the TMP component (75-100 mg/kg of SMX component) IV/PO in 3-4 divided doses for 21 days]. Clindamycin or dapsone (2 mg/kg/day) can be used in case of intolerance to cotrimoxazole. On laboratory confirmation, steroids can be added, as this has been shown to reduce inflammation and hasten recovery in adults. Prophylaxis with cotrimoxazole if known to decrease mortality due to PCP as well as other bacterial infections.

HIV Infection   313

6. How to select antiretroviral therapy (ART) in children?

Decisions about when to start therapy, what drugs to choose in antiretroviral-naïve children, and how to treat antiretroviral experienced children remain complex, and should be made in consultation with a specialist in pediatric and adolescent HIV infection. Treatment with ART depends on clinical condition, immune status of the child and HIV viral load. Before antiretroviral therapy is started, it is essential that parents, care-givers and patients are counseled regarding the importance of adherence to the prescribed treatment regimen. Triple combination therapy is recommended for treating all HIV infected children. Combination therapy slows disease progression, improves survival, results in greater and more sustained virologic and immunologic response and delays development of virus mutations which may lead to resistance. The choice of drugs depends on available formulations suitable for the individual child, taking into consideration age, developmental level and carer circumstances.

The current preferred first-line ART regimen for previously untreated children with no evidence of ARV resistance comprises two nucleoside reverse transcriptase inhibitors (NRTIs) with either a non-nucleoside reverse transcriptase inhibitor (NNRTI) or a ritonavir (RTV)-boosted protease inhibitor (PI). Lamivudine (3TC) and abacavir (ABC) are the NRTI backbone of choice for most children, based on long-term follow-up. Stavudine is no longer recommended. The preferred NNRTI is nevirapine (NVP) for children aged less than 3 years, and efavirenz (EFV) for older children. The preferred PI is ritonavir-boosted lopinavir for young children. Alternative boosted PIs may be considered for older children, including fosamprenavir/r and darunavir/r, atazanavir/r which are licensed from age 6 years, and saquinavir/r, which is not licensed in children, but may be suitable for adolescents.

7. What should be the ART in children with tuberculosis?

Concomitant rifampicin substantially decreases concentration of both Nevirapine (NVP) and PI due to induction of P450 enzyme. Plasma levels of NNRTIs are decreased by 25–35% and plasma levels of PIs are decreased by more than 80%. Thus, PIs should be avoided when a child is on rifampicin and rifabutin should be used as it does not induce the P450 enzymes and thus does not alter the levels of PIs. Dose of NVP should be increased by 20–30% when used concomitant with rifampicin to maintain the drug levels in the therapeutic range. However, a watch should be kept for hepatic toxicity.

Any child with active TB disease should begin TB treatment immediately, and start ART as soon as tolerated in the first 8 weeks of TB therapy, irrespective of CD4 count and clinical stage. The preferred first-line ARV regimen for infants and children less than 3 years of age, who are taking a rifampicin-containing regimen for TB, is 2 NRTIs + NVP. The preferred first-line ARV regimen for children more than 3 years of age, who are taking a rifampicin-containing regimen for TB, is 2 NRTIs + EFV. The preferred first-line ARV regimen for infants and children less than 2 years of age, who have been exposed to NVP and are taking a rifampicin-containing regimen for TB, is a triple NRTI regimen.

8. What are the situations when ART needs to be changed?

ART regimen may be changed in the following circumstances:
- Failure of current regimen
- Toxicity or intolerance to current regimen.

Poor adherence, inadequate drug levels, prior existing drug resistance or inadequate potency of the drugs chosen can all contribute to ARV treatment failure. Treatment failure is considered as either clinical failure, immunological failure or virological failure. Clinical failure is defined as recurrent, persistent or new HIV related illness after at least 3 months on ART. Also lack or decline of growth rate, development of encephalopathy or neuroregression is taken as clinical failure. Immunological failure is considered when there is persistently declining CD4 cell count measured on at least 2 separate occasions or failure to increase age related CD4 threshold despite an adequate trial of ART or developing or returning to the following age-related immunological thresholds after at least 24 weeks on ART, in a treatment-adherent child: CD4 count of ≤ 200 cells/mm^3 or %CD4+ ≤10% for a child more than 2 years to less than 5 years of age and CD4 count of ≤100 cells/mm^3 for a child 5 years of age or more. Virologic failure is defined when there is inability of viral load to below undetectable levels within 6 months of initiating therapy or when there is repeated detection of virus in plasma after initial suppression to undetectable levels.

9. How to prevent parent-to-child transmission of HIV? Should breastfeeding be continued in a baby born to HIV positive mother?

HIV transmission from infected mother to child is mainly prevented by antiretroviral drug (ARV) prophylaxis to mother and baby, replacement feeding and elective cesarean section (ECS). ARV prophylaxis acts by reducing viral load in the mother and as postexposure prophylaxis to the fetus and baby. Cesarean section before onset of labor or rupture of membranes has been used as an intervention for PPTCT to decrease risk of intrapartum transmission of HIV.

HIV has been detected in breast milk in cell-free and cell-associated compartments and there is now evidence that both compartments are involved in transmission of HIV through breast milk. Even if intrauterine and intrapartum transmission are significantly reduced, postnatal transmission through breastfeeding still is an additional risk for transmission of HIV. (Risk varies from 10–15%). This risk increases with high viral load in the breast-milk, maternal nipple lesions, mastitis and breastfeeding for longer than 15 months. Replacement feeding clearly abolishes the risk of breast milk transmission. However, replacement feeding increases the risk of diarrheal diseases and malnutrition. Exclusive breastfeeding for up to six months, however, is associated with a three to four fold decreased risk of transmission of HIV compared to non-exclusive breastfeeding. Mixed feeding, therefore, appears to be a clear risk factor for postnatal transmission.

The year 2009 was the turning point for the prevention of postnatal transmission of HIV where 3 randomized controlled trials found that antiretroviral prophylaxis in pregnant women and their infants coupled with breastfeeding could lead to a significant decrease in the vertical transmission of HIV. It has been clearly shown that when antiretrovirals are taken through the pregnancy and breastfeeding stage, there is a greatly reduced HIV infection rate of 2 percent. But there must be 100 percent adherence to taking the drugs correctly, otherwise there is a risk that the baby will become infected with HIV or resistant to the medication. There needs to be good support for mothers to help them adhere to an extended drug regimen as well as keeping to 6 months of exclusive breastfeeding. This approach offers new hope for mothers with HIV infection who cannot safely feed their babies with replacement. It will improve the chances of infants remaining healthy and free of HIV infection as breast milk provides optimal nutrition and protects against other fatal childhood diseases such as pneumonia and diarrhea.

World Health Organization rapid advise for use of antiretroviral drugs for treating pregnant women and preventing HIV infection in infants, 2010-2012:

Antiretroviral therapy in pregnant woman for her own health: In pregnant women with confirmed HIV serostatus, initiation of antiretroviral therapy for her own health is recommended for all HIV-infected pregnant women with CD4 cell count ≤ 350 cells/mm^3, irrespective of WHO clinical staging; and for all HIV-infected pregnant women in WHO clinical stage 3 or 4, irrespective of CD4 cell count irrespective of gestational age and continue throughout pregnancy, delivery and thereafter, infant born to these women should receive daily nevirapine (NVP) or zidovudine (AZT) from birth until 4 to 6 weeks of age.

Antiretroviral prophylaxis for all HIV-infected pregnant women who do not need treatment for their own health: ARV prophylaxis should be started from as early as 14 weeks gestation (second trimester) or as soon as possible when women present later in pregnancy or in labor or delivery. WHO has recommended 3 ARV prophylaxis options in the woman as shown in Table 3:

Table 3: ARV prophylaxis options

Option A	Option B	Option B+

For pregnant women
• Antepartum daily AZT
• Single dose NVP at onset of labor
• AZT + 3TC during labor and delivery
• Twice daily AZT + 3TC for 7 days postpartum (to reduce risk of NVP resistance in the mother)
	For pregnant women
	• Triple ARV drugs starting from as early as 14 weeks of gestation until one week after all exposure to breast milk has ended
	• Recommended regimens include:
	  − AZT + 3TC + LPV/r
	  − AZT + 3TC + ABC
	  − AZT + 3TC + EFV
	  − TDF + 3TC (or FTC) + EFV
		For pregnant women
		• Triple ARV drugs starting from as early as 14 weeks of gestation and **continued for life**

Contd...

Contd...

For infants	For infants	Same as option B
• If breastfeeding: Single dose NVP at birth and then daily administration of NVP to the infant from birth until one week after all exposure to breast milk has ended • If non-breastfeeding: Single dose NVP at birth and then daily administration of NVP or AZT from birth until 4 to 6 weeks of age	Daily administration of AZT or NVP from birth until 4 to 6 weeks of age	
Type of delivery Vaginal	**Type of delivery** Vaginal	**Type of delivery** Vaginal

AZT = Zidovudine, 3TC = Lamivudine, LPVr = Lopinavir/ritonavir, ABC = Abacavir, EFV = Efavirenz, TDF = Tenofovir.

Note: Single dose NVP and AZT+3TC intra-and postpartum can be omitted if the mother receives more than 4 weeks of AZT during pregnancy

WHO will release new, consolidated ARV-related guidelines in mid-2013. A rigorous and inclusive process is underway, incorporating systematic review of evidence; weighing values and preferences of providers and affected communities; and assessing ethics, safety, cost, and feasibility, including for Option B+.

Further Reading

1. Lyall H. Diagnosis, staging and clinical presentation of HIV in children. Clinical and laboratory diagnosis. Available from Tr@inforPedHIV. 2011 .
2. Review of opportunistic infections and treatment in children. MMWR. 2004; 53(RR14):1-63.
3. Scarlatti G. Pediatric HIV infection. Lancet. 1996;348:863-8.
4. Shah I, Dhabe H, Lala M, Katira B. Assessment of adherence to antiretroviral therapy in HIV infected children—A preliminary indian study. Pedicon. 2007, Mumbai, January 2007.
5. Shah I, Dhabe H, Lala M. Prevention of maternal to child transmission of HIV: A profile in indian children". 42nd National Conference of IAP (PEDICON - 2005), Kolkata, January 2005; JF/08(P).
6. Shah I, Katira B. Tuberculosis coinfection in HAART Naïve HIV infected children. Indian J Pediatr. 2009;76:966-7
7. Shah I. Adverse effects of antiretroviral therapy in HIV-1 infected children. J Trop Pediatr. 2006;52(4):244-8.
8. Shah I. Age related clinical manifestations of HIV infection in indian children. J Trop Pediatr. 2005;51(5):300-3.
9. Shah I. Efficacy of HIV PCR techniques to diagnose HIV in infants born to HIV infected mothers—An Indian perspective. JAPI. 2006;54:197-9.
10. Shah I. HIV and Pregnancy—Is vaginal delivery a safe and viable option? Indian Pediatrics. 2008;45:603-4.

11. Shah I. Is elective caesarian section really essential for prevention of mother-to-child transmission of HIV in the era of antiretroviral therapy and abstinence of breast feeding? J Trop Pediatr. 2006;52:163-5.
12. Shah I. Diagnosis of perinatal transmission of HIV-1 infection by HIV DNA PCR. JK Science. 2004;6:187-9.
13. World Health Organization (WHO). Rapid advice: Use of antiretroviral drugs for treating pregnant women and preventing HIV infection in infants. 2010. WHO.

Index

Page numbers followed by '*f*' and '*t*' indicate figures and tables respectively.

A

Abdominal pain 66
Absence of meningococcal disease 36
Active
   and passive immunization 147
   chorioretinitis 279
   meningococcal infection 36
Acute
   bacillary dysentery 220
   bacterial
      rhinosinusitis 200
      tonsillitis 303
   bilateral cervical lymphadenopathy 303
   cervical lymphadenopathy 302
   diarrheal diseases 45*t*
   encephalitis syndrome 190
   gastroenteritis
      etiology of 218
      indications of antibiotics 224
      laboratory investigations 222
      organisms 218
      parasites of 219
      stool test 223
      viruses of 219
   hepatitis 149, 152
   liver failure 149
   lymphangitis
      differential diagnosis 250
      scrofuloderma 251
      tuberculosis verrucosa cutis 251
   mastoiditis 204
   pancreatitis 62
   pharyngitis 13
   poststreptococcal glomerulonephritis 16
   rheumatic fever 13, 15, 18
   rhinosinusitis 200
   suppurative otitis media 202
   viral
      hepatitis 143
      pharyngitis 303
   watery diarrhea 45
Aerosol transmission 134
Afebrile 244
Agammaglobulinemia 220
Air-borne
   infections 51
   respiratory droplets 23
   spread 3
Allergic rhinitis 200
Amebiasis 178
Amebic dysentery 178
Amebic liver abscess 178, 179
Aminoglycoside 243, 293
Aminosidine 168
Amphotericin B 167
Anemia and thrombocytopenia 69
Anerobic coverage 243
Angular cheilitis 308
Anhidrotic ectodermal dysplasia 285
Anicteric form 72
Animal bites and rabies 134
Annual vaccination 114
Antibiotic regimens 18
Antibody detection 192
Antifungal therapy 295
Antigenic
   detection 192
   drift 111
   shift 112
Antimicrobial
   prophylaxis 230
   therapy 26, 37, 216
Antirabies vaccines, administration of 139
Antiretroviral
   naïve children 313
   prophylaxis 315
   therapy 313
Antistaphylococcal vaccine 10
Antiviral
   activity 115
   resistance 116
   therapy 279
Aortic valve stenosis 269
Aphthous stomatitis 95, 96
ART regimen 314
Artemisinin combination therapy 174
Arterial blood gas 292

Arthritis 62
Artificial heart valves 212
Assessment of dehydration status 45t
Associated hemophagocytic syndrome 107
Asymptomatic
    infection to dengue shock syndrome 121
    respiratory tract carriage 23
Atypical features 165
Auramine O 256
Aztreonam 243

B

Bacteremia 291
Bacterial
    infections
        brucella 302
        cat scratch disease 302
        rickettsia 302
        Salmonella typhi 302
        scarlet fever 302
        tubeculosis 302
    meningitis 185, 186
Bacteriological test in pediatric TB
    conventional
        culture techniques 257
        methods 256
    newer rapid growth techniques 258
    newer techniques 257
    polymerase chain reaction 258
Bacterium *Bordetella pertussis* 28
Bandemia 243
BCG test 258
Benign EBV-associated proliferations 107
Beta-lactam antimicrobial agents 57
Bite and scratch from infected animals 134
Blastomycosis 164
Blocks absorption of sodium 43
Blood and cerebrospinal fluid 194
Blood pressure 176
Bloody stools 178
Blueberry muffin 272
Body louse infestation 254
Bone
    and joint infections
        differential diagnoses of 246
        etiology of 246t
        infarction 246
    marrow
        cultures 54
        examination 165
        recipients 7
Bronchiolitis 118
Bronchoalveolar lavage 211, 312
Brucella 51
Bullous impetigo 249
Burkitt's lymphoma 107

C

C. diphtheriae spread 23
Candida 162
Candidiasis, clinical types of 157
Canine rabies endemic 141
Cardiac
    defects 269
    disease 13, 62
Cardiogenic shock 235
Cardiopulmonary abnormalities 118
Cardiovascular
    manifestations 52
    system 5, 60, 91
Castleman's disease 302
Cat scratch disease 303
Causative organisms of bacterial meningitis 185
Cefazolin and cefuroxime 9
Ceftriaxone 293
Cell culture
    rabies vaccine 135
    vaccines 140
Cellulitis and endophthalmitis 36
Central nervous system 5, 52, 60, 61, 91, 96, 187, 270
Cerebral malaria 176, 177
Cerebrospinal fluid
    culture 186
    findings in CNS infections 187t
    PCR 186
    study 185
Cervical lymphadenopathy 80, 90, 96
Chance detection of amebic or giardia cysts 181
Characteristic features of
    bronchiolitis 119
    influenza infection 112
    risckettsial diseases 68
Chediak-Higashi disease 288, 302

Chemoprophylaxis 37, 41, 48
Chikungunya, clinical presentation of 154
Children with
  Dengue, classifications of 121
  tuberculosis 313
Chlamydia pneumoniae 64
Cholera
  pandemics 43
  toxin 43
  treatment 46
Chorioretinitis correlates 274
Chronic
  cervical lymphadenopathy 303
  cryptosporidiosis 308
  granulomatous disease 285, 286, 302
  HBeAg
    negative hepatitis 150
    positive hepatitis 150
  HCV infection 152
  herpes simplex infection 308
  immune tolerant phase 149
  inactive HBsAg carrier 149
  pharyngeal carriers 12
  progressive panencephalitis 270
  pulmonary disease 13
  suppurative otitis media 202, 204
Ciliary dyskinesia 211
Cingulum 103
Ciprofloxacin plus coamoxyclav 299
Clarithromycin 70
Closed tube thoracostomy drainage 9
Cloxacillin 9
CMV
  antigen 274
  infection 272
  PCR 274
Coagulase-negative staphylococcal infection 6
Coagulation
  profile 292
  screen 298
Coccidioidomycosis 163
Cold agglutinin test 62
Common
  causative organisms 200
  fungal species 157
  fungi 157
  modes of transmission 134
  opportunistic fungal infections 160

organism of croup syndrome 205
organisms 199
sequelae of complications of JE 195
symptom of giardia infection 180
Community acquired pneumonia
  clinical features 207
  etiological agents 206
  laboratory diagnosis 208
  signs 207
  symptoms 207
Compartmentalized metastatic infections 36
Compensated cirrhosis 150
Complement
  defects 286
  fixation test 123
Complete blood cell count 125, 186, 286
Complication of
  ASOM 203
  bacterial meningitis 188
  diphtheria 26
  pertussis 30
  rickettsial infection 68
Confirmation of cholera 45
Confirmatory laboratory tests 165
Confirmed case of chikungunya fever 155
Congenital
  and neonatal manifestations 52
  CMV infection 271
  cutaneous candidiasis 158
  cytomegalovirus infection 268
  heart disease 212
  infections screening tests 268
  malformation of lung 211
  rubella, syndrome 92t, 269, 279
  syphilis 277
  toxoplasmosis 274, 276
  varicella 268
Conjugate vaccines 38
Contact with
  asymptomatic carriers 3
  contaminated objects 3
  infected persons 3
  PETs 4
Contaminated secretions 118
Control of
  convulsion 195
  temperature 195
Conventional culture techniques 257

Core body temperature 66
Corporis managed 254
Correction of hypovolemia 177
Corticosteroid therapy 57
Corynebacterium diphtheriae 23
Cotrimoxazole prophylaxis 307
Course of rabies vaccination 141
Coxsackie B 268
Coxsackie B enterovirus 96
C-reaction protein 77
Criteria for
    probable dengue 122
    severe dengue 122
Cryptococcus 163
Cryptorchidism 270
CSF examination 197
Cut off values for fast breathing 207
Cutaneous diphtheria 24
Cystic fibrosis 211
Cytomegalovirus (CMV) infection 308
Cytotoxic drugs 297

D

Daptomycin and tigecycline 8
Dark field microscopy 73, 75
Darkening of skin 165
Daytime cough 200
Decompensated cirrhosis 150
Demerits of rabies vaccines 139
Dengue
    serology 124
    shock syndrome 122, 125
    specific tests 123
    with warning signs 122
Detection of
    antiamebic antibodies 179
    dengue ribonucleic acid 123
    DNA 75
Development of
    brucella resistance 56
    vaccines 48
Diagnosis of
    acute bacterial sinusitis 200
    amebiasis 178
    bacterial meningitis 185
    brucellosis 53
    C. pneumoniae 65
    chikungunya fever 155
    cholera 44
    dengue infection 123

diphtheria 25
kala-azar 169
measles 79*t*
pertussis 29
rheumatic fever 19
rickettsial infection 69
Diaper dermatitis 158
Different rabies vaccines 139
Dimercaptosuccinic acid 229
Diphtheria disease 27
Direct fluorescent antigen testing 30
Directly observed treatment short-
    course (DOTS) strategy 260
Disseminated
    candidiasis 159
    infection 160
    intravascular coagulation 100, 235
Dose of
    acyclovir 198
    invasive fungal infections 162*t*
    rabies immunoglobulin 137
Down syndrome 285
Doxycycline and chloramphenicol 70
Drinking milk of rabid animal 139
Drug reaction 302
Drugs recommended for secondary
    prophylaxis 20*t*
Duke criteria
    diagnosis 215
    evidence of 214
    major 214
    minor 214
    pathological criterion 214
Duncan's syndrome 107
Dysentery in children cause of 178

E

Early trials of ribavirin 120
EBV infection 107
Effectiveness of therapy of kala-azar 169
Elective cesarean section 314
Embryogenesis 267
Empiric
    antibiotic therapy 187, 243, 294
    therapy for invasive fungal infections
        162
Empyema in young children 9, 211
Encephalitis 190
Encephalitis case classification 190
Endemic typhus and scrub typhus 66

Endocarditis
 diagnose of 213
 empirical antibiotic 215
 infective 213
 investigations 214
 neonatal 213
Entamoeba histolytica 178
Enteric
 fever 233
 infection 158
Enteroviral infections 268, 287
Enteroviruses 94, 96
Enzyme-linked
 immunospot 258
 immunosorbent assay 55, 63, 70, 192, 258
Epidemic typhus 66
Epidemiology of
 chikungunya 154
 cholera 43
 dengue 121
 diphtheria 23
 histoplasmosis 159
 JE 190
Epithelial cell malignancies 107
Epithelial cells 43
Epstein-Barr virus 107
Equine rabies immunoglobulin 137
Eradication of polio 94
Erysipelas 13
Erythematous
 base 249
 papular lesions 53
 papulovesicular lesions 95
Erythrocyte sedimentation rate 77, 292
Ewing's sarcoma 246
Examination of stool 178
Exposure to immunized pet animals 138
Extrahepatic manifestations 147
Extraintestinal amebiasis 178
Extrapulmonary
 manifestations 61
 tuberculosis 304, 308

F

Faine's criteria 73
Fanconi anemia 285
Fatal disease 78
Fatal RSV infection 119

Features of
 secondary infections 165
 the different hepatitis viruses 143
Febrile
 illnesses 69
 neutropenia 297, 298
Fetal infection 90
Fluconazole 253
Fluid
 and electrolytes and calories/
  nutrition 195
 management of a child 46
 therapy in various stages of dengue 126
Fluorescent polarization immunoassay 55
Fluoroquinolone 300
Focal necrotizing retinitis 276
Folinic acid 275
Follicular, inflammatory nodule 249
Food poisoning 6
Food-borne infections 51
Foreign body 211
Fracture and trauma 246
Fungal
 and protozoal infections 157
 endocarditis 216
 infections
  coccidiomycosis 302
  histoplasmosis 302
  neonatal intensive care unit 157
 skin infections 252

G

Gamma benzene hexachloride 254
Gangrene of the digits 68
GAS pharyngitis 13
Gastrointestinal
 manifestations 52
 symptoms 66
Gaucher's disease 246
Genitourinary
 complications 53
 manifestations 52
Genome detection 192
Genus rickettsia 66
Gestation 270
Giardia lamblia 219
Giardiasis, clinical manifestations of 180

Glomerulonephritis 13, 53, 62
Glycoprotein of dengue virus 124
Gram positive bacterium 23
Gram stain 186
Gram-positive coccoid-shaped bacteria 12
Granulomatosis infantiseptica 278
Group A streptococcal
   pharyngitis 17, 18
   infection 12
Guillain-Barré's syndrome 235

H

Haemophilus influenzae 78
Hallmarks of infectious mononucleosis 108
Hand hygiene 9
Haversian systems 245
HBV infection 147
Health care-related transmission 118
Hemagglutination inhibition (HI) test 123
Hemagglutination inhibition test 192
Hemagglutinin 111
Hematological
   neoplasias 107
   system 60
Hematopoietic stem cell transplantation 300
Hemolytic uremic syndrome 69, 225, 235
Hemophagocytic lymphohistiocytosis 302
Hepatitis A 143
Hepatitis A and B, enterovirus 302
Hepatitis B 143, 280
Hepatitis B immunoglobulin 147
Hepatitis C 143
Hepatitis D 144
Hepatitis E 143
Hepatobiliary manifestations 52
Hepatocellular carcinoma 143
Hepatology and nutrition 152
Hepatomegaly 165
Hepatosplenomegaly 270, 272
Herd immunity 84
Herpes simplex
   encephalitis 190, 196
   virus infection 307
Heterophile antibody tests 108
Histoplasma capsulatum 159
Histoplasmosis 163
HIV in children
   category A: mildly symptomatic 306
   category B: moderately symptomatic 306
   category C: severely symptomatic 306
   category N: not symptomatic 306
   diagnosis of 309
   infection 13, 166, 305
   transmitted in children 305
Hodgkin's disease 107
Home available fluids 46
Homeland of cholera 43
Household contacts 26
Human
   brucellosis 51
   diploid cell vaccine 140
   influenza A subtypes 111
   mucous membranes 23
   rabies immunoglobulin 137
Hydration and temperature 176
Hydrocephalus 267
Hydrops fetalis 267
Hyper IgE syndrome 288
Hyperbilirubinemia 272
Hyperparasitemia 177
Hypogammaglobulinemia 270
Hypoglycemia 177

I

Icteric form 73
Idiopathic thrombocytopenic purpura 69
Immune status 98
Immunity against pertussis 32
Immunochromatographic test 171
Immunocompetent pregnant 275
Immunofloroscence assay 70
Immunoglobulin 155
Impetigo 13
Implementation of infection control policy 10
Inactivated purified vaccine 195
Inactivated seasonal influenza vaccines 114
Incubation period 66
Indian Pediatric Nephrology group 229
Indications for hepatitis B immunoglobulin 147
Indications of steroids 109

Indwelling medical devices 7
Infectious
    dermatitis 204
    disease 102
    mononucleosis 107–109
Infective endocarditis
    clinical features 212
    nocardiac features 213
Influenza
    and parainfluenza
        type C 111
    viral infections 199
    virus circulation 113
    viruses 111
Initial antimicrobial therapy 201
Integumentary systems 52
Interferon gamma assay 258
Interferon gamma radioimmunoassay (IGRA) 258
Interpretation of HBV serology 144–146
Interpretation of serological markers in HAV and HEV infection 144
Interstitial
    pneumonitis 270
    epithelial cells 43
Intestinal
    lumen 43
    motility reducers 226
Intra-abdominal
    infections, different types of 243
    pathology 242
    sepsis 293
Intracellular
    parasites 298
    calcifications 267, 268, 274
    complications 204
Intracranial pressure 195
Intradermal (ID) regimen 140
Intramuscular (IM) regimen 140
Intratemporal complications 204
Intrauterine
    growth restriction 270
    infection 98
Intravenous
    therapy 47
    drug
        abusers 212
        use 13
    fluid therapy 133
    immunoglobulin 280, 295

Invasive
    aspergillosis 163
    fungal disease 157
    fungal infections 162
    GAS infections 12
    infections 4
    meningococcal disease 34
Isolation of rickettsia 70

J

Janeway lesions 213
Japanese B encephalitis 190
Jaundice 272

K

Kala-azar, clinical features of 166
Kaposi sarcoma 307, 308
Kawasaki disease 78, 302
Ketoconazole 253
Kikuchi Fujimoto disease 302
Klebsiella pneumoniae 291

L

Lactic acidosis 176
Laryngotracheobronchitis 24, 205
Larynx 24
Late onset pericarditis 36
Latent tubercular infection 258
Leptospira 72, 75
Leptospirosis 155
Leukemia 246
Leukocyte adhesion defect 288
Level of consciousness 176
Levofloxacin 299
Limitations of MAT 74
Listerial bacteremia diagnosis of 278
Live attenuated seasonal influenza vaccines 114
Liver
    and brain abscess 285
    and renal functions 292
    diseases or malignancy 220
    function tests 125
Lowenstein Jensen 257
Lower respiratory tract diseases, cause of 60
Lumbar puncture 185
Lung abscess 9

Lymph nodes 301
Lymphadenitis, different types of 301
Lymphadenopathy 52, 69, 301
Lymphocytic choriomeningitis virus 268
Lymphoid
　interstitial pneumonitis 107
　tissues 301
Lymphoproliferative disorders 107

M

M. pneumoniae infection 60
Macular lesions 276
Malabsorption syndrome 180
Malaria 171
　clinical and laboratory criteria for severe malaria 173*t*
　complicated malaria 175
　diagnosis of severe malaria 173
　epidemiology of malaria in India 171
　falciparum 155
　laboratory confirmation of malaria 172
　management of complications of malaria 176
Malignancy (lymphomas) 302
Malignant EBV-associated proliferations 107
Management of
　acute otitis media 202
　airways and breathing 195
　ASOM in different age groups 202
　circulation 195
　common cold 199
　congenital toxoplasmosis 276
　dengue infection 122
　hypotensive shock 132
　otitis media with effusion 205
　shock in dengue infection 127
　skin 8
Mantoux test 259
MASCC scoring index 299*t*
Mass chemoprophylaxis 48
Maternal antibody 12
Measles
　and enteroviral exanthemas 69
　immunoglobulin M 83
　vaccine 82, 83, 84
Mediterranean spotted fever 70
Meningism 66
Meningitis in geneva 33

Meningoccal disease 37
Meningococcal
　A epidemics 34
　belt 34
　disease 33, 36, 37
　infection 33, 34, 36, 37
　meningitis 33, 36
　pneumonia 36
　polysaccharide vaccines 38
　vaccination 37, 41
Meningococcemia 35, 69
Meningoencephalitis 68
Merits of rabies vaccines 139
Meropenem 243
Metabolic tests 125
Miconazole 253
Microbiological tests 208
Microcephaly 267
Microcornea 276
Microimmunofluorescence 65
Microscopic agglutination test (MAT) 74, 75
Micturating urethrogram 229
Middle ear effusion 205
Midstream clean catch 227
Miltefosine 168
Mixed infections 175
Mode of transmission 143
Molecular detection 55
Molluscum contagiosum
　clinical manifestations 251
　management of 251
Monitoring in a child with dengue 127
Monovalent serogroup c conjugate vaccines 39
Mucocutaneous complications 53
Mucocutaneous HSV infection 100
Multinational association for supportive care in cancer 299
Multiorgan dysfunction syndrome 290
Multiple
　nodular infiltration of the 165
　organ dysfunction syndrome 290
Mumps 85, 87, 88
Musculoskeletal infection 5
Myalgias and restlessness 66
Mycobacterium tuberculosis 258
Mycoplasma
　and giardia 287

infections 60, 63
pneumoniae infections 61
Myocarditis 213, 267

N

Nalidixic acid resistance *S. typhi* 238
Nasal
   diphtheria 24
   discharge 200
Nasogastric tube 176
Nasopharyngeal carcinoma 107
National Anti-malaria Program 175
National Center for Disease Control 34, 34*t*
National Institute of Communicable Diseases 33
National Vector Borne Disease Control Program 171
Necrotizing fasciitis 12
Neonatal
   hepatitis C infection 151
   herpes 98, 99, 268
   listeriosis clinical manifestation 278
   septicemia 6
   symptomatic disease 276
Neonates and young infants 290
Neuraminidase (NA) inhibitors 115
Neurological manifestations 52
Neutralization tests 123
Neutropenia
   mild 297
   moderate 297
   profound 297
   severe 297
Newer
   diagnostic tools 166
   techniques 257
Non-anaphylactic β-lactam allergy 201
Non-cardiogenic pulmonary edema 68
non-Hodgkin lymphoma 308
Non-malignant proliferations 107
Nonoccupational exposure 148
Non-polio enteroviruses 94, 96
Non-steroidal anti-inflammatory agents 130
Nontuberculous mycobacteria 303
Norwalk virus 210
Nosocomial fungal infection in intensive care unit 157

Nosocomial infection 291
NS1 antigen 124
Nucleoside reverse transcriptase inhibitors 313
Nystagmus 276

O

Obstructive uropathy 229
Occupational exposure 147
Oophoritis 86
Oral
   acyclovir 100, 101, 104
   hairy leukoplakia 107, 308
   rehydration salts solution 46
   therapy 104
   thrush 158
Orchiepididymitis 53
Organ transplantation 134
Organisms
   causing bronchiolitis 119
   responsible for common cold 199
Orolabial herpes 99
Oropharyngeal inflammation 27
Orthomyxoviridae family 111
Osteoarticular
   complications 52
   manifestations 52
Osteomyelitis and septic arthritis 245
Otitis media with effusion 202
Outbreak of
   disease 33
   response vaccine 196
Oxygen therapy 176

P

Palpable purpura 69
Pandemic influenza 112, 113
Papular pruritic eruptions 308
Para-colic gutter 243
Parapneumonic effusion 9
Parasite lactate dehydrogenase 171
Parasitemia 291
Parasitic
   infections
      filaviasis 302
      skin 253
      toxoplasmosis 302
Parenteral
   antibiotic therapy 244
   antibiotics 244

Parent-to-child transmission of HIV
prevent 314
Paronychia and onychomycosis 158
Parotid
glands 85, 86
swelling 85, 86
Parvovirus B19 155, 280, 302
Pathogenesis of cholera 43
Pathogens specific antimicrobial therapy 187
Patient wise box 260
Paucibacillary 257
Pediatric
autoimmune neuropsychiatric disorders 16
gastroenterology 152
hepatitis C infection 151
intensive care unit 157
oncology patients 7
Pediculosis
capitis (head louse infestation) 254
corporis 254
Pelvic inflammatory disease 36
Penicillin allergy 18
Pentavalent antimony drugs 167
Perianal dermatitis 13
Pericardial cavity 213
Perinatal
infections 267
transient viremia 152
Period of contagiousness 112
Periodic fever (PFAPA) 303
Perioral vesicular lesion 98
Periurethral inflammatory disorders 228
Persistent symptoms of viral URI 200
Person-to-person infection 51
Pertussis in
adolescents 28
burden 28
children 28
Petechiae 272
Petechial rash 67*f*
Peyer's patches 234
Phagocytic defects 286
Pharyngeal
diphtheria 303
infection 12
serotypes 13
strains 13
Phenylbutazone thiouracil 85
Pityriasis versicolor treatment 253

Plaque reduction neutralization test 194
Plasmodium
falciparum 171
vivax 171
Pleomorphic rash 102
Pleural effusions 9, 53
Pneumocystis
carinii pneumonia 307
jirovecii 312
Pneumocystis pneumonia 308
Pneumonia 118, 160
Polymerase chain reaction 30, 55, 63, 70, 77, 155, 186, 258
Polymerase chain reaction 45
Polymicrobial coverage 243
Polymorphonuclear leukocytosis 243
Polypeptide exotoxin 23
Polysaccharide vaccines 38
Post kala-azar dermal leishmaniasis 165
Postnatal rubella 89
Postpartum period 98
Poststreptococcal reactive arthritis 16
Prednisone 279
Predominance of polymorphonuclear leukocytes 186
Predominant T-cell deficiency 286
Predominantly antibody deficiencies 285
Predominat B-cell 286
Pre-exposure prophylaxis in children 141
Prevent mother to child transmission 147
Prevention of
cholera 48
RSV infections 120
seizures 177
transmission 37
Primary
immunodeficiency 285, 302
meningococcal conjunctivitis 36
Staphylococcal pneumonia 5
Probiotics 225
Procalcitonin 293
Prothrombin time 125
Psychomotor retardation 270
Pulmonary
complications 53
disease 119
infection 159
manifestations 52, 61

microvascular leakage 68
valvular stenosis 269
Purified
   chick embryo cell vaccine 140
   duck embryo vaccine 139, 140
   vero cell rabies vaccine 140
Purulent parotitis 85
Pyelonephritis, nephrotic syndrome 235
Pyrimethamine 275

Q

Quadrivalent conjugate vaccine 40
Quadrivalent meningococcal conjugate vaccines 39
Quantification of immunoglobulin levels 286

R

Rabies immunoglobulin 135, 137, 138
Rapid
   detection of mycobacterium isolates 257
   diagnostic tests 171
   point-of-care assays 55
   tests 55
Rare modes of transmission 134
Rash on soles 67*f*
Reactive treponemal test 277
Recognition of
   dengue hemorrhagic fever 125
   pertussis 29
Recommended drugs for chemoprophylaxis 42*t*
Recurrent episodes of skin 8
Reflex neurovascular dystrophy 246
Rehabilitation 195
Renal and liver function test 298
Renal and musculoskeletal system 60
Respiratory
   distress 119
   epithelial cells 9
   support 176
   syncytial virus 118, 300
   system 5
   tract obstruction 26
Reticuloendothelial
   cells 298
   system 239
Reverse transcription polymerase chain reaction 155

Rhabdomyolysis 62
Rheumatic fever 246
Rheumatic heart disease 15, 212
Rheumatological disorders 302
Rhinosinusitis 200
Ribonucleic acid 155
Rickettsia
   disease 67, 70
   infection 66, 69
   species 66
   vasculitis and thrombosis 68
Rifampin 8
Ritonavir 313
RNA viruses 94
Role of
   antiviral drugs 114
   corticosteroid in bacterial meningitis 188
   dorfman disease 302
   RDTs in the diagnosis of malaria 172
   tourniquet test 123
   vitamin A 82
Rotavirus 219, 221
Roth's spots 213
RSV
   bronchiolitis 120
   infections 118
Rubella 155
Rubella
   measles, adenovirus 302
   syndrome 79, 89-93
   vaccine 83, 87, 92

S

Salmonella typhi 238
Sarcoidosis 302
Scabies in children 253
Scarlet fever 13
Schedule of pre-exposure vaccination 141
Scintigraphy 229
Secondary syphilis 69
SEM disease 99
Sensorineural
   deafness 91
   hearing loss 268, 272, 273
Sensory motor neuropathy 289
Sepsis in immunocompetent child 290
Septicemia 246
Seroconversion 270, 272

Serodiagnosis 54, 258
Serogroup B vaccines 40
Serological
    diagnosis 155
    evidence of rickettsial infection 69
    markers of various hepatitis viruses 144
    tests 30, 236
Serum
    agglutination test 54
    lactate 292
    procalcitonin 186
Severe
    anemia 176
    β-lactam allergy 201
    combined immunodeficiencies 285
    illness with high fever 200
    in utero infection 278
    infantile RSV infection 120
    invasive disease 13
    invasive GAS infection 14
    vaso-occlusive disease 68
Shenton line 247
Shigella 222
Shingles 103
Shock and multiorgan failure 13
Short-term complications 188
Sickle cell disease 220, 246
Sinusitis 200
Sinusoidal vessels 245
Site of
    injection 140
    specific infections 291
Skin
    cellulitis and erysipelas 249
    ecthyma 249
    furunculosis 249
    impetigo 249
    infections 13, 249
    management 249
    manifestations 52
    secretions 23
Small isolated outbreak 33
Sodium stibogluconate 167
Soft tissue infection 8, 13
Sonography abdomen 55
Specific antitoxin 25
Specimen collection and handling 194
Spectrum of
    hepatitis B infection 148
    proliferative disorders 107

Spin-enhanced culture or shell vial 273
Splenectomy 169
Splenic puncture in kala-azar 166
Splenomegaly 165
Spotted fever 66, 69
    infection 8, 10
    pneumonia 9
    scalded skin syndrome 6
Staphylococci isolated 9
Staphylococcus aureus 3, 85
Steroids in sepsis 295
Stevens-Johnson syndrome 53
Streptococcal infection 15
Streptococcal toxic shock syndrome 12, 14
Subperiosteal needle aspiration 246
Subtypes of influenza virus 111
Sulfadiazine 275
Superficial
    candidiasis 158
    fungal infection 157
Supportive
    tests 125
    therapy 37
Supraclavicular lymph node 303
Suprapubic aspirate 227
Suspected case of
    acute meningitis 36
    chikungunya fever 155
Sustained viral response 152
Swollen glands 85
Syndromal causes 302
Syndrome of inappropriate antidiuretic hormone secretion 188
Systemic
    candidiasis 158
    fungal infection 157
    infections 183
    inflammatory response syndrome 290
    neutralizing antibodies 118
    steroid therapy 105
    viral infection 303

T

Techniques for diagnosing CMV 273
Terbinafine preparations 253
Tetralogy of Fallot 269
Thoracoscopy and formal thoracotomy 9
Thrombocytopenia 272
Thrombocytopenic purpura 270

Thymic hypoplasia 270
Tinea pedis
    diagnosis 253
    treatment 253
Tissue culture vaccines 196
Tonsillar and pharyngeal diphtheria 24
Tonsils and pharynx 24
Total leucocyte count 208, 286
Toxemia in children 291
Toxic
    cardiomyopathy 27
    neuropathy 27
    shock syndrome 5, 69
    synovitis 246
Toxoplasma gondii 274
Toxoplasmosis 279, 303, 311
Transmission
    and disease burden 121
    in healthcare settings 4
Transplacental
    infection 51, 278
    transmission 277, 278
Traveler's diarrhea 220
Treatment of
    anemia 177
    brucellosis 56*t*
    Chlamydia pneumoniae 65
    dengue case management 129*f*
    leptospirosis 75
    oral clindamycin 8
    P. vivax malaria 174
    RSV infection 119
    shock 131
    streptococcal pharyngitis 17
    uncomplicated falciparum malaria 176
    uncomplicated *P. falciparum* malaria 174
    upper respiratory tract infection 199
Trimethoprim-sulfamethaxazole 8
Trimethoprim-sulfamethoxazole 309
Tuberculin skin test 259
Tuberculosis
    abdominal 264
    antitubercular drugs
        ethambutol 259
        isoniazid 259
        pyrazinamide 259
        rifampicin 259
    bacteriological test 256
    daily versus intermittent therapy 259
    diagnosis 263
    high-risk factors for 256
    lymphadenitis 263, 304
    MDR 265
    pediatric dosages 261
    preventive therapy 262
    pulmonary 256
    symptoms 256
    treatment categories and regimens for children 261
Tympanic membrane perforation 204
Types of
    diseases 12
    influenza virus 111
Typhoid fever
    clinical features 235
    complications 235
    epidemiology of 233
    laboratory investigations 235
    transmitted 233
    treatment of 237*t*
Typhus 66
Typical rash of rickettsial fever 67
Typical triad of fever 66

U

Uncomplicated malaria 174
Unconscious child 176
Unexplained persistent parotid enlargement 308
Universal Program of Immunization 28
Upper respiratory tract infection (URTI) 13, 199
Upper respiratory tract pathogen 12
Ureteroceles 231
Urethral valves 231
Urinalysis components of 228
Urinary tract infection
    diagnostic tests 227
    symptoms of 227
Urine and sputum 298
Urticarial maculopapular lesions 96

V

Vaccination policy in the country 41
Vaccines for influenza 114
Vaginal infection 158
Vaginitis 14
Valganciclovir 279

Vancomycin therapy 299
Varicella
  infection 102
  vaccine 103, 104, 105
  zoster immune globulin 104
Vascular ring 211
Vehicle transmission 234
Ventricular septal defect 269
Vesicoureteric reflux 230, 232
Vibrio cholerae 43, 221
Video-assisted thoracoscopic surgery 9
Violaceous macule 249
Viral
  disease 103
  encephalitis in Asia, cause of 191
  hepatitis 143
  infections 200, 301, 310
  meningitis 86
Virchow's node 303
Viremia 291
Virulence of the organism 23
Virus isolation 123, 193
Visual disturbances 268
Vitreitis 276
Volkmann canals 245

W
Watery diarrhea 43
Weil's syndrome 73

Weil-Felix test 70
WHO Classification of Dengue 122, 123
WHO clinical staging of HIV/AIDS for children with confirmed HIV 307*t*
Widal test 236, 237
Widespread zoonosis 72
Wiskott-Aldrich syndrome 302
With late-onset disease 278
Wound management
  do's of 136
  don'ts of 136

X
X-linked
  agammaglobulinemia 287
  lymphoproliferative syndrome 107
X-ray 211

Y
Yellow-white cotton-like patches on the retina 276
Yersinia 219

Z
Ziehl-Neelsen stain 256
Zinc and antispasmodics 225
Zinc deficiency 225, 259